T0327422

EVALUATION OF DRUG CANDIDATES FOR PRECLINICAL DEVELOPMENT

EVALUATION OF DRUG CANDIDATES FOR PRECLINICAL DEVELOPMENT

Pharmacokinetics, Metabolism, Pharmaceutics, and Toxicology

Edited by

CHAO HAN
Centocor Research and Development Inc.

CHARLES B. DAVIS
GlaxoSmithKline

BINGHE WANG
Georgia State University

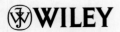

A JOHN WILEY & SONS, INC., PUBLICATION

Published by John Wiley & Sons, Inc., Hoboken, New Jersey
Published simultaneously in Canada

For general information on our other products and services or for technical support, please contact our Customer Care Department within the United States at (800) 762-2974, outside the United States at (317) 572-3993 or fax (317) 572-4002.

Wiley also publishes its books in a variety of electronic formats. Some content that appears in print may not be available in electronic formats. For more information about Wiley products, visit our web site at www.wiley.com.

Library of Congress Cataloging-in-Publication Data:

Evaluation of drug candidates for preclinical development : pharmacokinetics, metabolism, pharmaceutics, and toxicology / [edited by] Chao Han, Charles B. Davis, Binghe Wang.
        p. ; cm.
    Includes index.
    ISBN 978-0-470-04491-9 (cloth)
   1. Drug development.   2. Pharmacokinetics.   3. Drugs–Metabolism.   I. Han, Chao.   II. Davis, Charles B. (Charles Baldwin)   III. Wang, Binghe, PhD.
    [DNLM: 1. Drug Evaluation, Preclinical.   2. Drug Discovery.   3. Drug Industry–standards.   4. Pharmaceutical Preparations–metabolism.   5. Pharmacology–methods. QV 771 E917 2010]
    RM301.25.E93 2010
    615′.19–dc22

                                        2009035876

Printed in the United States of America

10 9 8 7 6 5 4 3 2 1

CONTENTS

PREFACE

In the past two decades, the pharmaceutical industry has experienced tremendous transformation. There have been significant scientific advances with the potential to revolutionize the treatment of human disease. Advanced technologies and automation have increased efficiency in the laboratory. Productivity of the industry as a whole, however, has not met the high expectations of society. As mature products lose patent protection pharmaceutical companies have struggled to fill gaps in their pipelines. Reorganization in the industry is commonplace; a wave of mega-mergers is under way as this book goes to press. Despite these challenges, small biotechnology companies and academic researchers continue to enter the fray, and competition in the industry remains fierce. Outsourcing of diverse discovery and development activities is increasingly common as the industry attempts to minimize infrastructure and maximize financial flexibility. These adaptations reflect the high attrition rates experienced during development, increasing costs, and the increased expectations of society that new medicines will be safe, effective, and affordable. It is in this complex and dynamic context that we edit this book on the preclinical evaluation of drug candidates.

We believe that selecting the "right" drug candidate for development is key to success. To lower attrition rates during early clinical development, pharmaceutical as well as pharmacological properties of the molecule should be optimized. This undertaking requires good science, perseverance, and often luck. There is precedence that the evaluation and optimization of pharmacokinetic properties early in drug discovery has a positive impact on the effort to lower attrition rates. We believe this example can be extended further and that a comprehensive evaluation of candidate developability at an early stage is an essential step.

This book presents three major scientific areas: pharmacokinetics and drug metabolism, pharmaceutical development, and safety assessment. The various properties of a new chemical entity are typically evaluated by groups of scientists with diverse backgrounds and exquisite specialization, often working in isolation. Given the great potential for experimental findings in one discipline to profoundly influence outcomes in another, integration is essential. Our goal is not to emphasize the leading edge of science and technology but rather to stress the integration of activities and information essential for the advancement of new medicines during drug development. We expect this book will enhance the formulation of appropriate strategies for compound progression and improve decision-making. We hope this book will be valuable to readers from academia, industry, and service organizations, and thank the contributors for their dedication and patience.

CHAO HAN
Centocor Research and Development Inc.

CHARLES B. DAVIS
GlaxoSmithKline Pharmaceuticals

BINGHE WANG
Georgia State University

CONTRIBUTORS

RAMESH B. BAMBAL, Absorption Systems, Exton, Pennsylvania

DION R. BROCKS, University of Alberta, Edmonton, AB, Canada

BARRY S. BROWN, Department of Safety Pharmacology, GlaxoSmithKline

BRUCE D. CAR, Bristol-Myers Squibb Research and Development

KHURAM W. CHAUDHARY, Department of Safety Pharmacology, GlaxoSmithKline

STEPHEN E. CLARKE, Preclinical Development, Drug Metabolism and Pharmacokinetics, GlaxoSmithKline Pharmaceuticals, Ware, United Kingdom

CHARLES B. DAVIS, Cancer Research, GlaxoSmithKline Pharmaceuticals

JINQUAN DONG, Johnson & Johnson PRD

PENG DUAN, Department of Pharmaceutics, Rutgers University

WILLIAM R. FOSTER, Bristol-Myers Squibb Research and Development

XIANGMING GUAN, South Dakota State University, College of Pharmacy, Department of Pharmaceutical Sciences

CHAO HAN, Centocor Research and Development Inc., Johnson & Johnson

LIAN HUANG, Johnson & Johnson PRD

SHYAM KARKI, Johnson & Johnson PRD

VIKRAM RAMANATHAN, Drug Metabolism and Pharmacokinetics and Clinical Pharmacology, Advinus Therapeutics Pvt. Ltd., Bangalore, India

VITO G. SASSEVILLE, Bristol-Myers Squibb Research and Development

NIMISH VACHHARAJANI, Drug Metabolism and Pharmacokinetics and Clinical Pharmacology, Advinus Therapeutics Pvt. Ltd., Bangalore, India

GUOFENG YOU, Department of Pharmaceutics, Rutgers University

FANFAN ZHOU, Department of Pharmaceutics, Rutgers University

CHAPTER 1

INTRODUCTION

CHARLES B. DAVIS
GlaxoSmithKline Pharmaceuticals, Collegeville, PA

The challenges faced by the pharmaceutical industry in the twenty-first century are potentially overwhelming. Nonetheless, there remains substantial demand for new medicines to address unmet medical needs. The global market for pharmaceuticals is growing. For cardiovascular, endocrine, metabolic, respiratory, neurological, infectious diseases, and oncology, the market is expected to exceed $500 billion by 2012.[1] The cost of drug development also is continuing to increase. The R&D expenditures for a single new chemical entity approach $1 billion.[2] Overall, attrition during drug discovery and development remains high. Thousands of compounds may be profiled before a development candidate emerges and only 1 or 2 in 10 that initiates testing in humans, is expected to reach the market.[3] The process overall may take 10–15 years. Despite R&D expenditures of $48 billion by Pharmaceutical Research and Manufacturers of America member companies in 2007, US drug approvals were the lowest in 24 years.[4]

Today, scientists in pharmaceutical R&D face unprecedented pressure from payers, regulators, ethicists, and the public, to bring to market safe and effective drugs while reducing costs. As recent events attest, even after having received regulatory approval, idiosyncratic drug reactions or infrequent adverse safety events may lead to "black-box" warning labels or potentially the removal of a drug from the market all together.[5,6] Serious adverse events may be extremely difficult to detect during the course of drug development given the numbers of patients

Evaluation of Drug Candidates for Preclinical Development: Pharmacokinetics, Metabolism, Pharmaceutics, and Toxicology, Edited by Chao Han, Charles B. Davis, and Binghe Wang
Copyright © 2010 John Wiley & Sons, Inc.

involved in pivotal clinical trials and the relative homogeneity of these patient populations. Despite numerous challenges, sponsors need to anticipate the most likely asset profile, as early as possible, to make intelligent investment and portfolio decisions. Resource must be minimized for compounds less likely to progress through development. Given the increased costs associated with late phase development terminations, "fail early and fail cheap" has become the mantra for many in drug discovery.

Routine use of absorption, distribution, metabolism, and elimination (ADME) screening in drug discovery has successfully reduced attrition due to poor human pharmacokinetics from about half of all development failures in 1990,[7] to approximately 10% presently.[3] Experimental ADME screening remains a cost effective and robust way to assure a thorough understanding of the desired and undesired biological effects of a new chemical entity in animals and humans. For this, sufficient free drug concentrations must be maintained at the site of action, for an appropriate period of time, to enable a thorough evaluation of biological effects. This finding is as critical for comprehensive animal toxicology studies as it is for successful, decision-making clinical investigation.

This book describes powerful experimental approaches employed today by modern laboratories within pharmaceutical R&D, biotechnology companies, and academia to characterize ADME properties of drugs with a focus on small molecules. The primary *in vivo* and *in vitro* tools used to characterize a drug candidate are discussed. Included are theoretical and practical aspects of preclinical pharmacokinetics (in Chapter 2), the important role of transporters (Chapter 3) and the cytochromes P450 (Chapter 4), the role of metabolism and metabolite identification in drug discovery (Chapter 5), plasma protein binding (in Chapter 6), and the prediction of human pharmacokinetics (Chapter 7). Effort has been made to integrate the subject matter to account for important interdependencies. The concepts should be applied in a cross-functional manner and with due consideration of the context including potential clinical implications.

One of the most important sources of development termination today is animal safety. Our ability to predict toxicological effects of new drugs, particularly those that develop over time, continues to be limited due to the enormous complexity and dynamic nature of biological systems. Therefore, in conjunction with ADME, successful drug discovery depends on experimental toxicology. Chapters 9 and 10 of this book discuss general, genetic, and cardiovascular toxicology as it is applied in the drug discovery setting. Central to the field of safety assessment is the consideration of the therapeutic window of a drug: the difference between exposure associated with the desired therapeutic benefit and exposure associated with adverse effects. Preferably, there is substantial separation between these drug exposures (a large therapeutic window) to permit safe and effective treatment for a heterogeneous patient population. The therapeutic window may decrease as the duration of dosing increases. Acute effects (desired and undesired) may differ from those observed with intermittent or chronic drug administration. The therapeutic window may or may not be conserved between preclinical species and humans (one reason to study multiple preclinical species). Different species may have different sensitivity to drug treatment (same effect at different exposures) or the biological effects themselves may differ from one species to another. The many challenges of early safety assessment include the provision of cost-effective *in vitro* and *in vivo* technologies that can be integrated into the drug discovery process and are predictive of clinical outcomes.

Additionally we included a chapter (Chapter 8) on pharmaceutics, encompassing theoretical and practical aspects of the physical characterization of drug substance, the importance of selecting an appropriate version (parent or salt) of the chemical for development and formulation considerations for definitive animal safety studies, and initial clinical trials. When fully integrated within a drug discovery program, drug metabolism and pharmacokinetics, safety assessment, and pharmaceutical development will play a crucial role. Together, they will assure the best chance of success by building the appropriate properties into the drug molecule as early as possible in the process. They will help to identify potential liabilities as the asset progresses, as well as areas for further specialized study. This is the nature of the developability assessment.

It is important not to underestimate the interrelatedness of these developability activities in drug discovery. Understanding and addressing issues at the interfaces can have a significant impact on the development plan, the time and resource involved in the activities, as well as the success of the program overall. For example, as previously indicated, animal safety studies will need to be performed to evaluate the full range of biologic effects including exaggerated pharmacology and off-target effects, acute and chronic, to appropriately manage potential liabilities. In many cases, prerequisites for this will include low to moderate *in vivo* clearance and acceptable oral bioavailability from a solid dosage form. This in turn will require well-characterized drug substance, a suitable formulation, and an understanding of factors influencing the rate and extent of dissolution of drug at the absorption site.

Although some aspects of the process and strategy will be very similar from program to program, others will not. Development hurdles will differ depending on the therapeutic area, the availability of existing treatments, and ultimately the level of risk that may be acceptable given the potential benefit to the patient (the risk/benefit ratio). Therefore, the lead optimization strategy, including the staging of assays and the acceptance criteria will adjust accordingly. An analgesic or antibiotic may require relatively higher free drug concentrations thus rapid dissolution, high intestinal permeability, and low protein binding may be required. Some drugs will need to effectively penetrate the blood–brain barrier (e.g., an anticonvulsant). For other drugs, it may be desirable to have limited brain penetration. On this basis, assays to assess central nervous system (CNS) penetration may be included in the screening cascade.

Drugs administered intravenously will require relatively higher solubility and will need to have limited hemolytic potential. An asthma drug may be inhaled directly into the lungs and therefore relatively higher metabolic clearance may be desirable to minimize potential systemic effects. Others drugs will be used to treat a chronic condition (e.g., osteoporosis) and may be taken for many years on a regular basis. In this case, a longer biological half-life may be desirable. Some drugs will be taken in combination with others [e.g., antiretrovirals for human immunodeficiency virus (HIV) infection]. For these, it may be particularly important to study cytochrome P450 enzymology, to minimize the potential for drug–drug interactions. For diseases where there are limited or no therapeutic alternatives, convenience of administration will be less important. For life-threatening illnesses, there may be less of a concern regarding manageable side-effects, long-term or reproductive toxicities. Therefore, drug discovery strategy should be customized following thoughtful consideration of the desired product profile.

How does this complex process begin? In the earliest phase of drug discovery, a biological target (receptor, enzyme) is identified and its relationship to the disease process is elucidated. As confidence builds that inhibition of the target represents a valid approach for therapeutic intervention, assays are developed and a high-throughput screen is conducted. Libraries containing potentially millions of chemicals are tested for their ability to inhibit the target and hits are identified. When hits are deemed an appropriate starting point, lead optimization begins. During lead optimization, the structure of chemical leads is modified to optimize potency, selectivity, cell-based activity, pharmaceutical, and ADME properties while assuring structural novelty that will form the basis of successful patent applications.

Patents provide market exclusivity for the innovator for a defined time period after which generic drug companies can manufacture and sell the same active ingredient. They must establish bioequivalence with the innovator's product (a statistical analysis of the rate and extent of absorption in humans). In so doing, they avoid conducting extensive clinical trials to evaluate safety and efficacy, which have been demonstrated previously by the innovator. The situation is more complicated for biologics since these products tend to be heterogeneous, and it is generally not possible to demonstrate chemical identity to the innovator's product. Regulatory agencies around the world are developing strategies for approval and marketing of well-characterized biologics given the potential for substantial savings and increased benefit to patients and society.

During lead optimization, a team of scientists including chemists, biologist, and drug metabolism and PK experts will work closely together to develop an appropriate screening cascade. This is a series of assays of various priority and throughput that are performed sequentially to optimize compound properties. Higher throughput assays designed to measure and incorporate the most critical attributes of the molecule are typically performed earlier in the screening cascade and require relatively smaller amounts of compound for testing. More detailed and resource intensive studies take place subsequently on a more limited number of promising compounds. These studies often require a larger quantity of drug for testing. It always requires some work to be performed in parallel, at risk, to avoid unnecessary delay. Turn-around time becomes critical in such a cascade because test results influence the subsequent round of chemical synthesis and biological testing, the order that compounds may be studied subsequently, and their priority for scale-up and further evaluation.

Assays with insufficient capacity to accommodate leads that have passed previous tests have the potential to become a bottleneck. Although assays may be redeveloped or resources redeployed to improve the situation (or acceptance criteria changed), bottlenecks often persist or may move to other areas within the screening cascade. Scientists involved in profiling compounds during lead optimization will require perseverance and creativity to adjust their experimental approaches to meet the needs of the program. Appropriate distinctions will be made between assays used for more definitive assessments and predictions, compared to those used primarily for rank ordering or screening compounds. Thus, drug discovery assays will be fit for this purpose.

During lead optimization there will be occasions when a particular challenge presents itself and the team will need to pull together to address the challenge. Changes may need to be made in the screening cascade temporarily to solve a particular problem. Or, a parallel screening cascade may need to be put in place temporarily. Identifying and addressing these challenges will be critical for the success of the team, which requires strong leadership, excellent working relationships among team members, and thoughtful integration of data and information.

Various organizational models have proven successful in promoting collaboration and efficient decision making. In one model, the line functions [e.g., chemistry, biology, drug metabolism and pharmacokinetics, pharmaceutical development, and safety assessment] are separately managed. In this case, individuals are appointed to represent their discipline on a matrix program team and senior line management assures resources are aligned in a manner that is consistent with the overall strategic intent of the organization. In another model, smaller drug discovery units are dedicated to a therapeutic area or therapeutic approach and have, more or less, ring-fenced resource and potentially considerable autonomy. Typically, these drug discovery units include the minimal essential complement of scientists required considering the phase and maturity of the program (for lead optimization, often chemistry, biology, and DMPK). Ideally, these scientists are colocated to facilitate frequent discussion, interaction, and collaboration.

The former model may be more bureaucratic, accountability may be less clear, and loyalty may be split between the line function and the team. On the other hand, the larger line functions will likely have more specialized expertise and may be better able to respond to peaks and troughs in activity by reassigning staff to the most active and/or highest priority projects. In the latter model, the entrepreneurial model, there may be a greater sense of ownership, empowerment, and engagement. Of course, another model that has developed recently matches various aspects of the above with an aggressive outsourcing strategy. In this case, much of the laboratory work is performed by contract research organizations (CRO). More often than not, the CRO is located in a market where the cost of labor may be substantially lower than in the United States or western Europe.

In any case, it is inevitable that as teams advance compounds further into development, substantially more resource will be required and more discussion and debate will take place to assure organizational consensus, as well as continued commitment to the project and the underlying development plans. Most teams will eventually require expertise and resource outside of their direct control and thus the importance of skilled matrix management and team work should not be underestimated. The most successful teams will take full advantage of expertise on and off the team, tapping into know-how and experience where ever it may exist. Transparency and communication will be critical as issues often arise within one area that have the potential to impact strategy and planning in another.

One of the major challenges discovery and development teams will face is to assure that there is an appropriate balance between what needs to be done now and what can be done later. The critical path must be well defined and there must be consensus around what activities are most essential in advancing the program to the next major decision point. What activities need to be completed when and at what cost? What activities can be postponed without affecting the critical path? What kinds of enabling activities need to be considered? What are the issues and risks associated with delaying a resource intensive study? What is the asset profile and how does it compare to the desired product profile? In a world of limited time and resource, these types of questions need to be considered proactively and on an on-going basis as new data and information become available.

On behalf of my co-editors, Dr. Chao Han and serial editor, Dr. Binghe Wang, I would like to take this opportunity to thank the contributing authors for sharing their considerable scholarly expertise, for their tireless effort preparing their contributions, and for their patience as this monograph was compiled. We hope our readers find this book to be relevant if not insightful and we wish you the best of fortune in your journey to bring important new medicines to patients.

REFERENCES

1. Pfizer Annual Report, 2007.
2. Adams, C. P.; Brantner, V. V. Health Aff. 2006, 25(2), 420–428.
3. Kola, I.; Landis, J. Nat. Rev. Drug Discov. 2004, 3(8), 711–715.
4. Hughes, B. Nat. Rev. Drug Discov. 2008, 7(2), 107–109.
5. Wadman, M. Nature (London) 2005, 438(7070), 899–899.
6. Cressey, D. Nature (London) 2007, 450(7173), 1134–1135.
7. Prentis, R. A.; Lis, Y.; Walker, S. R. Br. J. Clin. Pharmacol. 1988, 25(3), 387–396.

PART I

PHARMACOKINETICS AND DRUG METABOLISM IN DRUG DISCOVERY

CHAPTER 2

PHARMACOKINETICS IN PRECLINICAL DRUG DEVELOPMENT: AN OVERVIEW

DION R. BROCKS

University of Alberta, Edmonton, AB, Canada

2.1 INTRODUCTION

At its most basic level, the interaction of a drug with its target receptor for activity is almost always associated with a definable concentration

Evaluation of Drug Candidates for Preclinical Development: Pharmacokinetics, Metabolism, Pharmaceutics, and Toxicology, Edited by Chao Han, Charles B. Davis, and Binghe Wang
Copyright © 2010 John Wiley & Sons, Inc.

versus response relationship. Usually, these target receptors take the form of macromolecular entities, usually proteins. Other entities including messenger ribonucleic acid (mRNA), or other forms of nucleic acid [e.g., deoxyribonucleic acid (DNA) as part of genes and chromosomes], may also be the foci of a pharmacodynamic change in response to presence of a drug. In most cases these drug–receptor interactions occur within cells of the body, which with the exception of the blood cells, are usually fixed as part of tissue structures. For this reason, a precise tissue drug concentration versus effect relationship may not be readily discernable due to the practical issues involved in obtaining tissue samples after dosing. Such study designs are by nature destructive and are not ideal for *routine* characterization of a drug–receptor interaction and response.

In tandem with this reality, there is also a relationship between the concentrations of the drug in the blood and the concentrations of the drug in the tissues in which the target pharmacologic receptors might reside. This relationship is possible because in order for a drug to be considered to possess systemic availability, it must first find its way into the posthepatic blood. Blood is an important compartment in the body because it is the primary fluid that connects all tissues of the body as a circuit. It transports nutrients (including oxygen) to the cells, and removes byproducts of cellular metabolism. It also helps to maintain homeostasis by performing its essential buffering functions. Another role is to act as a transport pathway for hormones, which allows specific endocrine tissues to influence the biochemical processes of anatomically far removed tissues. In a manner akin to hormone transport, the blood also serves as a conduit by which drugs can be introduced directly, as in the case of intravenous administration, or absorbed from the intestinal tissues (oral route), skin (transdermal route), or depots (intramuscular or subcutaneous injection) into the blood, where it can be transported to the tissue possessing receptors. This cascade is illustrated in Figure 2.1.

The processes that dictate the magnitude of plasma concentrations in response to a given dosage of a drug fall into the general realm of pharmacokinetics (PK). Pharmacokinetics encompasses the processes that are related to what the body does to the drug when the two come into contact with one another. The four basic PK processes are absorption (input) of drug into the body, distribution of drug through the body, metabolism of drug by the body, and excretion of the drug from the body. The moniker usually used to denote the processes is "ADME"; namely, the absorption, distribution, metabolism, and excretion of drugs. In recent times, another subset of processes has been

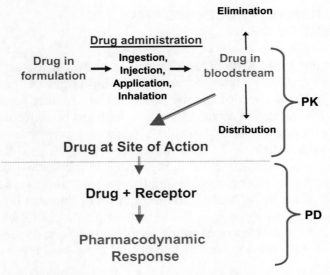

Figure 2.1. The link between pharmacokinetics (PK) and pharmacodynamics (PD).

introduced into this scenario and the moniker ADMET has been coined, wherein the "T" represents the transport of drug across cell membranes, facilitated by specialized protein. Conceptually, however, transport processes might be considered to be part of the subprocesses involved under the wider umbrellas of absorption, distribution, and excretion of drugs. Hence, the use of the term ADMET could be viewed as being superfluous.

Pharmacokinetics incorporates a wide body of knowledge, and borrows extensively from many disciplines including biochemistry, physiology, mathematics, physical pharmacy, and chemistry. The underlying foundation for the need for PK information during the development of new drug candidates is the concentration in blood fluids versus effect relationship. Pharmacokinetic information may aid in the decision-making processes pertinent to selection of a lead compound for further development.

The purpose of this chapter is to provide an introduction to PK in a general sense, including a discussion of the different processes involved in the PK of a drug, with special focus on the use of pharmacokinetics in preclinical studies. The chapter will begin with some basic PK concepts and follows with some discussion of the place of PK data in lead selection decision making.

2.2 BASIC KINETIC PROCESSES INVOLVED IN MOVEMENT OF DRUG

Drug movement into, through, and from the body can be separated into zero- and first-order types of processes. The nature of the differences between these sorts of kinetic processes are readily seen when dealing with PK data, which typically takes the form of concentrations measured in blood, plasma, or serum at different time points after administration of a dose.

Zero-order processes are those that proceed at a constant rate and are independent of concentration. When the concentration versus time data are plotted on linear scaled graphs, a straight line can be drawn through the concentration or amount versus time data points (Fig. 2.2). If the same data is plotted on semilog graph paper (i.e., paper where the x-axis plot representing time is linear, and the y-axis representing

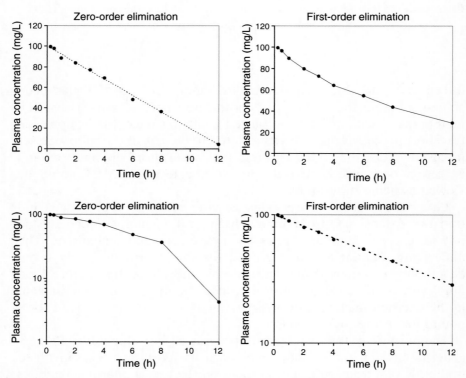

Figure 2.2. Differences between zero (constant rate) and first order (concentration-dependent rate) elimination kinetics are readily apparent when concentration versus time data are plotted on linear (top panels) or semilog graph paper (lower panels). Dotted lines represent best-fit lines extrapolated using regression analysis.

concentration is log-transformed), then curvature is observed (Fig. 2.2).

In contrast to zero-order processes, first-order processes proceed at a rate that is fractional in nature (Fig. 2.2). As an example of a first-order process, let us assume that we have 100 mg/L of drug in the body, and over each hour, 10% of the drug present in the body at the beginning of the hour is removed. The net result is a curved line through the data points when plotted on a linear plot, but a linear line through the data points when plotted on semilog graph paper.

In PK, first-order decline in blood fluid concentration versus time is most frequently observed. In first-order kinetics, the mechanism is either one of passive movement of drug, or one that involves a facilitative protein/enzyme for transport or metabolism, but where the concentrations are so low that the majority of the protein-binding sites are unoccupied with drug. In essence, the concentrations of drug are far below the concentration where the process occurs at maximal rate (i.e., far below the Michaelis–Menten (k_m) affinity constant of the process).

Mechanistically, zero-order processes always require an energy-consuming facilitative protein/enzyme to proceed, which are capable of transporting drug against a concentration gradient. Further, they are observed only when the concentrations are at a high enough level whereby essentially all of the binding sites on the protein are occupied by the drug. In contrast to first-order processes, there are few drugs that behave according to true zero-order concentrations after therapeutic doses of a drug. A good example of a compound that displays zero-order elimination with ingestion of normal dose levels in humans is ethanol.[1]

2.3 PHARMACOKINETIC METHODOLOGY

2.3.1 Compartmental Models

In order to allow for an understanding of the processes involved in the constitution of the pharmacokinetics of a drug, or to allow for predictions of blood fluid concentrations in the presence of altered conditions or changes in dosage, compartmental models can be used to quantitatively describe drug disposition (Fig. 2.3). The rationale for classical compartmental modeling is based on differences in rates of tissue uptake of drug, which is related to permeability and physicochemical properties of the drug, and perhaps even more importantly, differences in blood perfusion through organs. If a drug has good permeability

Classical compartmental model

Physiologically based model

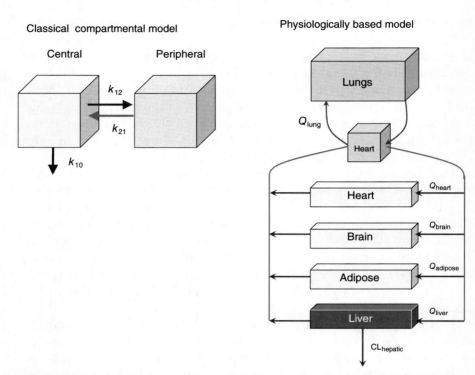

Figure 2.3. Examples of two basic types of PK models. Classical compartmental models "lump" tissues that behave similarly from a distribution perspective into nonspecific compartments. Intercompartmental transfer events are described by micro-rate constants. Physiologically based models typically represent specific tissues as discreet compartments with varying volume terms. Rather than rate constants, these models include blood flows into and out of the organs. Although both have their advantages and disadvantages, both can be used to predict the relationship between dose and plasma concentrations.

characteristics into most of the tissues into which it will be taken up, and if the blood flow going through those tissues is high, then a rapid uptake of drug will ensue. In this case, uptake is almost instantaneous, and as a consequence, if the drug follows first-order kinetics, a single straight line can best describe the decline in concentrations when a semilog concentration versus time plot is used. This hallmark presentation of a drug follows a one-compartment open model. On the other hand, many drugs penetrate significantly not only into well-perfused tissues, but also medium or poorly perfused tissues. In these cases, curvature will be present in the log concentration versus time plot. These sorts of models are multicompartmental. The number of compartments involved (i.e., the number of different tissue types based on blood flow) can be identified using, most reliably, nonlinear curve-fitting programs, or by manual graphical manipulation (method of residuals). The judge of model fit can be made using visual assessment of predicted to actual data, and objective statistical criteria, such as Akaike Information Criterion, Schwartz Criteria, and sum of least squares, or a combination of all of these.[2]

Once an appropriate model is selected, the compartmental estimates of PK parameters are based on the estimated data points from the model fitting, rather than the actual measured data as reported by the drug analysis laboratory. There are a number of compartmental equations that are used for estimation of volume of central compartment, area under the concentration versus time curve, area under the concentration versus time curve (AUC), clearance, and so on. Compartmental modeling is a very useful tool for obtaining data that can be used to predict plasma concentrations in response to a change in a rate constant, or for predicting plasma concentrations obtained with repeated dosing of a drug.

A unique type of modeling used in PK, which is arguably more rational than classical compartmental modeling, is physiologically based modeling (Fig. 2.3). This approach still makes use of compartments in the model structure. However, rather than lumping tissues in a compartment in an empirical way based on similarities in rate of tissue penetration, physiological-based PK modeling uses compartments to represent specific organs.[3] Actual organ volumes may be incorporated into the model, with unknowns being the unbound fraction in the tissues. Another difference from classical compartmental modeling is that the physiologically based model links compartments by blood flows into and from the organ. In contrast, classical compartmental modeling typically links tissues in a mammillary design with arrows representing movement into and out of compartments, with the arrows representing a rate or rate constant. Conceptually, physiologically based models are more true to the actual situation, although there level of complexity raises some issues with respect to validation of the model.

2.3.2 Noncompartmental Methods

Because compartmental methods require a derived model that may or may not be valid, in most applications of PK, especially for drug discover in pharmaceutical R&D, it is most common to see the use of noncompartmental methods to estimate parameters. This approach is truly descriptive, and its major advantage is that the actual data is used, with no need to worry about model choice. Noncompartmental approaches to PK require AUC to be calculated by the trapezoidal rule, which in turn is used to calculate clearance (CL) and volume of distribution of drug at steady state (V_{dss}) using an approach that does not rely on any specific predefined model. This finding is a major advantage, in that validation of a model is not necessary; one simply uses the data as is to gain the important parameters that best describe the PK properties of the drug (CL and V_{dss}). It must be recognized that noncompartmental methods are not useful for the purpose of predicting a plasma concentration versus time curve. This result is best achieved by use of an appropriate PK model and compartmental fitting.

2.4 PHYSIOLOGICAL PROCESSES AND RELATED CONSIDERATIONS INVOLVED IN PHARMACOKINETICS

2.4.1 Absorption of Drug

With the exception of the intravenous (iv) and intraarterial (ia) routes, all other routes of drug administration are associated with an absorption step. These include parenteral injection via the subcutaneous, intramuscular and intraperitoneal routes, inhalation, transdermal, and most importantly due to its ease, safety and frequency of use, the oral route.

The half-life ($t_{1/2}$) of a drug after iv or ia administration is a reflection of the distribution and elimination properties of a drug. A theoretical terminal half-life is determined when the distribution phase is complete. However, after dosing by a route with an absorption step it is possible for the terminal phase $t_{1/2}$ to represent the absorption rate constant, rather than elimination rate constant of the drug. This finding is often referred to as the "flip–flop" phenomenon.

2.4.1.1 Absorption and Nonoral Routes of Administration. In the intramuscular and subcutaneous routes, the drug is directly injected into the muscle or under the layers of the skin, respectively, from where it is absorbed into either the adjoining capillaries or the lymphatic drainage.[4] Highly lipophilic or large molecules tend to gravitate toward lymphatic absorption. When a drug is injected into the peritoneal cavity, it is mostly absorbed by the mesenteric blood system lining the serosal side of the intestinal tract. Although the normal absorption steps and enteric metabolism or efflux is largely avoided, the drug is

still directly transported into the liver via the hepatic portal vein, which still allows for the first pass extraction of drug by the liver.

The transdermal pathway of absorption is an alternate means of allowing systemic availability of drug. This pathway requires the use of specialized formulations that take the form of an adherent patch. They contain ingredients that promote the transfer of drug from the patch matrix to and through the skin into the bloodstream. Examples include hormonal replacement patches,[5] patches for motion sickness,[6] and nicotine patches for smoking cessation therapy.[7] One of the interesting PK aspects of this form of drug delivery is that in many cases residual drug in the skin is minimal, which results in rapid decline of plasma concentrations if the patch is removed from the skin.

2.4.1.2 Oral Absorption.

Absorption by the oral route is complex and involves a number of steps (Fig. 2.4). Before a drug can be absorbed across the mucosal surfaces of the cells lining the gastrointestinal (GI) tract, it must be solubilized within the fluids of the GI tract. Therefore if the drug is given as a solid tablet formulation, the tablet must first disintegrate into smaller pieces. This provides a larger surface area for contact with fluids of the GI tract, which in turn enhances the disintegration process and enhances the ability of the drug to be dissolved in the fluids. The speed at which disintegration occurs is dependent on the excipients used in the formulation, and by physiological factors, such as GI motility and peristalsis.

Once dissolved, the drug can be absorbed by the cells lining the stomach, intestines, or colon. The absorbable uptake of the drug is

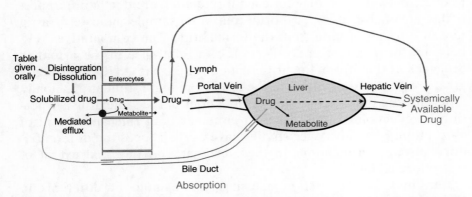

Figure 2.4. Schematic diagram showing the complex steps associated with drug entry into the systemic circulation following oral administration of a drug from a tablet formulation.

dependent on numerous physicochemical properties of the drug, such as size, charge, intrinsic lipophilicity, and salt form. The major collective sites of drug absorption comprise the intestinal segments, which includes the duodenum, jejunum, and ileum. These segments possess a huge surface area within which drug has the ability to come into contact with mucosal cells and be absorbed. After its entry into the cells, it is possible for the drug to be metabolized thus limiting its absorption. The intestinal tract contains several phase I and II metabolizing enzymes, including notably CYP3A isoforms.[8] Also present in various regions of the intestinal tract specialized transport proteins, such as P-glycoprotein, which can force drug movement from the intestinal cells back into the lumen.[9] Drug can be considered absorbed by the oral route after the drug has successfully moved intact from the dosage form administered through the enterocytes into the mesenteric blood circulation. In general, the rate of absorption is highest for solution formulations, followed by capsules and finally tablets, which tend to have the slowest disintegration rates.

Within the context of drug absorption, we are usually interested in describing the speed of absorption, and the extent of drug absorption from the formulation. There are several PK indexes that can be measured, which have different meanings in relation to the speed and extent of absorption. These include the maximal blood fluid concentration after a dose was administered (C_{max}), the time at which this concentration occurred (T_{max}), and the AUC. The relative bioavailability of two formulations is calculated by the ratio of a test formulation AUC to a reference formulation, with dose normalization.

In comparing two or more oral formulations of the same drug, differences between the tmax for each formulation are due to differences in the rate of absorption. A shorter tmax, for example, indicates a faster rate of drug absorption from the formulation. The comparative AUC between formulations is a reflection of a difference in the extent of drug absorption from the formulation. A higher AUC indicates a greater extent of absorption of the drug from that formulation. Finally, differences in the C_{max} between formulations of the same drug are possibly a reflection of differences in either or both rate and extent of absorption. Bioequivalence studies have as their focus the differentiation between formulations in these estimates of rate and extent of systemic availability.

Care must be exercised in assessing the meaning of a difference in each of these indexes of absorption (e.g., C_{max}, AUC) when looking at differences between two or more different chemical entities, such as a series of new drug candidates. Each of the parameters is a reflection of a combination of PK parameters, including clearance and volume of distribution, which may differ between compounds. Consequently, differences between drugs in either of the C_{max}, T_{max}, or AUC may not necessarily be due to a difference in rate or extent of absorption. This will only be the case when one is comparing the parameters between different formulations of the same drug.

2.4.2 Distribution

Upon entry of drug into the systemic circulation, it is transported to tissues by the blood, which facilitates distribution through the body to tissues permeable to the drug. As indicated above, it is possible for some tissues to take up the drug more readily than others, in which case multiple compartments may be visualized in the blood concentration versus time curves. Although in most tissues the intracellular entry of drug is passive in nature, for some drugs it is known that their cellular influx and/or efflux can be mediated by specialized transport proteins.[10]

The extent of drug penetration into the tissues is characterized by the volume of distribution (V_d). Different types of V_d can be determined from blood concentration versus time data. These include the V_c, which represents the volume of the central compartment. This measure of volume is truly a compartmental PK parameter, and represents drug distribution into those tissues readily permeable to drug, and well perfused with blood. For an estimate of drug distribution to tissues throughout the body, there are also descriptors called the $V_{d\lambda n}$ or $V_{d\beta}$ (also called V_{area}), which relies heavily upon the terminal phase half-life, and the V_{dss}, that may be calculated. The V_{ss} is considered to be a superior measure of overall drug distribution because mathematically it can be demonstrated that it is only dependent on drug transfer into and out of the tissues. On the other hand, mathematically V_{area} is dependent not only on intercompartmental distribution of drug, but also drug elimination. Hence, a change in an elimination process can significantly influence the estimate of V_{area}, even when no true change in distribution has occurred. For a drug that follows a one compartment model, the V_c, V_{area}, and V_{dss} are all approximately the same. In contrast, for other types of drugs, the rank order is normally $V_{area} > V_{ss} > Vc$.

One must consider that the V_d is a proportionality constant, and is not usually a physiologically relevant constant. The larger the value of V_d, the greater is the amount of drug in the tissues compared to the blood compartment. The only case in which the volume of distribution is directly physiologically relevant is when the V_d has a value equal to plasma volume, which is the smallest possible value of V_d that is possible.

In general, the V_d of a drug in most preclinical species correlates well with the human condition.[11] Although the value of V_{dss} or $V_{d\beta}$ tells us something about the relative distribution of a drug to tissues, it is not possible to use the value to gain insight into the amount of drug that might be present at the site of action of the drug, in a specific tissue type. For this purpose, the best experimental approach is to look at tissue concentrations of drug as part of a well-defined, formal tissue distribution study. Because tissues cannot be routinely harvested in humans, preclinical studies play an invaluable role in gaining insight into the ability of drug to permeate into specific tissues. Again, usually these preclinical findings correlate well to humans.

The actual processes determining the magnitude of the volume of distribution are tissue permeability, which is related to physicochemical properties of the drug and the cellular membranes of different tissues, and perhaps most importantly, the affinities of the drug to plasma and tissue proteins. The unbound fraction in plasma, which can be readily determined by methods, such as ultrafiltration or equilibrium dialysis, does not always allow for a prediction of whether a drug will have a high or a low V_d (Table 2.1). A general model for drug movement between proteins in tissues and plasma, and between unbound drug is presented in Figure 2.5. One can liken the equilibrium ratio of drug in plasma to tissue to a tug of war, the winner of which is dictated by whether plasma or tissue proteins possess a higher affinity for drug.

The proteins involved in the binding of drugs include albumin, α1-acid glycoprotein, lipoproteins, and various steroid-binding globulins. Each of these proteins binds drugs in a specific manner, sometimes with

TABLE 2.1. The Unbound Fraction in Plasma (f_u), Expressed as a Percentage, and the V_d of a Number of Drugs[a]

Drug	V_d (L/kg) (L Based on a 70 kg Man)	$f_u\%$
Warfarin	0.14 (9.8 L)	1.0
Ketoprofen	0.15 (10.5 L)	0.8
Kanamycin	0.26 (18 L)	100
Nifedipine	0.78 (55 L)	4.0
Nicardipine	1.1 (77 L)	0.5
Ketoconazole	2.4 (168 L)	1.0
Imipramine	23 (1610 L)	10

[a]It is clear that plasma unbound fraction alone does not dictate the V_d of a drug.

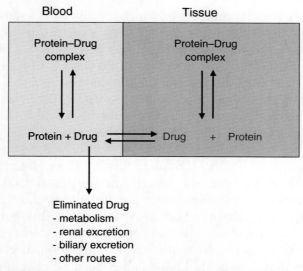

Figure 2.5. A model that describes the relationship between steady-state blood and tissue concentrations of drug, tissue binding relationships, and movement of drug between blood and tissues. Note that in this model, only the unbound drug may be transported across cell membranes.

more than one binding site per protein molecule. For example, acidic drugs tend to have a higher affinity to albumin than basic drugs, the converse being true of binding of such drugs to α1-acid glycoprotein. Lipoproteins are most apt to bind to lipophilic molecules. The steroid-binding globulins, as the name suggests, selectively bind to drugs possessing a specific chemical structure. These proteins may vary in concentration and binding affinities to drugs in a species specific manner. There are also a number of different clinical conditions and disease states that may specifically increase or decrease the circulating concentrations of these proteins, and hence influence the unbound fraction in plasma and the distribution and elimination of the drugs to which they bind. Protein binding and the methodology for its determination will be discussed in Chapter 6.

2.4.3 Elimination of Drug from the Body

2.4.3.1 Metabolism. Most drugs undergo some measure of biotransformation from the parent drug to metabolism. This metabolism may take the form of phase-I metabolism, which is most often facilitated by enzymes of the cytochrome P450 superfamily, and which results in oxidative or reduced metabolites. The other major category of drug metabolism is phase II metabolism, which usually adds a sizable molecular group or molecule to the parent drug structure by conjugation. These processes will be discussed in detail in Chapter 5. Metabolism may impart some unique considerations into the PK of a drug.

One important consideration of drug metabolism is the actual site of metabolism. Most drug metabolism occurs in the liver. From an anatomical perspective, taking into account blood flow, the liver is a uniquely situated organ (Fig. 2.4). With the exception of very small portions of the entire GI tract from the mouth to the anus (e.g., the sublingual route), all of the blood flow flowing through the capillaries of the various tissues empties eventually into the portal vein. The portal vein then directs all of the blood from the mesenteric circulation to the liver. For an orally administered drug, therefore, this permits drug metabolism to occur between the GI tract and the systemic circulation. Only that fraction of drug escaping first-pass metabolism in the liver is normally considered as being bioavailable, because only that fraction of the dose is able to reach tissues possessing target receptors for drug action. The exception, of course, is a drug that might have the liver as its target for pharmacological action.

Other tissues possessing metabolic activity may also contribute toward a decrease in drug bioavailability. One obvious site is the GI tract. As discussed above under drug absorption, the GI tissue possesses drug metabolizing enzymes (e.g., CYP3A and CYP1A1). These activities may contribute to a decrease in bioavailability as well. One other site that is often ignored is the lungs. Pulmonary tissue possesses the ability to metabolize drugs. Because from the perspective of blood flow it lies in series following the liver, in the presence of significant drug metabolizing activity, pulmonary metabolism my contribute to a lowering in bioavailability by decreasing the amount of drug that is passed on to the post left ventricular heart tissues. Indeed, iv bioavailability, which is often considered to be equal to one, may be less than ia injection in the presence of significant pulmonary drug metabolism.

Metabolism can lead to the circulation of metabolites possessing less or more of the desired pharmacological activity than parent drug. These metabolites may also present with a qualitatively different type of pharmacological activity than the parent drug. In many cases, this may take the form of an undesirable activity, leading to toxicity or side effects. In such cases, it is important to characterize the PK of not only the parent drug, but also its active metabolites, to provide a full consideration of the relationship between drug concentrations and effect. Pharmacokinetic modeling may be extremely helpful in assisting in the prediction of drug concentration versus effect, by incorporation of the exposure data of active metabolites.

The PK of metabolite may be complex. Specific PK equations and experimental designs have been developed to allow for a prediction of formation and excretory rates of metabolites. In some cases, the drug may be sequentially metabolized to other secondary metabolites that may possess pharmacological activity. In other cases, metabolism can be reversible. Again, estimation of the PK of metabolites subject to these conditions can be assessed using specialized methods.[12,13]

2.4.3.2 *Direct Excretion.*

The most common physiological mechanisms of drug excretion are afforded by the kidneys, via the processes of glomerular filtration and tubular secretion, and the liver via biliary secretion. Other pathways of drug removal from the body are possible (e.g., sweat, tears, breastmilk, saliva, and even hair), but these pathways are, from a practical, mass balance perspective, relatively unimportant.

i Renal Excretion. The functional unit of the kidney is the nephron, which consists of the glomerulus, proximal and distal tubules, and the Loop of Henle. The kidney plays numerous important physiologic functions in the body, including regulation of water, plasma pH, blood pressure regulation, thirst response, and elimination of waste products. The kidneys afford several mechanisms of drug removal from the body. Metabolism is possible, and cells of the kidney possess cytochrome P450, as well as other phase II metabolizing enzymes. In general, however, this activity is much lower than that present in the liver. Small peptides, however, may be subject to significant hydrolysis to substituents amino acids by renal tubular cells.

For drugs with a molecular weight of <45,000 Da, drug that is not bound to plasma proteins is freely filtered by the glomerulus. The glomerulus is comprised of a specialized network of fenestrated, high-pressure capillaries contained within the Bowman's capsule of the nephron. The high-pressure creates a force that drives filtration of the plasma through the fenestrations. Drug that is bound to plasma proteins is not normally filtered, because in normal kidneys the fenestrations in the capillaries selectively retain proteins of molecular weight (MW) > 45,000 Da.

Another major mechanism involved in the renal excretion of drug is by the active tubular section of drug from the capillaries lining the proximal and/or distal tubules to the luminal space containing the forming urine. This mechanism requires the presence and function of transport proteins that may reside on the basolateral and brush border membrane surfaces of the tubular cells.[10] Such proteins include organic anion and cation transport proteins, P-glycoprotein, and other adenosine triphosphate (ATP) binding cassette proteins, and peptide transporters. Usually, the transport occurs from the capillary to the luminal side, although in some cases, such as those involving the peptide trasnporters, the net flux can be from the lumen brush border side into the tubular cells. In Chapter 3, the categories and function of these transporter proteins will be discussed specifically. Nevertheless, the process of tubular secretion is usually one that increases the renal clearance beyond that of the filtration process. Because only a finite number of binding sites for drug will be available on the membrane surfaces, this process may become saturated at high drug plasma concentrations, possibly leading to disproportionate increases in drug plasma AUC with increases in dose.

The glomerular filtrate is directed through the proximal tubules, the Loop of Henle, the distal tubules, collecting ducts, and eventually into the urine unless the drug undergoes tubular reabsorption. This latter process is usually passive, and unlike tubular secretion does not consume energy, does not involve specialized transport proteins. It works along the direction of a concentration gradient. Functionally, tubular reabsorption works against renal clearance, and may reduce the calculation of renal clearance to less than that of filtration clearance. This process is dependent on urine pH in the cases of weakly acidic and/or basic drugs.

ii Biliary Secretion. Another potentially important pathway of drug excretion is biliary secretion. In this process drug is actively secreted from the blood, across the hepatocytes, and into the canalicular spaces. Like renal secretion, this process is dependent on transport proteins,[10] usually requires cellular energy, and can be saturated at higher concentrations. Biliary secretion is more common for higher molecular weight compounds, particularly conjugates of drugs formed by phase II metabolism. Biliary secretion is sometimes associated with unusual multiple peaking phenomenon in the plasma concentration versus time curve, because upon secretion into the bile, drug is transported to the duodenum by the biliary duct, which includes in some species (human and dog, but not rats) a gall bladder. Once in the duodenum, intact drug or drug reformed by deconjugation of Phase II metabolite may result in reabsorption of the drug. The time lag in the process of extrusion of drug into bile and entry into the duodenum, followed in some cases by cleavage of the conjugated metabolite to release free drug, is the cause of this double peaking phenomenon. This process of "futile cycling" is known as enterohepatic recirculation.

Preclinical animal species, in particular rodents, are much more adept at secretion of drugs into bile than are larger mammalian species (e.g., human). Consequently, evidence of enterohepatic recycling in a plasma concentration versus time profile is more commonly seen in rodents than in humans.

2.4.4 Clearance Concepts: Hepatic Clearance and Extraction Ratio

As drug enters the liver from the portal vein, a proportion of the drug will be removed due to metabolism and/or biliary secretion before it will pass through the organ into the hepatic vein (Fig. 2.6). The portion removed is known as extracted drug, and that which passes through unscathed is known as the hepatic bioavailable fraction. The factors that determined the amount of drug extracted are the rate at which the drug enters the organ, which is dictated by the rate of hepatic blood flow, the unbound fraction in the blood, and the intrinsic clearance of the unbound drug. The intrinsic clearance concept and related methods will be briefly discussed in Chapter 7. For a drug that is exclusively metabolized by the liver, the intrinsic clearance of the unbound drug is really the quotient of the maximal rate of metabolism, V_{max}, to the k_m constant.

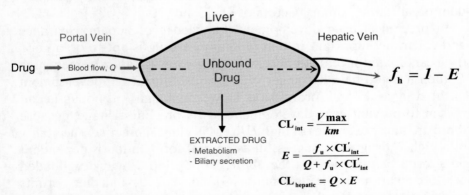

Figure 2.6. Steps involved in hepatic clearance, including relevant mathematical relationships (Q = hepatic blood flow; V_{max} = maximal rate of metabolism; km = affinity constant; E = extraction ratio; f_u = unbound fraction in blood; CL'_{int} = intrinsic clearance of unbound drug; $CL_{hepatic}$ = hepatic clearance; f_h = hepatic bioavailability).

For a drug with a major component of clearance being attributed to hepatic elimination or metabolism, calculation of extraction ratio is of major importance (Fig. 2.6). Knowledge of this value will tell us what the major dependencies are in the determination of hepatic clearance. The hepatic extraction ratio may be determined by the ratio of hepatic clearance to hepatic blood flow, for which an average value may be substituted. The reader is referred to a very useful review of physiological constants by Davies and Morris,[14] which summarizes hepatic blood flows from a number of species.

Drugs with an extraction ratio of 0.7 or above are categorized as being highly extracted. The hepatic blood flow is the major determinant of the hepatic clearance of a high E drug. Indeed, for such a drug, the hepatic clearance will be close to that of hepatic blood flow. On the other hand, the bioavailability of orally absorbed drugs with high E will be dependent on hepatic blood flow, unbound fraction in the blood, and the intrinsic clearance of the unbound drug. An increase in Q, for example, would allow a greater fraction of the drug entering the liver to avoid first pass metabolism and hence oral bioavailability would increase. On the other hand, an increase in f_u or CL'_{int} would enhance first pass extraction, and hence decrease systemic bioavailability after administration by the oral route.

Drugs with low E have a calculated E of <0.3. In such cases, the major determinant of hepatic clearance will be the product of f_u and intrinsic CL of the unbound drug. For such drugs the oral bioavailability is already near 1, and as such a change in Q, f_u, or CL'_{int} will not cause a notable change in oral bioavailability. For drugs with E ranging from 0.3 to 0.7, hepatic clearance and oral bioavailability will be dependent on all three primary factors of Q, f_u, and CL'_{int}.

In preclinical drug development, knowledge of hepatic clearance and E can be important in determining if a drug is apt to be a good drug candidate for oral administration. If a drug has an extremely high E, then it could be a harbinger of a serious difficulty in development of the drug as an oral formulation. However, a high E is not sufficient reason to prevent drug development at the preclinical stage, because there are many examples of high E drugs in clinical practice. The ability of a high E drug to be successful as an oral formulation is dependent on several factors, such as the ability to develop a high drug-loaded oral formulation that causes minor GI side effects, and that permits sufficient amount of a drug to gain access to the systemic circulation to permit a suitable level of drug access to pharmacological receptors at the site of action. If the drug has a low V_d and a high E, the likelihood of being able to achieve this is low. Having a high E and small binding affinity constant for pharmacological receptor interaction may make the low F associated with a high E drug a minimal problem. High E drugs also will possess a significant degree of first pass metabolism; if the metabolites possess beneficial pharmacological activity, then they could potentially partially or fully counterbalance the loss in activity due to loss of parent drug bioavailability.

2.4.5 Nonlinear Kinetics

In the presence of linear PKs, as the dose increases there will be a proportional increase in the measures of plasma concentration, which are usually the C_{max}, AUC, or trough concentrations in repeat dose modes of administration (Fig. 2.7). This in turn infers that primary PK parameters of CL, V_d, and F remain constant as the dose is increased. In practice, this is usually the case, especially for marketed drugs where it is desirable to have a predictable dose versus plasma concentration relationship. However, during preclinical evaluations, particularly in those involving dose levels intended to demonstrate safety in toxicological assessments, it is not uncommon to see a dose dependent change in CL, V_d, and/or F. In this situation, there is saturation in a process

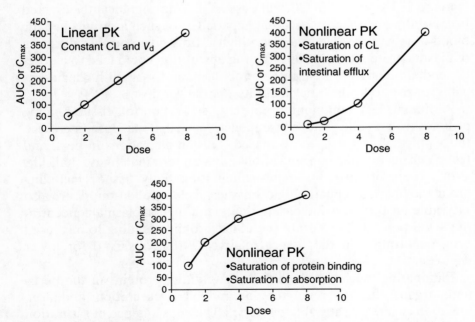

Figure 2.7. Nonlinearity in PK ensues from a saturation of absorption, elimination, or distribution mechanisms.

leading to altered pharmacokinetics; this occurrence is commonly termed as being nonlinear PKs.

Saturation in the absorptive process may be the result of the solubility of the drug being exceeded in the GI tract with high oral doses. Another cause of nonlinearity in absorption is a saturation of uptake or efflux transport proteins localized on the mucosal aspect of enterocytes. Saturation of these processes can have opposite outcomes on the plasma drug concentration versus time relationship. Saturation of binding to circulating proteins may also impact on the bioavailability of a drug, as is described below.

Nonlinearity in drug distribution is most often facilitated by saturation of drug binding to proteins either in the plasma or in the tissues. Most typically, saturation will occur at the level of plasma protein binding. The outcome of saturation of plasma protein binding on PK is complex, and depends to a large extent on how much and how rapidly the drug is metabolized by the liver.

In cases of drugs with low and moderate hepatic extraction ratio, saturation of plasma protein binding will cause increases in the fraction of drug available for metabolism and distribution, and the V_d and the CL of the drug will increase as the dose increases. For high E drugs with a significant proportion of drug CL being due to hepatic CL, an increase in V_d, but not in CL, will ensue; CL is not significantly affected because the main factor affecting hepatic CL of such a drug is hepatic blood flow. At the same time, for a high E drug given orally, saturation of plasma protein binding during drug absorption could lead to a dose-dependent change in first pass metabolism, and as such higher doses will give rise to lower bioavailability than lower doses.

Although less commonly reported, saturation of tissue-binding proteins is possible. The consequences are that as dose increases, the V_d of the drug will be decreased, causing alterations in peak and trough drug plasma concentrations and in terminal phase half-life. Efflux transport proteins in noneliminating body tissues, including brain and heart, or in pathological tissues, such as solid tumors, are also saturable. In this case, increasing doses and higher plasma concentrations will potentially saturate the efflux proteins, leading to increased drug penetration in the tissues relative to that observed for lower dose levels.

Eliminating mechanisms, such as drug efflux proteins in the pertinent organs, through renal tubular and biliary secretion, and drug metabolism, are all saturable processes. The consequence of saturation of these eliminating mechanisms will be a greater than proportional increase in drug plasma concentrations with increasing dose levels, and a potentially great change in the nature of the drug dose versus response relationship.

The most common occurrence of nonlinear PK in marketed drugs is typically at the level of plasma protein binding. For low E drugs, saturation of plasma protein binding will result in lower than expected total (bound + unbound) drug concentrations due to the greater CL and V_d, although $t_{1/2}$ will not change. Although lower plasma total drug concentrations will be realized, a linear dose versus effect relationship is still expected because the unbound concentrations still increase in a dose proportional manner. In contrast, for a high E drug, a change in plasma unbound fraction will not result in a change in AUC of total drug because CL is not affected. However, the dose versus effect relationship will change because relatively more drug is unbound and can distribute to tissues without the compensatory increase in CL.

For already marketed drugs, few examples of nonlinearity in metabolism over the therapeutic range of doses are available. Saturation of eliminating mechanisms is a potentially dangerous situation because even a small increase in dose level can result in a much greater than expected increase in effective plasma concentrations. One well-known example is phenytoin, the metabolism of which may be saturated. The drug also has a narrow therapeutic range of concentrations, which necessitates diligent therapeutic monitoring. In cases of saturation in preclinical studies, one must be aware that clinical dose levels are likely to be much smaller. As such caution should be exercised in the assumption of nonlinearity in the human population for the drug in question.

2.5 WHY USE ANIMALS IN PRECLINICAL PHARMACOKINETIC ASSESSMENTS?

There are two major reasons for performing preclinical (i.e., before human testing) PK assessments of a new drug candidate in a nonhuman species. The first is to provide, hopefully, for a rudimentary assessment of what might be expected of the PK characteristics of the drug if it were given to humans. This includes each of the major subcategories of ADME. Indeed, preclinical assessments of pharmacokinetics in a whole body system, provided by an animal experiment, provides the only ability to preview what the plasma concentrations of a drug might look like if given to humans. Although *in vitro* studies examining plasma protein binding, or the rates of metabolism by drug metabolizing enzymes or cells, are helpful for this purpose, such systems lack the influence of tissue protein binding and organ blood flows that are integral contributors to the resultant plasma concentrations attained *in vivo*.

Special relationships can be identified between the body mass of a mammalian species and the PK parameters of clearance and volume of distribution. These methods, which are known as allometric interspecies scaling techniques, have shown that for many drugs a linear relationship exists between the log normalized body weight and clearance or volume of distribution. The basis for this relationship is observational, although it can be conceptually linked to body surface areas, body masses, and cellular respiration and heat loss.[15] Because of this linear relationship, it might be possible from the preclinical clearance and volume of distribution to predict plasma concentrations in humans given the drug. This approach, called interspecies scaling, is potentially advantageous in rationally setting the initial dose levels of a new drug candidate in phase I first administration to human studies.

In general, interspecies scaling seems to work well in predicting the volume of distribution between species. It is not as successful for prediction of clearance, particularly when a high percentage of the drug clearance is via metabolism. In cases where the majority of drug clearance is afforded by glomerular filtration in the kidneys, classical allometric scaling for clearance has proven to be successful. Some authors have included into their scaling equations considerations of brain mass, maximum life potential, and enzyme kinetic parameters from *in vitro* studies. The latter approach worked very well for improving the prediction of clearance of the endothelin antagonist, bosentan.[16]

The second major reason for conducting preclinical PK is to provide a context by which the toxicology data collected in preclinical testing can be rationalized. For example, if given orally, it is important to know if systemic availability of the drug has been achieved with the doses used. Further, because of the high doses used in toxicology studies, nonlinear PK in absorption, distribution, and elimination are all potential considerations. In essence, in order to place the toxicological findings in line with the dose regimens used, the nature of the plasma concentrations, measured as C_{max} or AUC, must be known. In drug discovery, it carries another weight that is delivering the drug to animal models.

Not all preclinical ADME studies have a high priority or are essential for preclinical lead optimization. For example, the need for specific radioactive balance, biliary recirculation, and protein-binding interaction studies at the pre-Phase I stage have been questioned.[17]

2.6 PRECLINICAL PHARMACOKINETIC/DYNAMIC MODELING

The use of *in vitro* receptor binding studies is common during pharmacological assessment, and permits identification of chemical entities with a promise as new drug candidates. Indeed, in pharmacological assessments, modeling of these relationships is common practice to identify maximal binding capacities and affinities of the agents for the receptor. Although this is typically reserved for application in a clinical study, a similar approach can be used as part of a preclinical PK study to identify the plasma concentration versus effect relationship for a potential new drug candidate. In addition to the basic PK properties used to assess differences between new drug candidates at an early stage, inclusion of some sort of preclinical assessment of maximal effect and affinity based on plasma concentration versus effect profiles can be exceedingly informative. For example, a drug could have perfectly ideal PK properties of half-life and clearance, which would predicate administration of an appropriate dose regimen in a future human study. However, if the drug does not penetrate the target organ efficiently, despite any favorable PK properties associated with the drug, poor effect might be the result. Knowledge of preclinical PK–PD relationships could thus be very informative, and could greatly add to the body of knowledge required for decision making during lead optimization.

2.7 PRECLINICAL DEVELOPMENT DECISION MAKING BASED ON PHARMACOKINETIC DATA

The decision to proceed with new drug candidates beyond the preclinical stage is a critical step for a pharmaceutical company, due to the resultant enormous costs and scientific and clinical workload. Preclinical PK data generated during this process of lead optimization is an important consideration. Although some PK parameters are critical, care must be taken not to oversimplify or take unnecessary or unwarranted leaps of faith in viewing the PK data in making this vital decision. All decisions must be carefully weighed keeping in mind not just the PK data, but all of the preclinical toxicology and pharmacological assessments. Some example situations that might be encountered, and a brief discussion, are included here. In Table 2.2 a number of scenarios from preclinical studies are presented to highlight the issues.

Systemic availability is perhaps the most important consideration in deciding upon the fate of a drug as a new drug candidate, based on

TABLE 2.2. Perceived Problematic PK Issues Identified During Preclinical Drug Development

Primary PK Variable	Effect on Secondary PK Variable	Possible Difficulty Posed	Comments
Combination of high CL and low Vd	Rapid disappearance of drug from plasma with short $t_{1/2}$	Low level of drug effect Suboptimal dose regimen (high-dose frequency)	For iv route use infusion Might be able to develop a sustained release oral product or alternate administration route (sc/im/transdermal) with rate of input < rate of output to increase half-life CL is often lower in humans than animals
Low absorption from the GI tract	Low systemic exposure (low AUC)	Low level of drug average plasma concentration and effect	Increase dose to overcome problem Preclinical formulation may be suboptimal If problem is permeability, less chance of formulation improving absorption
High level of intestinal metabolism or P-glycoprotein mediated efflux	Low systemic exposure (low AUC)	Low level of drug average plasma concentration and effect	Increase dose to overcome problem Human metabolic/transport rate may be less than preclinical species Consider adding a P-glycoprotein inhibitor in the formulation
High level of hepatic clearance	Low systemic exposure (low AUC) due to high CL and low bioavailability	Low level of drug average plasma concentration and effect	Increase dose to overcome problem Human metabolic rate may be less than preclinical species Understand plasma protein binding between species *in vitro* Take drug with a meal to increase hepatic blood flow and increase oral bioavailability

TABLE 2.2. *Continued*

Primary PK Variable	Effect on Secondary PK Variable	Possible Difficulty Posed	Comments
Nonlinear elimination	Disproportionate changes in concentrations/ response versus change in dose	Dose regimen design may be problematic	May not occur in humans due to differences in rates of metabolism or transport processes
			In vitro metabolism date from preclinical and human species are important.
			May not occur within the therapeutic range of concentrations required in humans
			Use of therapeutic drug monitoring might be an option in humans
Low volume of distribution	—	Low tissue concentrations at the site of action	May be a nonissue; depends on uptake in the tissue containing receptors for activity.
			Could be a desirable property if uptake of drug into target tissues is good, and permeability into tissues where side effects originate is poor.
			Increase dose to overcome problem
			Examine carefully plasma protein binding *in vitro* between species
High-plasma protein binding	Low unbound fraction in plasma	Potential for low tissue uptake and response	Often is a nonissue; tissue uptake depends largely on tissue permeability and binding of drug in tissue as well as plasma
Formation of active metabolites	None	Possibility of unpredicted effect and or toxicity	Humans may not metabolize the drug to the same extent as preclinical species
			In vitro metabolism studies using animal and human microsomes are important.

primarily PK factors. If the drug is to be given orally, and bioavailability is poor, the underlying reasons for the poor bioavailability must be clearly identified. If the cause of the poor bioavailability is extensive presystemic metabolism, and from *in vitro* experiments both animals and humans display high intrinsic clearance from *in vitro* studies, it is very unlikely that this problem could be overcome by dosage form modification. On the other hand, if the drug candidate otherwise has a strong pharmacological profile, and no other suitable candidate is available, it might be worthwhile to consider the entity for administration by an alternate route of administration. In these cases, a preclinical PK–PD study is especially desirous, as even with poor bioavailability by the oral route, the concentration versus effect relationship still might provide an acceptable level of pharmacological response.

If poor absorption due to physicochemical properties of the drug is apparent, then modification of the formulation is a possibility, assuming that permeability is not an issue. There is more hope for such a drug as an oral formulation than a drug with extensive first pass effect, because the poor bioavailability can potentially be overcome by a nonphysiological-based modification.

One might be tempted to use a low f_u in plasma or blood as a reason for rejecting a candidate during lead optimization decision making. This could be a serious mistake. It must be kept in mind that even with a low f_u in plasma or blood, acceptable levels or even high concentrations of drug might be present in the tissues. The amount of drug penetrating into the tissues is dependent on not only plasma protein binding, but also bindings to tissue proteins (Fig. 2.5). A more useful criterion for this decision might be the *in vivo* uptake of drug into the target organs, relative to the penetration of drug into tissues that are related to toxicities of the drug. This finding could be part of a formal tissue distribution study.

A high clearance of drug might be a factor to consider in lead optimization. A high hepatic clearance, for example, will be associated with high hepatic extraction and low bioavailability when the drug is administered orally. On top of this, whatever is bioavailable will be rapidly cleared, causing the drug to have especially low AUC after oral dosing. This finding is not necessarily going to result in low pharmacological activity, however, because if the drug is metabolized to active metabolites the activity could be significant. Similarly, the liability posed by this occurrence could be minimized if the drug has a high V_d and high affinity to the target receptors for PD effect.

Although terminal phase $t_{1/2}$ is a PK parameter dependent on volume of distribution and clearance, it should be a relevant consideration for lead optimization. In repeated dose regimens, the terminal phase $t_{1/2}$ may be an important consideration in permitting maximal, minimal, and average plasma concentrations that maximize the effect of the drug over the dosing regimen at steady state. Especially short terminal phase $t_{1/2}$ are potentially problematic from the perspective of design of a repeated dose regimen, because they make it difficult to arrive at an appropriate dosing regime that permits therapeutic concentrations over a workable dosing interval. Another problem may be development of a convenient repeated dose regimen. Problematic short $t_{1/2}$ are most common when the CL is very high and the V_d is very low.

It is important to evaluate the $t_{1/2}$ after the same dosing route of administration as that intended in follow-up studies. For example, the oral terminal phase $t_{1/2}$ should be evaluated if the drug is intended for oral administration. For example, if a drug is given intravenously and has a very short $t_{1/2}$, this alone should not be used to judge the potential applicability of the drug. Rather, the preclinical $t_{1/2}$ data after oral administration could be more informative. The $t_{1/2}$ after oral administration is more important to consider, because terminal phase $t_{1/2}$ after oral dosing is dependent on the slower of the combined elimination–distributive processes and the absorptive processes, the latter of which is not involved after iv doses. As discussed under drug absorption, it is possible for the $t_{1/2}$ after oral doses to be longer than that after iv doses (flip–flop phenomenon). Even in cases where the oral formulation used in preclinical studies has a short $t_{1/2}$, it should be recognized that tailoring the formulation to provide a more prolonged release rate could result in a longer $t_{1/2}$.

The critical question becomes; based on PK variables, when is it prudent to proceed, and when to "pull the plug" on the new drug candidate at the preclinical stage? The answer inevitably lies with the nature of the PK–PD relationship of the drug. In the absence of this critical information, it cannot be known with certainty if the decision to proceed or stop further development of the compound based on PK considerations alone is rational and/or appropriate.

REFERENCES

1. Norberg, A.; Jones, A. W.; Hahn, R. G.; Gabrielsson, J. L. *Clin. Pharmacokinet.* **2003**, 42, 1–31.
2. Imbimbo, B. P.; Martinelli, P.; Rocchetti, M.; Ferrari, G.; Bassotti, G.; Imbimbo, E. *Biopharm. Drug Dispos.* **1991**, 12, 139–147.

3. Dixit, R.; Riviere, J.; Krishnan, K.; Andersen, M. E. *J. Toxicol. Environ. Health. B Crit. Rev.* **2003**, 6, 1–40.

4. Porter, C. J.; Charman, S. A. *J. Pharm. Sci.* **2000**, 89, 297–310.

5. Brocks, D. R.; Meikle, A. W.; Boike, S. C.; Mazer, N. A.; Zariffa, N.; Audet, P. R.; Jorkasky, D. K. *J. Clin. Pharmacol.* **1996**, 36, 732–739.

6. Nachum, Z.; Shupak, A.; Gordon, C. R. *Clin. Pharmacokinet.* **2006**, 45, 543–566.

7. Gorsline, J.; Okerholm, R. A.; Rolf, C. N.; Moos, C. D; Hwang, S. S. *J. Clin. Pharmacol.* **1992**, 32, 576–581.

8. Kaminsky, L. S.; Zhang, Q. Y. *Drug Metab. Dispos.* **2003**, 31, 1520–1525.

9. Benet, L. Z.; Cummins, C. L.; Wu, C. Y. *Int. J. Pharmacol.* **2004**, 277, 3–9.

10. Ayrton, A.; Morgan, P. *Xenobiotica* **2001**, 31, 469–497.

11. Mahmood, I. *J. Pharmacol. Sci.* **1999**, 88, 1101–1106.

12. Pang, K. S.; Gillette, J. R. *J. Pharmacokinet. Biopharm.* **1979**, 7, 275–290.

13. Hwang, S; Kwan, K. C.; Albert, K. S. *J. Pharmacokinet. Biopharm.* **1981**, 9, 693–709.

14. Davies, B.; Morris, T. *Pharmacol. Res.* **1993**, 10, 1093–1095.

15. Mordenti, J. *J. Pharmacol. Sci.* **1986**, 75, 1028–1040.

16. Lave, T.; Coassolo, P.; Ubeaud, G.; Brandt, R.; Schmitt, C.; Dupin, S.; Jaeck, D.; Chou, R. C. *Pharmacol. Res.* **1996**, 13, 97–101.

17. Campbell, D. B. *Eur. J. Drug Metab. Pharmacokinet.* **1994**, 19, 283–293.

CHAPTER 3

THE ROLE OF MEMBRANE TRANSPORTERS IN DRUG DISPOSITION

FANFAN ZHOU, PENG DUAN, and GUOFENG YOU
Department of Pharmaceutics, Rutgers University, Piscataway, NJ

3.1 INTRODUCTION

Transporters are membrane proteins whose primary functions are to transport nutrients or endogenous substrates, such as sugars, amino acids, nucleotides, and vitamins. However, the specificity of these transporters is not restricted strictly to their physiological substrates. Drugs that have similar structures to the physiological substrates have the potential to be recognized and transported by these transporters. Consequently, these transporters also play roles in governing drug absorption, distribution, and elimination in the body, and are considered potential causes of drug–drug interactions and individual differences in pharmacokinetic (PK) profiles. Examples of membrane

Evaluation of Drug Candidates for Preclinical Development: Pharmacokinetics, Metabolism, Pharmaceutics, and Toxicology, Edited by Chao Han,
Charles B. Davis, and Binghe Wang
Copyright © 2010 John Wiley & Sons, Inc.

transporters, which also function as drug transporters, include organic cation transporters (OCT, OCTN), organic anion transporters (OAT), organic anion transporting polypeptides (OATP), peptide transporters (PEPT), monocarboxylate transporters (MCT), nucleoside transporters (CNT, ENT), bile acid transporters (NTCP, BSEP, ASBT), multidrug resistance proteins (MDR), multidrug resistance-associated proteins (MRP), and breast cancer resistance protein (BCRP). Detailed information on these transporters is described in a recently published book entitled *Drug Transporters*.[1]

Most drug transporters are expressed in tissues with barrier functions, such as the liver, kidney, intestine, placenta, and brain. Cells at the border of these barriers are usually polarized into apical membrane and basolateral membrane and are separated by a tight junction. Transporters expressed on the apical membrane and on the basolateral membrane concertedly determine the direction of net transcellular transport of drug substrates and, ultimately, govern their PK profiles in the body. Although most transporters are specifically expressed on the apical membrane or the basolateral membrane, some exceptions have been observed. For example, human organic anion transporter 4 (OAT4) is expressed on the apical membrane of the kidney proximal tubule cells[2] and on the basolateral membrane of the placental syncytiotrophoblasts.[3] Rat organic anion transporting polypeptides 2 (Oatp2) is expressed on both the apical and the basolateral membranes of the blood–brain barrier.[4]

Most drug transporters can be classified as a member of the ABC (ATP-Binding Cassette) transporter family or the SLC (solute carrier) transporter family based on sequence similarity by the Human Gene Nomenclature Committee. The ABC transporters are primary active transporters. These transporters move molecules against their electrical–chemical gradient through the hydrolysis of adenosine triphosphate (ATP). The SLC transporters are the secondary active transporters. These transporters utilize ion gradients, such as sodium or proton gradients, across the membrane produced by the primary active transporters and transport substrates against an electrochemical difference. The best-studied drug transporters, which are classified as ABC transporters, are MDR, MRP, and BCRP. Most drug transporters belong to SLC transporters.

3.2   REGULATION OF DRUG TRANSPORTERS

Given the critical roles that drug transporters play in the absorption, distribution, and excretion of a diverse array of clinically important drugs, alteration in the activity of these drug transporters plays an important role in the PK of substrate drugs, and therefore, intra- and interindividual variability of the therapeutic efficacy. As a result, the activity of drug transporters must be under tight regulation so as to carry out their normal duties. Factors involved in the regulation of transporters could be physiological (hormones, cytokines, development), pathological (disease conditions), or pharmacological (drug treatment). Diverse regulatory mechanisms are involved in these regulations, which include transcription, messenger ribonucleic acid (mRNA) stability, translation, and post-translational modification. The control mechanism governing the activity of each transporter is different. Regulation of transporter activities at the gene level usually occurs within hours to days and is therefore classified as long term or chronic regulation. Long-term regulation usually occurs when the body undergoes massive change, such as during development or the occurrence of diseases. Regulation at the post-translational level usually occurs within minutes to hours and is therefore classified as short term or acute regulation. Short-term regulation usually occurs when the body has to deal with rapidly changing amounts of substances as a consequence of variable intake of drugs, fluids, or meals as well as metabolic activity. In addition to the regulation at gene expression level,[5–9] post-translational modification is one of the most encountered regulations of drug transporter activities. Post-translational modification includes several types: glycosylation, ubiquitination, phosphorylation, disulfide bond formation, and oligomerization.

Glycosylation is the most common and diverse form of post-translational modifications for newly synthesized proteins. It is a process in which sugars are covalently added to a nascent polypeptide in the endoplasmic reticulum (ER), followed by a series of trimming and modification of the added sugars in the ER and Golgi. The newly synthesized glycoproteins then exit the Golgi and are transported to their final destination. Glycosylation has been demonstrated to play critical roles in the regulation of membrane targeting,[10,11] protein folding,[12,13] the maintenance of protein stability (resistance to proteolysis),[14,15] and providing recognition structures for interaction with diverse external ligands.[16,17] Many drug transporters are found to possess consensus sites for glycosylation in their amino acid sequences. For example, multiple potential sites for N-linked glycosylation were identified in all members of the OAT family. Mutagenesis studies on OAT1[10] and OAT4[12] in cultured cells revealed that disruption of N-glycosylation caused retention of these transporters in an intracellular compartment, suggesting that addition of sugars to the transporters plays a critical role in the targeting of these transporters to the plasma membrane. Addition of oligosaccharides may also bring in spatial hindrance or conformation changes to the substrate-binding sites of OATs, and thereby affect the substrate recognition of OATs. Mutation of a glycosylation site Asp-39 in either hOAT1 or mOAT1 disrupted their functions through change in substrate binding without affecting their membrane trafficking. Furthermore, it was shown that the substrate recognition of hOAT4 prefer the structure the of N-acetylglucosamine form to relative simpler oligosaccharides structure mannose-rich type.[12]

Ubiquitination is another form of post-translational modulation of transporters. Ubiquitination is a three-step process. In the first step, ubiquitin, an 8-kDa polypeptide, is activated by an ubiquitin-activating enzyme. The activated ubiquitin is subsequently transferred to an ubiquitin carrier protein. Finally, ubiquitin–protein ligase catalyzes the covalent binding of ubiquitin to the target protein. Ubiquitination of cellular proteins usually serves to tag them for rapid degradation, and therefore can modulate their stability and activity. It was found that transfection of multidrug-resistant cells with wild-type ubiquitin increased the ubiquitination of P-glycoprotein (Pgp), an efflux pump, and increased Pgp degradation, which resulted in reduced function of the transporter, as demonstrated by increased intracellular drug accumulation and increased cellular sensitivity to drugs transported by Pgp.[18]

The activity of many drug transporters is also regulated by reversible phosphorylation. Phosphorylation is the covalent attachment of one or several phosphate groups to the hydroxyl side chains of serine, threonine, or tyrosine on proteins. Phosphorylation influences the conformation and charge of the protein, thereby also its activity (either up or down), cellular location or association with other proteins. Phosphorylation is catalyzed by protein kinases, which move a phosphate group from an ATP molecule to the protein. However, the phosphate group can also be removed from the protein by a process called dephosphorylation. This process is catalyzed by protein phosphatases. The amount of phosphate that is associated with the protein is thus determined by the relative activities of relevant kinases and the phosphatases. Together, protein kinases and protein phosphatases act in an exact opposite fashion to regulate a population of target proteins by controlling their phosphorylation states. It was shown that in HEK293 cells stably expressing rat organic cation transporter rOCT1, stimulation of protein kinase C (PKC) by sn-1, 2-dioctanoyl glycerol resulted in a significant increase in the transport affinity of rOCT1 for its substrates tetraethylammonium, tetrapenthylammonium, and quinine.[19] Such an increase in transport affinity was accompanied by serine phosphorylation of the transporter. It was therefore proposed that the phosphorylation of rOCT1 by PKC resulted in conformational changes at the substrate-binding site. Similarly, increasing phosphorylation of mOAT1 inhibited the uptake of PAH mediated by mOAT1.[20]

Membrane transporters need to be presented correctly in the cell membrane for normal function. Therefore, the activity of many drug transporters could be regulated by any process altering their membrane trafficking process (internalization and recycling). For example, the enhanced or reduced internalization of drug transporters from the cell membrane would decrease or increase the amount of transporters available in the cell membrane, which results in down- or upregulation of the drug transporters. Activation of PKC was shown to regulate the function of OAT1,[20,21] OAT3,[22] or OAT4[23] by redistribution of these transporters between cell membrane and intracellular compartments. The hOAT1 was shown to constitutively trafficking back and forth between cell membrane and intracellular compartments in COS-7 cells, a process partly through a dynamin- and clathrin-dependent pathway. Activation of PKC accelerated the internalization of hOAT1 without significantly affecting its recycling,[21] thereby reducing the free transporters available in the cell membrane able to carry substrates. Proteins associated with hOAT1 during the membrane trafficking process are most likely the targets subjected to the regulation of PKC and are need to be identified and elucidated in future studies.

The formation of a disulfide bond is also involved in the regulation of many transporters. A disulfide bond is a strong covalent bond formed by oxidation of two sulfhydryl groups (—SH) present in the cysteine residue. Reducing conditions can reverse the formation of disulfide bonds. These conditions may include the presence of agents with free sulfhydryl groups, such as dithiothreitol (DTT), β-mercaptoethanol, or glutathione. A disulfide bond that links two peptide chains together is called an intermolecular disulfide bond, whereas a disulfide bond that links different parts of one peptide chain is called an intramolecular disulfide bond. Disulfide bonds are very important to the folding, subunit assembly, and function of the proteins. The greater the number of disulfide bonds, the less susceptible the protein is to denaturation by forces (detergents, heat, etc.). Breast cancer resistance protein (BCRP/ABCG2) is believed to depend on both inter- and intramolecular disulfide bonds for its structural and functional integrity.[22] Unlike most other ABC transporters, which usually have two nucleotide-binding domains and two transmembrane domains, ABCG2 consists of only one nucleotide-binding domain and one transmembrane domain. Thus, ABCG2 has been thought of as a half-transporter that may function as a homodimer. Three extracellular cysteines (Cys-603, Cys-608, and Cys-592) have been identified in this transporter. It has been found that the transporter migrates as a dimer in sodium dodecyl sulfate–polyacrylamide gel electrophoresis (SDS–PAGE) under non-reducing conditions. Mutation of Cys-603 to Ala (C603A) caused the transporter to migrate as a single monomeric band. Therefore, Cys-603 forms an intermolecular disulfide bond. However, this mutation had no effect on efficient membrane targeting and the function of the trans-porter. In contrast to C603A, both C592A and C608A displayed impaired membrane targeting and function. Moreover, when only Cys-592 or Cys-608 were present (C592A/C603A and C603A/C608A), the transporter displayed impaired plasma membrane expression and func-tion. These data suggest that Cys-592 and Cys-608 form an intramo-lecular disulfide bridge in ABCG2 that is critical for its function.

Single polypeptides can associate with each other through intermo-lecular disulfide bonds as discussed above. A more common and widely occurred association of single polypeptides with one another to form larger protein complexes is through noncovalent forces, such as hydro-phobic interactions. Individual polypeptides in such complexes are referred to as *subunits*. The geometrically specific arrangements and stoichiometry of the composition of the complexes is crucial for the activity of these proteins. Oligomerization can be *homomeric (self-association)* or *heteromeric* (association with a different polypeptide). The heteromeric composition of most protein complexes gives the cells an additional level of diversity and complexity, which the cell can use for its activities. Often, heteromeric compositions of protein complexes are tissue specific or developmental specific and multiple genes can control the activity of a single heteromeric protein complex. Oligomerization plays critical roles in various aspects of transporter function. Several subunits in an oligomer may be required to form a single pore for the substrate to be translocated, as in K^+ channels.[23] In addition to such a functional role, oligomerization is also believed to play a role in membrane trafficking and stability of the transporters. After synthesis in the endoplasmic reticulum (ER), proteins undergo a strict process of quality control. Newly synthesized transporters may contain retention signal and are thereby retained in the ER. Oligomerization may shield/hide such a retention signal, and therefore is essential for the progress of the transporters from ER for subsequent targeting to the plasma membrane.[24–26] One example for the homo-oligomerization of drug transporters is human organic anion trans-porter OAT1.[27] The hOAT1 exists in the plasma membrane of kidney

LLC-PK1 cells as a homo-oligomer, possibly trimer, and higher order of oligomer. However, the functional consequence of such oligomerization remains to be elucidated. Drug transporters are often seen to form hetero-oligomers with their associating proteins. These interactions determine the polarized localization of transporters on the specific cell surface domain, their stability at the specific cell surface and their shuttling between the specific cell surface and the intracellular compartments when responding to stimuli. The PDZ proteins, for example, are one of the most common interacting partners with transporters. These PDZ proteins contain multiple PDZ domains ranging from 80 to 90 amino acids in length and typically bind to proteins containing PDZ consensus binding sites, the tripeptide motif (S/T)X (X = any amino acid and = a hydrophobic residue) at their C termini.[28] These multi-domain molecules not only target and provide scaffolds for protein–protein interactions, but also modulate the function of receptors and ion channels with which they associate.[29,30] The disruption of the association between PDZ proteins and their targets contributes to the pathogenesis of a number of human diseases, most likely because of the failure of PDZ proteins to appropriately target and modulate the actions of associated proteins.[31,32] Examples of such protein–protein interactions are found in urate-anion exchanger URAT1 and hOAT4, two members of the OAT family.[33] Interactions of URAT1 and hOAT4 with PDZ proteins augment the transport activity of these transporters in HEK-293 cells though an increased surface expression level of these transporters. In addition to PDZ proteins (proteins like caveolin-1), the members of caveolae, which is the small flask-shaped component in the plasma membrane, was colocalized rOAT3[34] in rat kidney and hOAT4[35] in primary cultured human placental trophoblasts. Caveolin-2, another member of caveolae, was associated with rOAT1[36] in rat kidney. This protein–protein interaction was found to upregulate the OATs mediated uptake in Xenopus oocytes or Chinese Hamster Ovary (CHO) cells. Based on the above findings, it seems that in different tissues or host cell types, different sets of proteins might be involved in their association with membrane transporters.

3.3   CLINICAL IMPLICATION OF DRUG TRANSPORTERS

3.3.1   Gene Polymorphisms and Their Implications in Diseases

Genetic polymorphism of drug transporters is a potential determinant of interindividual variability in drug absorption, disposition, and elimination. The coding region polymorphism can be classified as synonymous variants, which do not cause amino acid changes, and nonsynonymous variants, which do cause amino acid changes. The difference in the specific genotype, age, ethnicity, and sex of the patients may contribute to the variants in genetic polymorphisms. In most cases, polymorphism arises from people of different ethnic origins and/or reflects acquired changes during infancy. Nonsynonymous variants can lead to completely altered transporter functions or partially modified transporter functions. Sometimes, such variants have no effects on functions. Those variants causing dramatic functional change have been targets of major studies. Transporters in liver, kidney, intestine, and brain are the greatest source of variability, which results in different drug disposition profiles. Thus the consequences of polymorphism of these transporters have received considerable attention in recent clinical studies or personalized drug therapy researches.

The multidrug resistance associated protein MRP2 belongs to the ATP binding cassette (ABC) family of transporter proteins, which mediate ATP dependent transfer of solutes. As an important canalicular transport protein, MRP2 is responsible for the hepatic excretion of drugs–metabolites. A mutation on the MRP2 gene at codon 1066 from CGA to TGA, which changes arginine to stop-codon, has been proven to cause the rare autosomal recessive liver disorder, Dubin–Johnson syndrome (DJS) in humans.[37] Patients with DJS have chronic conjugated hyperbilirubinemia caused by impaired hepatobiliary transport of nonbile salt organic anions.

Another important canalicular transport protein for drugs–metabolites, the bile salt export pump BSEP, is involved in progressive familial cholestasis (PFIC-2) in a subgroup of infants and children. The disease is characterized as a cholestatic disorder causing extreme pruritus, growth failure, and can progress to cirrhosis in the first decade of life.[38] Mutations on the BSEP gene, such as 890A $\to$ G (E297G) and 2944G $\to$ A (G982R), result in a dysfunction of the transport protein, which is characterized by impaired active transport of bile acids across the hepatocyte canalicular membrane into bile.

Organic anion transporters are a family of transporters expressed in multiple organs. Due to their ability to transport a large number of the most commonly prescribed drugs, they played a critical role in maintaining endogenous homeostasis, are implicated in several clinical disorders, and are important modulators of drug efficacy and toxicity.[39] Urate transporter 1 (URAT1) is a member of the organic anion transporter family. Studies showed that URAT1 was involved in the hereditary disease renal hypouricemia. This disease is more prevalent in

Japanese and non-Ashkenzai Jews than in other ethnic groups. Patients with this disease have low serum urate levels. They have no renal or systemic diseases except for the development of nephrolithiasis or exercise-induced acute renal failure. Some patients with this disease have defects in URAT1.[40–42] The most frequently found mutation W258Stop of URAT1 results in a premature truncated protein, which is devoid of the transporter function due to deficiency in targeting to cell membrane.[40] Several studies have demonstrated that the single-nucleotide polymorphisms (SNPs) or regulatory SNP (rSNPs) sometimes could result in interindividual variation in mRNA expression of OATs and could potentially regulate the drug PKs in human tissues or animal models.[43–45] However, some conflicting data on the effects of polymorphisms on the function of drug transporters such as OAT3 or OAT1 may highlight that some SNP might be substrate or race specific.

As one important member of the ABC superfamily, Pgp has been one of the most studied membrane transporter proteins. Overexpression of Pgp is involved in multidrug resistance (MDR) in cancer.[46–48] Due to the fact that Pgp is responsible for protecting tissues and organs from toxicants, its malfunction may contribute to the progression of various diseases. It has been reported that patients with ulcerative colitis have a higher frequency of the nonsynonymous polymorphism of Pgp (C3435T genotype), which results in a decreased expression of Pgp in the intestine.[49]

3.3.2 The Involvement of Drug Transporters in Other Diseases

Recently studies showed that the development of some pathophysiological conditions was accompanied by the redistribution of OAT1 or OAT3 from cell membrane to intracellular compartments. In a rat model with bilateral ureteral obstruction (BUO), a disease characterized by the development of hemodynamic and tubular lesions, a redistribution of rOAT1 from cell membrane to intracellular compartments was found and contributed to the down-regulation of rOAT1 mediated PAH uptake.[50] During the progress of BUO, the expression level of angiotensin II (Ang II) is elevated. It was shown that treatment of Ang II in COS-7 cells could down-regulate the function of hOAT1 by decreasing its surface expression,[51] which indicates that the altered function of OATs regulated by Ang II may be potentially responsible for the abnormal drug elimination found in BUO patients.

Another example of the involvement of OATs in the progression of diseases is acute renal failure (ARF), which is a clinical condition contributed to >50% of mortality rate.[52] Both mRNA and protein level of OAT1 and OAT3 was revealed to be down-regulated in ischemic acute renal failure (iARF) rats, which might contribute to the impaired secretion of PAH found in iARF.[53,54] Organic anion transporters play an important role in the renal drug clearance, the functional inhibition of OAT1 and OAT3 would likely have a substantial impact in the renal retention and elimination of organic anions in iARF patients.

There are various drug transporters expressed in the brain, which are responsible for the complex transport system of xenobiotics into the brain. Altered expression of drug efflux transporters at the blood–brain barriers and in brain parenchyma is related to many central nervous system (CNS) diseases. For example, a large number of studies have shown the correlation between polymorphisms of Pgp and diseases, such as pharmacoresistant epilepsy[55,56] and Parkinson's disease.[57–59] On the other hand, as a feedback, neurological diseases and pathological conditions of the CNS may also lead to altered expression of functional drug transporters, which leads to increased complexity of related CNS diseases and refractory to therapy.

3.3.3 Drug–Drug Interactions

Since many drug transporters can accept multiple drugs and/or xenobiotics as substrates, there is a high likelihood that coadministration of drugs and/or xenobiotics can competitively inhibit each other's transport. This may result in drug–drug interactions at the transport level.[60]

Organic anion transporters are important transporters involved with renal drug elimination. Coadministration of their substrates can lead to different pharmacokinetics of each drug due to modified transport. A notable example is the coadministration of an OAT substrate, the anti-cancer drug methotrexate, with OAT inhibitors/substrates including non-steroidal anti-inflammatory drugs (NSAIDs), penicillins, and probenecid. Such coadministration leads to diminished transport of methotrexate by OAT and can lead to altered drug concentrations with undesirable pharmacological consequences. For example, coadministration of methotrexate with probenecid, an OAT inhibitor, resulted in severe suppression of bone marrow through inhibition of the tubular secretion of methotrexate.[61]

The breast cancer resistance protein BCRP also belongs to the ABC transporter family. The BCRP protein can reduce the intracellular concentration of potential harmful substances through efflux. At the same time, it also can cause drug resistance by eliminating useful drugs from cells. Coadministration of topotecan, a BCPR substrate, with elacridar (GF120918), a BCRP/Pgp inhibitor, significantly increases the oral bioavailability of topotecan in animal model studies.[62] The same phenomenon has also been observed in a recent clinical study in cancer patients.[63] In another study, coadministration of GF120918 (an inhibitor for both BCRP and Pgp) with a potent antagonist of the N-methyl-D-aspartate receptor, GV196771, for the treatment of neuropathic pain can increase the bioavailability of GV196771.[64] Overall, coadministration of BCRP substrates and its inhibitor has been shown to result in drug–drug interactions due to modified transport capabilities. These data also clearly indicated that drug transporter plays an important role governing the absorption of substrate molecules.

Other examples of drug–drug interactions at the transport level involve the organic cation/carnitine transporters (OCTNs). It has been reported that competition between cephaloridine (β-lactam antibiotic) and carnitine transport at the level of OCTN2 can lead to renal mitochondrial damage.[65,66] In another study, the plasma concentration of sulpiride (a dopamine D2 receptor antagonist) decreased after concomitant oral administration with OCTN1 and OCTN2 substrates and/or inhibitors in rats.[67] Considering its wide tissue distribution in liver, intestine, kidney, brain, heart, and placenta, drug–drug interactions involving OCTNs can have broad impacts on the reabsorption, distribution, and elimination of their substrates and have profound clinical implications in our daily life.

The effect of drug transporter-related drug–drug interactions on bioavailability, tissue distribution, and pharmacological or toxicological functions of drugs can lead to altered therapeutic efficacy, unexpected adverse effects, and even toxicity. Understanding the interaction of the drug molecule with drug transporters, and the consequences of coadministration of multiple drugs has tremendous clinical implications.

3.4 CONCLUSION

Drug transporters as a group of critical membrane proteins play important roles in drug absorption, distribution, and elimination in the human body. Because of their wide tissue distributions, diverse functional characters, broad substrate spectra, and complicated regulation mechanisms, drug transporters need to be carefully studied. A thorough understanding of all aspects of transporter proteins is very important to drug design and evaluation.

As discussed in this chapter, drug transporters are under complicated regulation mechanisms and have important clinical significance due to their genetic polymorphism, their potential involvement in pathophysiological conditions, such as BUO and ARF, as well as transporter-mediated drug–drug interactions. All these have left us an expansive space to develop novel strategies by targeting drug transporter for the improvement of drug efficacy and reduction of toxicological side effects.

REFERENCES

1. G.Y.a.M.E. Morris. *Drug Transporters*, **2007**, Wiley & Son Inc.
2. Ekaratanawong, S.; Anzai, N.; Jutabha, P.; Miyazaki, H.; Noshiro, R.; Takeda, M.; Kanai, Y.; Sophasan, S.; Endou, H. *J. Pharmacol. Sci.* **2004**, 94, 297–304.
3. Ugele, B.; St-Pierre, M. V.; Pihusch, M.; Bahn, A.; Hantschmann, P. *Am. J. Physiol. Endocrinol. Metab.* **2003**, 284, E390–E398.
4. Gao, B.; Stieger, B.; Noe, B.; Fritschy, J. M.; Meier, P. J. *J. Histochem. Cytochem.* **1999**, 47, 1255–1264.
5. Scotto, K. W. *Oncogene* **2003**, 22, 7496–7511.
6. Labialle, S.; Gayet, L.; Marthinet, E.; Rigal, D.; Baggetto, L. G. *Biochem. Pharmacol.* **2002**, 64, 943–948.
7. Gerk, P. M.; Vore, M. *J. Pharmacol. Exp. Ther.* **2002**, 302, 407–415.
8. Haimeur, A.; Conseil, G.; Deeley, R. G.; Cole, S. P. *Curr. Drug Metab.* **2004**, 5, 21–53.
9. Terada, T.; Inui, K. *Biochem. Pharmacol.* **2007**, 73, 440–449.
10. Tanaka, K.; Xu, W.; Zhou, F.; You, G. *J. Biol. Chem.* **2004**, 279, 14961–14966.
11. Lee, T. K.; Koh, A. S.; Cui, Z.; Pierce, R. H.; Ballatori, N. *Am. J. Physiol. Gastrointest. Liver. Physiol.* **2003**, 285, G371–G381.
12. Zhou, F.; Xu, W.; Hong, M.; Pan, Z.; Sinko, P. J.; Ma, J.; You, G. *Mol. Pharmacol.* **2005**, 67, 868–876.
13. Kameh, H.; Landolt-Marticorena, C.; Charuk, J. H.; Schachter, H.; Reithmeier, R. A. *Biochem. Cell Biol.* **1998**, 76, 823–835.
14. Buck, T. M.; Eledge, J.; Skach, W. R. *Am. J. Physiol. Cell Physiol.* **2004**, 287, C1292–C1299.
15. Khanna, R.; Myers, M. P.; Laine, M.; Papazian, D. M. *J. Biol. Chem.* **2001**, 276, 34028–34034.
16. Ott, R. J.; Hui, A. C.; Giacomini, K. M. *J. Biol. Chem.* **1992**, 267, 133–139.

17. Bernardo, A. A.; Kear, F. T.; Arruda, J. A. *J. Membr. Biol.* **1997**, 158, 49–57.

18. Zhang, Z.; Wu, J. Y.; Hait, W. N.; Yang, J. M. *Mol. Pharmacol.* **2004**, 66, 395–403.

19. Mehrens, T.; Lelleck, S.; Cetinkaya, I.; Knollmann, M.; Hohage, H.; Gorboulev, V.; Boknik, P.; Koepsell, H.; Schlatter, E. *J. Am. Soc. Nephrol.* **2000**, 11, 1216–1224.

20. You, G.; Kuze, K.; Kohanski, R. A.; Amsler, K.; Henderson, S. *J. Biol. Chem.* **2000**, 275, 10278–10284.

21. Zhang, Q.; Hong, M.; Duan, P.; Pan, Z.; Ma, J.; You, G. *J. Biol. Chem.* **2008**, 283, 32570–32579.

22. Henriksen, U.; Fog, J. U.; Litman, T.; Gether, U. *J. Biol. Chem.* **2005**, 280, 36926–36934.

23. MacKinnon, R. *Nature* **1991**, 350, 232–235.

24. Ellgaard, L.; Helenius, A. *Nat. Rev. Mol. Cell Biol.* **2003**, 4, 181–191.

25. Veenhoff, L. M.; Heuberger, E. H.; Poolman, B. *Trends Biochem. Sci.* **2002**, 27, 242–249.

26. Scholze, P.; Freissmuth, M.; Sitte, H. H. *J. Biol. Chem.* **2002**, 277, 43682–43690.

27. Hong, M.; Xu, W.; Yoshida, T.; Tanaka, K.; Wolff, D. J.; Zhou, F.; Inouye, M.; You, G. *J. Biol. Chem.* **2005**, 280, 32285–32290.

28. Biber, J.; Gisler, S. M.; Hernando, N.; Murer, H. *J. Membr. Biol.* **2005**, 203, 111–118.

29. Kato, Y.; Watanabe, C.; Tsuji, A. *Eur. J. Pharm. Sci.* **2006**, 27, 487–500.

30. Perego, C.; Vanoni, C.; Villa, A.; Longhi, R.; Kaech, S. M.; Frohli, E.; Hajnal, A.; Kim, S. K.; Pietrini, G. *Embo. J.* **1999**, 18, 2384–2393.

31. Raghuram, V.; Hormuth, H.; Foskett, J. K. *Proc. Natl. Acad. Sci. USA* **2003**, 100, 9620–9625.

32. Shenolikar, S.; Voltz, J. W.; Minkoff, C. M.; Wade, J. B.; Weinman, E. J. *Proc. Natl. Acad. Sci. USA* **2002**, 99, 11470–11475.

33. Anzai, N.; Miyazaki, H.; Noshiro, R.; Khamdang, S.; Chairoungdua, A.; Shin, H. J.; Enomoto, A.; Sakamoto, S.; Hirata, T.; Tomita, K.; Kanai, Y.; Endou, H. *J. Biol. Chem.* **2004**, 279, 45942–45950.

34. Kwak, J. O.; Kim, H. W.; Song, J. H.; Kim, M. J.; Park, H. S.; Hyun, D. K.; Kim, D. S.; Cha, S. H. *IUBMB Life* **2005**, 57, 109–117.

35. Lee, W. K.; Choi, J. K. Cha, S. H. *Exp. Mol. Med.* **2008**, 40, 505–513.

36. Kwak, J. O.; Kim, H. W.; Oh, K. J.; Kim, D. S.; Han, K. O.; Cha, S. H. *Exp. Mol. Med.* **2005**, 37, 204–212.

37. Paulusma, C. C.; Kool, M.; Bosma, P. J.; Scheffer, G. L.; ter Borg, F.; Scheper, R. J.; Tytgat, G. N.; Borst, P.; Baas, F.; Oude Elferink, R. P. *Hepatology* **1997**, 25, 1539–1542.

38. Thompson, R.; Strautnieks, S. *Seminars Liver Diss.* **2001**, 21, 545–550.

39. Eraly, S. A.; Bush, K. T.; Sampogna, R. V.; Bhatnagar, V.; Nigam, S. K. *Mol. Pharmacol.* **2004**, 65, 479–487.

40. Ichida, K.; Hosoyamada, M.; Hisatome, I.; Enomoto, A.; Hikita, M.; Endou, H.; Hosoya, T. *J. Am. Soc. Nephrol.* **2004**, 15, 164–173.

41. Komoda, F.; Sekine, T.; Inatomi, J.; Enomoto, A.; Endou, H.; Ota, T.; Matsuyama, T.; Ogata, T.; Ikeda, M.; Awazu, M.; Muroya, K.; Kamimaki, I.; Igarashi, T. *Pediatr. Nephrol.* **2004**, 19, 728–733.

42. Tanaka, M.; Itoh, K.; Matsushita, K.; Matsushita, K.; Wakita, N.; Adachi, M.; Nonoguchi, H.; Kitamura, K.; Hosoyamada, M.; Endou, H.; Tomita, K. *Am. J. Kidney Dis.* **2003**, 42, 1287–1292.

43. Ogasawara, K.; Terada, T.; Motohashi, H.; Asaka, J.; Aoki, M.; Katsura, T.; Kamba, T.; Ogawa, O.; Inui, K. *J. Human Gen.* **2008**, 53, 607–614.

44. Zair, Z. M.; Eloranta, J. J.; Stieger, B.; Kullak-Ublick, G. A. *Pharmacogenomics* **2008**, 9, 597–624.

45. Maeda, K.; Sugiyama, Y. *Drug Metab. Pharmacokinet.* **2008**, 23, 223–235.

46. Ambudkar, S. V.; Sauna, Z. E.; Gottesman, M. M.; Szakacs, G. *Trends Pharmacol. Sci.* **2005**, 26, 385–387.

47. Teodori, E.; Dei, S.; Martelli, C.; Scapecchi, S.; Gualtieri, F. *Curr. Drug Targets* **2006**, 7, 893–909.

48. Varadi, A.; Szakacs, G.; Bakos, E.; Sarkadi, B. *Novartis Found Symp.* **2002**, 243, 54–65; discussion 65–68, 180–185.

49. Schwab, M.; Schaeffeler, E.; Marx, C.; Fromm, M. F.; Kaskas, B.; Metzler, J.; Stange, E.; Herfarth, H.; Schoelmerich, J.; Gregor, M.; Walker, S.; Cascorbi, I.; Roots, I.; Brinkmann, U.; Zanger, U. M.; Eichelbaum, M. *Gastroenterology* **2003**, 124, 26–33.

50. Villar, S. R.; Brandoni, A.; Anzai, N.; Endou, H.; Torres, A. M. *Kidney Int.* **2005**, 68, 2704–2713.

51. Li, S.; Duan, P.; You, G. *Am. J. Physiol. Endocrinol. Metab.* **2009**, 296, E378–E383.

52. Uchino, S.; Kellum, J. A.; Bellomo, R.; Doig, G. S.; Morimatsu, H.; Morgera, S.; Schetz, M.; Tan, I.; Bouman, C.; Macedo, E.; Gibney, N.; Tolwani, A.; Ronco, C. *JAMA* **2005**, 294, 813–818.

53. Schneider, R.; Sauvant, C.; Betz, B.; Otremba, M.; Fischer, D.; Holzinger, H.; Wanner, C.; Galle, J.; Gekle, M. *Am. J. Physiol.* **2007**, 292, F1599–F1605.

54. Kwon, O.; Wang, W. W.; Miller, S. *Am. J. Physiol. Renal Physiol.* **2008**, 295, F1807–F1816.

55. Volk, H. A.; Potschka, H.; Loscher, W. *Epilepsy Res.* **2004**, 58, 67–79.

56. Soranzo, N.; Goldstein, D. B.; Sisodiya, S. M. *Expert Opin. Pharmacother.* **2005**, 6, 1305–1312.

57. Lin, T.; Islam, O.; Heese, K. *Cell Res.* **2006**, 16, 857–871.

58. Mealey, K. L. *J. Vet. Pharmacol. Ther.* **2004**, 27, 257–264.

59. Marzolini, C.; Paus, E.; Buclin, T.; Kim, R. B. *Clin. Pharmacol. Ther.* **2004**, 75, 13–33.

60. Mizuno, N.; Sugiyama, Y. *Drug Metab. Pharmacokinet.* **2002**, 17, 93–108.

61. Hosoyamada, M.; Sekine, T.; Kanai, Y.; Endou, H. *Am. J. Physiol.* **1999**, 276, F122–F128.

62. Jonker, J. W.; Smit, J. W.; Brinkhuis, R. F.; Maliepaard, M.; Beijnen, J. H.; Schellens, J. H.; Schinkel, A. H. *J. Natl. Cancer Inst.* **2000**, 92, 1651–1656.

63. Kruijtzer, C. M.; Beijnen, J. H.; Rosing, H.; ten Bokkel Huinink, W. W.; Schot, M.; Jewell, R. C.; Paul, E. M.; Schellens, J. H. *J. Clin. Oncol.* **2002**, 20, 2943–2950.

64. Polli, J. W.; Baughman, T. M.; Humphreys, J. E.; Jordan, K. H.; Mote, A. L.; Webster, L. O.; Barnaby, R. J.; Vitulli, G.; Bertolotti, L.; Read, K. D.; Serabjit-Singh, C. J. *Drug Metab. Dispos.* **2004**, 32, 722–726.

65. Ganapathy, M. E.; Huang, W.; Rajan, D. P.; Carter, A. L.; Sugawara, M.; Iseki, K.; Leibach, F. H.; Ganapathy, V. *J. Biol. Chem.* **2000**, 275, 1699–1707.

66. Ohashi, R.; Tamai, I.; Yabuuchi, H.; Nezu, J. I.; Oku, A.; Sai, Y.; Shimane, M.; Tsuji, A. *J. Pharmacol. Exp. Ther.* **1999**, 291, 778–784.

67. Watanabe, K.; Sawano, T.; Jinriki, T.; Sato, J. *Biol. Pharm. Bull.* **2004**, 27, 77–81.

CHAPTER 4

CYTOCHROME P450: STRUCTURE, FUNCTION AND APPLICATION IN DRUG DISCOVERY AND DEVELOPMENT

RAMESH B. BAMBAL
Absorption Systems, Exton, PA

STEPHEN E. CLARKE
Preclinical Development, Drug Metabolism and Pharmacokinetics, GlaxoSmithKline Pharmaceuticals, Ware, United Kingdom

Evaluation of Drug Candidates for Preclinical Development: Pharmacokinetics, Metabolism, Pharmaceutics, and Toxicology, Edited by Chao Han, Charles B. Davis, and Binghe Wang
Copyright © 2010 John Wiley & Sons, Inc.

4.1 THE CYP ENZYMES

4.1.1 Localization

Cytochrome P450s (CYPs) are heme (iron-protoporphyrrin IX complex) containing proteins (Fig. 4.1, structure **A**) that exists in mammals, other animal species, plants, and bacteria.[1,2] The CYP enzymes are responsible for the oxidation of many lipophilic compounds including drugs, environmental chemicals, and endogenous substrates. The CYPs play an important role in the elimination of lipophilic drugs from the body by transforming them into more polar and water soluble metabolites by the process known as biotransformation. Due to this critical role in the metabolism, and thereby clearance of many pharmacological important drugs, CYPs are regarded as one of the most important adsorption, distribution, metabolism, and elimination (ADME) enzymes for drug discovery and development.

The CYPs are membrane-bound proteins located in the endoplasmic reticulum (microsomes) of the cells, although there are CYP enzymes that are located in the mitochondria of cells, where they play an important role in steroid hormone biosynthesis and vitamin D metabolism. The heme site in the protein is nearly an independent entity linked to the reminder of the apoprotein with only one or two amino acids that serve as axial ligands. The fifth axial ligand to the heme in CYP enzymes

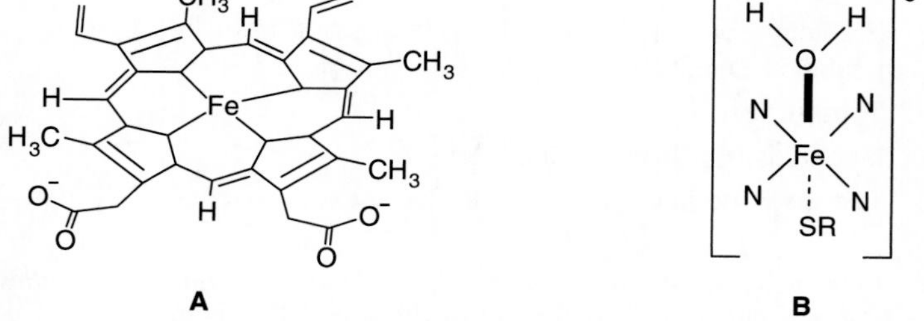

A   B

Figure 4.1. Structure A is an Iron-protoporphyrrin IX complex and structure B is iron ferric (Fe^{3+}) in the resting state of the enzyme with water bound as a sixth ligand.

is a cysteine thiolate. In the resting state of the enzyme, the iron is in the ferric state (Fe^{3+}) and the sixth ligand is the water molecule (Fig. 4.1, structure **B**).[3,4] When reduced to the ferrous (Fe^{2+}) state, CYP can bind ligands, such as oxygen (O_2) and carbon monoxide (CO). The complex between ferrous CYP and CO absorbs light maximally at 450 nm, from which CYP derived its name—cytochrome P450.[5] The highest amounts of CYPs are found in the liver. However, they are also found throughout the body, especially in tissues, such as intestine, lung, and kidney.[6,7]

Of the CYP enzymes identified in humans, only a handful are significantly involved in the metabolism of drugs. In humans, xenobiotics are metabolized primarily by three CYP families (CYP1, CYP2, and CYP3).[8] The enzymes of CYP3A subfamily are of major importance, since collectively they are by far the most quantitatively significant of all the human CYP enzymes and their substrate specificities are extremely broad. In early Drug Discovery processes it has been suggested that just five of the hepatic CYPs, namely, CYP1A2, CYP2C9, CYP2C19, CYP2D6, and CYP3A4, need to be considered with respect to enzymology and drug–drug interaction.[9]

4.1.2 The Catalytic Cycle of CYP

CYP catalyzes the oxidation of the substrate in which one atom of oxygen is incorporated into a substrate designated RH (where RH is an organic chemical), and the other is reduced to water with a reducing equivalent derived from reduced nicotinamide adenine dinucleotide phosphate (NADPH), as follows:[5]

$$\text{Substrate}(RH) + O_2 + NADPH + H^+ \rightarrow \text{Product}(ROH) + H_2O + NADP^+$$

The catalytic cycle of CYP is shown in Figure 4.2. In the resting state, the enzyme is in the ferric (Fe^{3+}) state with a water molecule acting as a sixth ligand. In the first step, the substrate binds to the enzyme in the hydrophobic pocket near the catalytic site [B] (step a). Substrates are quite distinct from the ligands that directly bind to the iron atom. Upon substrate binding, CYP changes from a low- to a high-spin state displacing the water molecule as a sixth ligand. Following the binding of the substrate to the CYP enzyme, the heme iron is reduced from the ferric (Fe^{3+}) to the ferrous (Fe^{2+}) state by the addition of a single electron from NADPH [C] (step b). The electrons from NADPH are transferred to cytochrome CYP by a flavoprotein enzyme localized in endoplasmic reticulum know as NADPH–CYP reductase.[10,11] Molecular

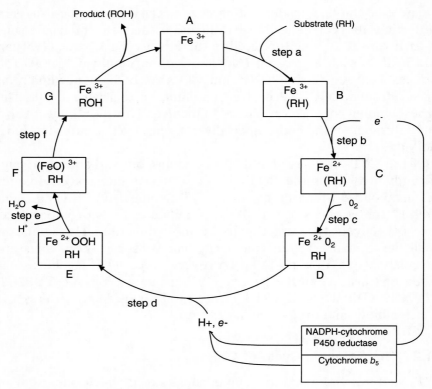

Figure 4.2. Catalytic cycle of the CYP enzyme.

oxygen has a strong affinity for the reduced form of CYP and binds to it in the ferrous state to form a ferrous dioxygen complex $Fe^{2+}O_2$ [D] (step c). The next step is the addition of a second electron to the $Fe^{2+}O_2$ complex. A second electron must be delivered rapidly, otherwise the $Fe^{2+}O_2$ complex dissociates with release of super oxide. Addition of a second electron can occur from NADPH via NADPH–cytochrome P450 reductase or from NADH–cytochrome b_5 reductase. With the addition of the second electron and a proton (H^+), the Fe^{2+}–O_2 complex is converted to the hydroperoxy cytochrome P450 complex $Fe^{2+}OOH$ [E] (step d). Faster input of the second electron via cytochrome b_5 can result in formation of more of the hydroperoxy complex. There is also a direct interaction of cytochrome b_5 with NADPH:cytochrome CYP reductase.[12] The hydroperoxy cytochrome P450 complex $Fe^{2+}OOH$ cleaves to produce water and a ferryl-oxo heme complex $(FeO)^{3+}$ [F] (step e). In the final step, the oxygen atom from ferryl-oxo heme complex $(FeO)^{3+}$ gets transferred to the substrate [G] (step f). This final substrate oxidation step occurs either by single-electron transfer (SET) or by hydrogen atom transfer (HAT). Release of oxidized substrate returns CYP to the initial ferric (Fe^{3+}) resting state. If the cycle is interrupted following introduction of the first electron, oxygen is released as a super oxide anion (O_2^-). If the cycle is interrupted after introduction of a second electron, oxygen is released as hydrogen peroxide (H_2O_2).

In mitochondrial CYP, the electron transfer from NADPH to CYP occurs via two proteins—an iron–sulfur containing protein called ferrodoxin and an flavin mononucleotide (FMN) containing flavoprotein called ferrodoxin reductase. The functional role of mitochondrial cytochrome b_5 in monooxygenase reaction is unclear. There is evidence for participation of mitochondrial cytochrome b_5 in reduction of cytosolic semiascorbate via the transport of electrons from NADH to NADH:cytochrome b_5 reductase and semidehydro reductase ascorbate.[13]

For each molecule of NADPH–cytochrome P450 reductase in rat liver microsomes, there are 5–10 molecules of cytochrome b_5 and 10–20 molecules of CYP. The NADPH-cytochrome P450 reductase can transfer electrons much faster than CYP can use them, which more than likely accounts for the low ratio of NADPH–cytochrome P450 reductase to CYP in liver microsomes.

4.1.3 Nomenclature

The CYP enzymes are now known to have a broad and overlapping substrate specificity, which precludes naming them by the reactions they catalyze. Instead, CYP enzymes are classified into families and subfamilies broadly based on the similarities between their gene and gene products. The amino acid sequence of numerous CYP enzymes has been determined largely by recombinant DNA techniques.[14–16] The root for all cytochrome P450 genomics and cDNA sequence names is an italicized *CYP*. A family is defined as having amino acid sequence similarity >40% (e.g., gene families) and denoted by Arabic numerals 1, 2, 3, 4 and so on.[17] Mammalian CYP enzymes with a >55% amino acid sequence similarity are classified within the same subfamily and designated with letters (2A, 2B, 2C, 2D, 2E, etc). Finally, an individual enzyme is designated with an Arabic number assigned on an incremental basis (i.e., first come, first served). Enzymes within each subfamily have a >70% amino acid sequence identity. Thus, for example, CYP3A4 is the fourth member of subfamily A of family 3. Human CYP drug metabolizing enzymes mainly belong to the gene families CYP1, CYP2, and CYP3. For a more detailed treatment of CYP nomenclature and links to other cytochrome P450 resources, see the cytochrome P450 home page at http://drnelson.utmem.edu/CytochromeP450.html.

Human liver microsomes contain more than 35 CYP enzymes. Some drug metabolizing enzymes from families 1, 2, and 3 in humans are CYP1A1, 1A2, 1B1, 2A6, 2B6, 2C8, 2C9, 2C18, 2C19, 2D6, 2E1, 3A4, 3A5, 3A7, 4A9, and 4A11. A handful out of these, such as, CYP1A2, 2C8, 2C9, 2C19, 2D6, 3A4, and 3A5, are quantitatively important for metabolism of pharmacological agents.

4.1.4 Tissue Distribution and CYP Enzyme Abundance in Humans

The CYP is most abundantly found in liver and intestinal epithelia and these are the main sites for drug clearance and drug–drug interactions. Although CYP is found in all organs and tissues throughout the body, it is unlikely to play an important role in overall drug elimination in all these tissues.[6] In human liver, CYP3A4 is quantitatively the most abundant enzyme representing ~34% of the total CYP in the liver.[18] The CYP1A2 represents 13%, CYP2A6 is 5%, CYP2B6 is 3%, CYP2C8 is 6%, CYP2C9 is 17%, CYP2C19 is 0.3%, CYP2D6 is 2%, CYP2E1 is 15%, and CYP3A5 is 2% of the total CYPs.[19] The CYP3A4 is responsible for the metabolism of 50% of oxidatively metabolized drugs, while CYP2D6, although representing only 2% of the total hepatic CYP, metabolizes 25% and CYP2C8, CYP2C9, and CYP2C19 together metabolizes 15% of the drugs. Other enzymes, such as CYP1A2 and CYP2E1, contribute to a lesser extent. Several CYPs also exist in animal species intestine including human. The CYP2C9, CYP2D6, and CYP2E1 enzymes are present at measurable levels in human intestine; however, the most significant enzyme in human intestine is CYP3A4 (at ~1% of the hepatic levels, but specifically located within the epithelial cells at high concentration) and is of significant concern for drug–drug interaction in the gut.

4.1.5 Structure of CYP Enzymes

Mammalian CYPs are membrane-bound proteins embedded in endoplasmic reticulum or the mitochondria. The CYPs are promiscuous enzymes with broad and overlapping substrate specificities. Knowledge of active site topology and ligand- or substrate-binding specificities of

CYP enzymes is essential for the understanding of novel drug substrate metabolism and in the design of new drugs. Due to the membrane bound nature of the enzymes, it has been challenging to obtain single crystals of CYP enzymes for X-ray structure determination. Until recently, our knowledge of active sites of CYP enzymes were mostly based on homology modeling built by site-directed mutagenesis. Recently, the crystal structures of three most important human enzymes CYP2C9, CYP2D6, and CYP3A4, have been determined. This determination was made possible by truncation of the membrane bound N-terminal domain and, in some cases, the introduction of small mutations that helped to solubilize the protein. Based on homology modeling, it was proposed that CYP2C9 preferentially binds small lipophilic substrates through basic residues in an anionic-binding active site. The crystal structure, however, shows that there are no basic residues in this site that could interact with substrate. Indeed the residues proposed to participate in anionic binding actually point away from the true binding site, which contain two acidic residues potentially capable of ligand interaction.[20,21] The CYP2C9–warfarin bound structure revealed that the binding pocket is large enough to accommodate the binding of additional small molecules at the same time as warfarin. This information could be useful in understanding the drug–drug interaction.

The crystal structure of CYP2D6 shows the characteristic P450-fold as seen in other members of the CYP family. The CYP2D6 structure has a well-defined active site cavity above the heme group, which could be defined as having the shape of a right foot, the volume of the cavity is ~540 Å. The active site contains many important residues that have been implicated in substrate recognition and binding, including Asp-301, Glu-216, Phe-483, and Phe-120.[22] While, Asp-301, Glu-216, and Phe-483 can act as substrate-binding residues, Phe-120 is involved in controlling the orientation of the aromatic ring found in most substrates with respect to heme.

The crystal structure of arguably the most important enzyme in drug metabolism, i.e. CYP3A4, has been published recently.[23] One key feature of the active site is the Phe cluster of seven phenylalanine residues that form a hydrophobic core pointing toward the active site. The presence of the cluster means that the accessible volume of the active site is much smaller than would be expected considering the large molecular size of some CYP3A4 substrates. It is suggested that the conformational change of a Phe cluster could reposition the Phe residue resulting in an extended active site that is capable of binding more than one substrate. In addition, the active site in CYP3A4 has greater access to a heme moiety. This proximity could enable two substrate molecules to have access to reactive oxygen, potentially providing the means for CYP3A4 to metabolize more than one substrate simultaneously showing allosteric behavior. Such binding can lead to atypical enzyme kinetics and substrate-dependent drug–drug interaction data. Furthermore, it is suggested that the movement of the Phe cluster could facilitate the transfer of substrate from the peripheral site to the active site by forming a substrate access channel. The crystal structures of other human enzymes, CYP2C8 and CYP2B6, have been published recently.[24,25]

4.1.6   Interindividual Variability and Polymorphism

Allelic variants, which arise by point mutations in the wild-type gene, are the source of interindividual variation in the CYP activity. Amino acid substitutions can result in an increase or more commonly a decrease in CYP activity. Environmental factors known to affect CYP levels include medications (e.g., barbiturates, anticonvulsants, rifampin, troglitazone, isoniazide), foods (e.g., cruciferous vegetables, charcoal broiled beef), social habits (e.g., alcohol consumption, cigarette smoking), and disease status (diabetes, inflammation, viral and bacterial infection, hyperthyroidism, and hypothyroidism.[5] Due to recessive inheritance of gene mutation, some CYP enzymes can be absent or poorly expressed in a certain percentage of the population leading to increased pharmacological response or toxic effects of drugs.[26–28] The two major polymorphically expressed enzymes are CYP2C19 and CYP2D6. The poor metabolizer phenotype of CYP2C19 is found in 2–3% of Caucasians and African–Americans and up to 20% of Asians.[29] Poor metabolism of (S)-mephenytoin to 4′-hydroxy mephenytoin in these phenotypes has resulted in limited clinical use of this drug.[30] Other drugs metabolized by this enzyme, such as omeprazole, have a reduced rate of drug clearance and the anxiolytic agent diazepam have increased the occurrence of toxicity following the administration of such agents. The CYP2D6 poor metabolizer phenotype is detected in ~6% of Caucasians, but is less common in Asian and African populations occurring at a frequency of <1%.[31,32] It has significant impact on the *in vivo* metabolism of several common pharmaceuticals that are metabolized by CYP2D6, including tricyclic antidepressants, haloperidol, metoprolol, codeine, and dextromethorphan.[33] In most clinical situations, administration of a standard dose of CYP2D6 substrate results in elevated blood levels in poor metabolizers accompanied by increased risk of toxicity.

4.1.7 The CYP Catalyzed Reactions

The CYP mediated oxidation occurs by the insertion of oxygen from ferryl-oxo heme complex $(FeO)^{3+}$ to the substrate. The primary oxidative reactions catalyzed by cytochrome P450s includes the following:

1. Insertion of oxygen into C–H bond of aliphatic and aromatic carbon to form C–OH. The newly formed C–O bond remains intact.
2. Insertion of oxygen into aliphatic and aromatic C=C to form epoxides. Formation of an epoxide by chemical or enzymatic reaction undergoes hydrolysis to the diols or aromatizes to phenol.
3. Insertion of oxygen into heteroatoms (e.g., N and S) to form N- and S-oxide and N-hydroxylation.
4. Heteroatom (N, S, and O) dealkylation. When aliphatic carbon is attached to the heteroatoms (e.g., as N, S, and O), the end products of C-hydroxylations are the heteroatom dealkylation due to instability of newly generated carbinol amine, ketal, or a thioketal, resulting in the cleavage of a heteroatom–C bond.
5. Dehydrogenation. Two hydrogens are abstracted from the substrate with the formation of a double bond (C=C, C=N, C=O).
6. Oxidative group transfer. Oxygenation of the substrate is followed by a rearrangement reaction leading to loss of the heteroatom (oxidative group transfer).

In addition, CYP also carries out such reactions as, reduction of azo and nitro groups, isomerization, and cleavage of a C–C bond in endogenous steroid synthesis.

Although CYP enzymes have broad and overlapping substrate specificity, many of the CYP hydroxylation reactions are regio- and stereoselective. For example, the oxidation of testosterone to 6-beta hydroxylation of testosterone by CYP3A4 is stereoselective[34] (Scheme 4.1). The deuterium isotope effect studies suggested that only the

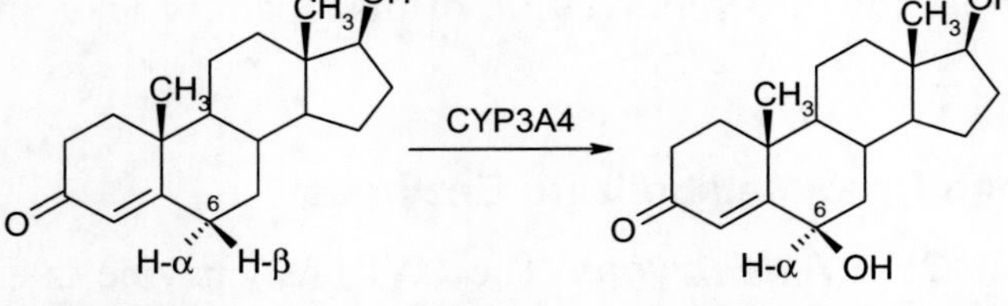

Scheme 4.1. Stereoselective abstraction and rebound at the 6-β hydrogen of testosterone.

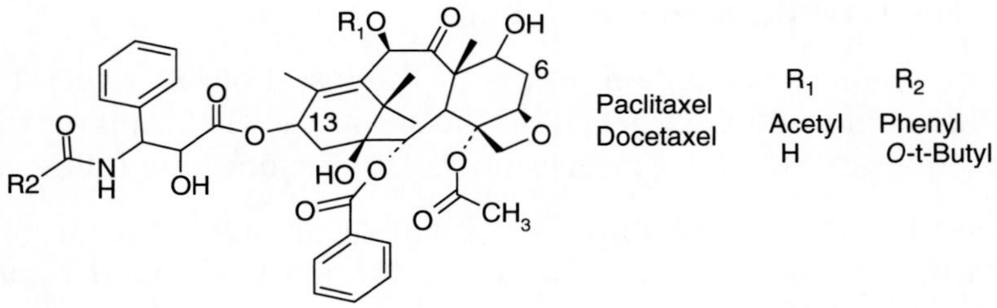

Figure 4.3. Structure of paclitaxel, docetaxel, and their metabolites.

6-beta-hydrogen is removed by CYP3A4 and not the 6-alpha-hydrogen. This finding indicat that CYP abstracts hydrogen and rebounds oxygen only at the beta face.

Structurally close analogues can be metabolized by different enzymes at different positions. For example, paclitaxel is hydroxylated at the 6-position of the taxane ring by CYP2C8, while the close structural analogue docetaxel is hydroxylated on the *tert*-butyl group of the lateral side chain in the C13 position by CYP3A4, as shown in Figure 4.3.[35]

Small structural changes in the molecule play an important role in determining the regioselective oxidation by the CYP enzymes. Drug can be metabolized by a single enzyme through multiple pathways, but with different affinities. For example, midazolam is metabolized by CYP3A4 to 1'-hydroxymidazolam with four times higher affinity than to 4'-hydroxymidazolam.[36] Dextromethorphan is metabolized by CYP2D6 through a selective O-demethylation pathway forming dextorphan, and by CYP3A4 and 2B6 by a selective N-demethylation pathway, leading to the formation of 3-methoxymorphinan,[37] as shown in Scheme 4.2.

Alternatively, more than one enzyme may be involved in the metabolism of the drug by the same pathway. For example, N-demethylation of diazepam is catalyzed by two human CYP enzymes, CYP2C19 and CYP3A4. However, the reaction is catalyzed by CYP3A4 with such a low affinity that the N-demethylation of diazepam *in vivo* appears to be dominated by CYP2C19.[38]

4.1.8 Human Drug Metabolizing Enzymes

4.1.8.1 The CYP1A2 Enzyme. The CYP1A2 enzyme is expressed primarily in liver, with little expression in extrahepatic tissues.[39–41] The CYP1A2 is inducible by its substrates and metabolizes carcinogenic

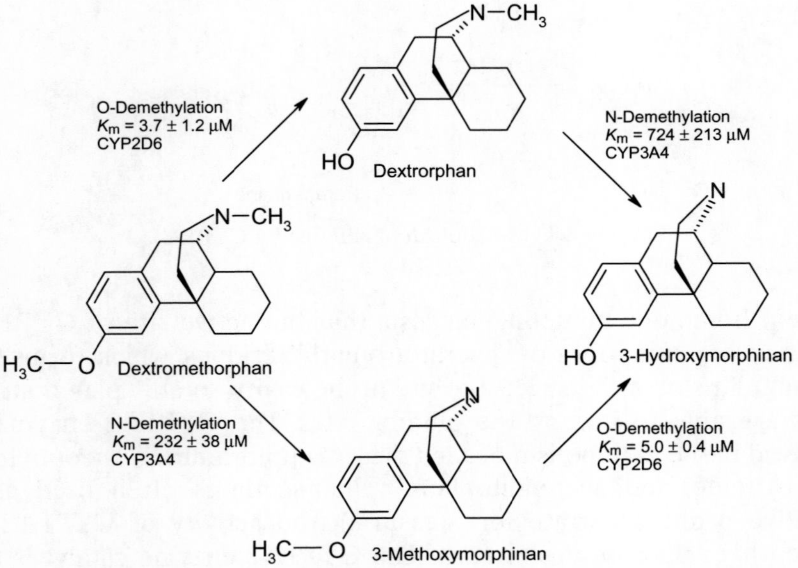

Scheme 4.2. Dedxtromethorphan demethylation pathways catalyzed by recombinant human CYP2D6 and CYP3A4.

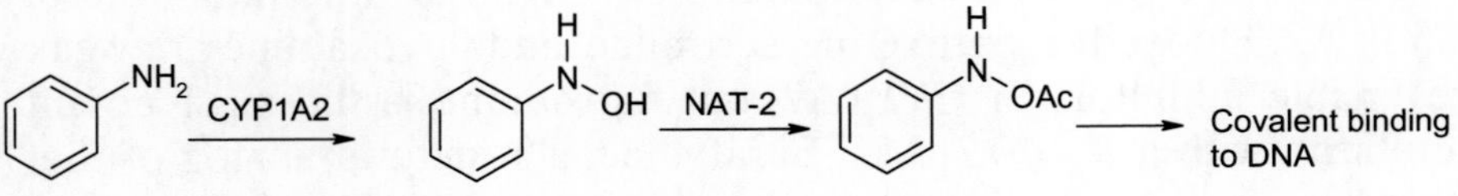

NAT-2 = N-Acetyltransferase -2

Scheme 4.3. Proposed metabolic pathway for metabolism of aromatic amines by CYP1A2 in liver.

aromatic and heterocyclic amines found in cigarette smoke and in charred food by N-oxidation.[42] In many cases, this represents an initial step in the conversion of aromatic amines to tumorigenic metabolites that form adducts with DNA (Scheme 4.3). Human exposure to these compounds has been implicated as a risk factor for colorectal cancer.[43]

Thus the induction of human CYP1A2 is paid considerable attention in drug development due to its association with the etiology of several cancers that are thought to arise through the formation of adducts between DNA and the oxidized products of CYP catalyzed reactions. However, omeprazole, which is a very successful and general is recognized as a safe drug, has been shown to induce CYP1A2 in humans.[44]

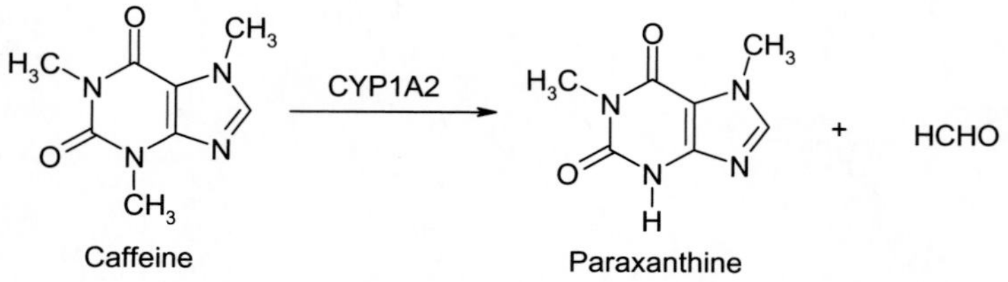

Scheme 4.4. Metabolism of caffeine by CYP1A2.

Protein homology modeling suggests that the active site of CYP1A2 enzymes are composed of several aromatic residues, which forms the rectangular slot and restricts the site of the cavity, so only planar structures are able to occupy the binding sites. The CYP1A2 enzyme is involved in the metabolism of such drugs as imipramine,[45] theophylline and caffeine, and acetaminophen.[46] Phenacetin is often used as a selective probe substrate for measuring the activity of CYP1A2 in human liver microsomes *in vitro*. The CYP1A2 enzyme catalyzes the N-demethylation of caffeine to paraxanthene and N-demethylation of caffeine is used as an *in vivo* probe to measure the activity of CYP1A2 in humans, as shown in Scheme 4.4.

Selective serotonin uptake inhibitors (SSRIs) are the inhibitors of CYP1A2. Fluoxetine, paroxetine, sertraline, and fluvoxamine are weak reversible inhibitors of CYP1A2, but fluoxamine is the most potent inhibitor, with a $K_i = 0.2\,\mu M$.[47] Furafylline, a structural analog of theophylline, is a metabolism-dependent inhibitor of CYP1A2.[48,49]

4.1.8.2 The CYP2C9 Enzyme. The CYP2C9 enzyme is the most highly expressed member of the CYP2C subfamily in hepatic tissues and catalyzes the metabolism of several important drugs including the antidiabetic agent tolbutamide, torsemide, the anti-inflammatory drug ibuprofen, diclofenac, the anticoagulant warfarin, the barbiturate hexabarbital, and anticonvulsants, such as phenytoin and trimethadon.[50–56] Due to a narrow therapeutic margin of some of the CYP2C9 substrates including warfarin, this enzyme is an important target for drug interaction issues. The frequency of CYP2C9 polymorphism is very low at 0.25% in Caucasians and even lower in the Asian population. However, the clinical consequences of these rare poor metabolizer polymorphisms can lead to life-threatening bleeding episodes following administration of warfarin and severe toxicity with phenytoin administration.

In human liver microsomes, diclofenac is metabolized to 4'-hydroxydiclofenac and diclofenac is a widely used selective probe *in vitro*. Tolbutamide, phenytoin, diclofenac, and flurbiprofen are used as

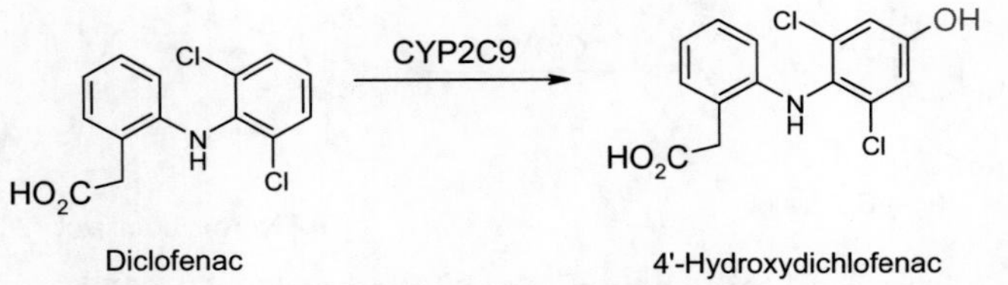

Scheme 4.5. Metabolism of dichlofenac by CYP2C9.

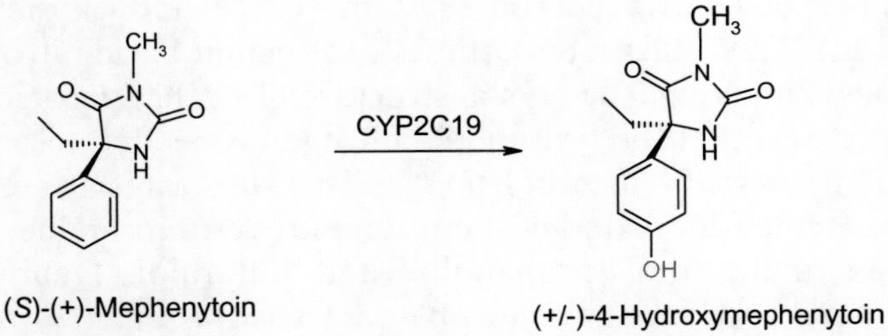

(S)-(+)-Mephenytoin   (+/-)-4-Hydroxymephenytoin

Scheme 4.6. Metabolism of (S)-(+)-mephenytoin by CYP2C19.

in vivo probes to measure the activity of CYP2C9 in humans,[57] as shown in Scheme 4.5.

Sulphaphenazole is a potent and selective inhibitor of CYP2C9 in both *in vitro* and *in vivo*, however, it has been less commonly used *in vivo*.[58] Tienilic acid is an irreversible and metabolism-dependent inhibitor of CYP2C9. The thiophene ring in tienilic acid is oxidized to thiophene sulfoxide by CYP2C9, which can react with either water or nucleophilic amino acids in CYP2C9[59] to form a covalent protein adduct that inactivates the enzyme.

4.1.8.3 The CYP2C19 Enzyme. The substrates for this enzyme include the anxiolytic and sedative drug diazepam, the proton-pump inhibitor omeprazole, and antidepressant drug imipramine. The anticonvulsant drug mephenytoin is a selective substrate for CYP2C19 used to measure the activity of CYP2C19 in human liver microsomes *in vitro*. Mephenytoin is oxidized to 4′-hydroxymephenytoin, as shown in Scheme 4.6.

Hydroxylation of mephenytoin is stereoselective and this 4′-hydroxylation of (S)-mephenytoin is 3–10-fold faster than that of the (R)-enantiomer in extensive metabolizers, but the ratio is ~1 or less in poor metabolizers.[60] There are few clinically relevant inhibitors of CYP2C19, the most significant being selective serotonin reuptake inhibitors (SSRIs). Fluvoxamine inhibits CYP2C19 *in vivo*, but it is not a selective inhibitor of CYP2C19.

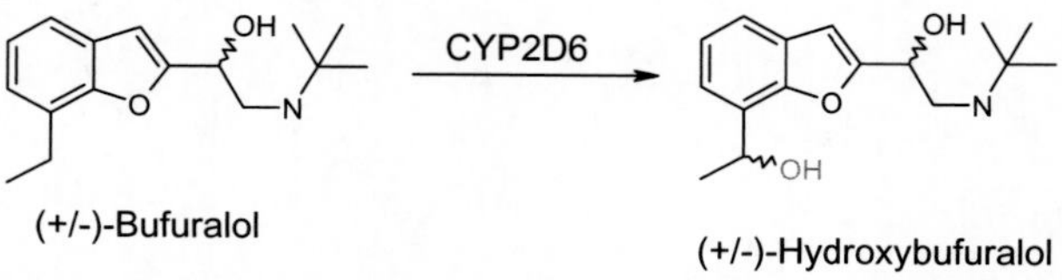

Scheme 4.7. Metabolism of (+/−)-bufuralol by CYP2D6.

4.1.8.4 *The CYP2D6 Enzyme.*

The CYP2D6 enzyme metabolizes a large number of central nervous system (CNS) and cardiovascular drugs. The CYP2D6 substrates contain protonated basic nitrogen and a planner aromatic ring. The crystal structure of CYP2D6 corroborates the previous view that the protonated nitrogen is needed to be 5–10 Å away from the site of metabolism.[61–63] The substrates for CYP2D6 include sparteine, debrisoquine, imipramine, desimipramine, dextromethorphan, metoprolol, propanolol, and bufuralol. Debrisoquine, desimipramine, and dextromethorphan are used as *in vivo* probes in human drug interaction studies and bufuralol and metoprolol are often used as selective *in vitro* probes as shown in Scheme 4.7. The poor metabolism phenotype of CYP2D6 is characterized clinically by a marked deficiency in metabolism that can result in drug toxicity or reduced efficacy.[64] Quinidine is a potent inhibitor of CYP2D6, but it is not metabolized by CYP2D6. Fluoxetine and several other SSRI inhibitors are also potent competitive inhibitors of CYP2D6,[65–67] as shown in Scheme 4.7.

4.1.8.5 *The CYP3A4 Enzyme.*

It has been estimated that 50% of the marketed drugs that are oxidatively metabolized are substrates for CYP3A4.[68,69] These drugs belong to a broad range of therapeutic categories and represent a wide range of molecular sizes and structures. For example, CYP3A4 can metabolize small molecules like quinidine, a medium sized molecule like midazolam, and a large molecule like cyclosporine. In general, many CYP3A4 substrates are either neutral or weakly basic with a relatively high molecular weight and lipophilicity. Most possess a hydrogen-bond donor–acceptor capability and an aromatic ring system.[70] Some of the common drugs metabolized by CYP3A4 include acetaminophen, amiodarone, amprinavir, benzphetamine, carbamazepine, digioxin, diazepam, erythromycin, indinavir, nifedipine, midazolam, omeprazole, taxol, verapamil, and warfarin. In addition to the xenobiotics, CYP3A4 is also known to play an important role in the metabolism of endogenous steroid substrates including testosterone, progesterone, and androstenedione.[64,71] Metabolic activity for CYP3A4 is variable in the human population (>10-fold) without the need for polymorphisms. Such variability can impact the safety and efficacy of drugs that are metabolized by this enzyme. Because of its ability to metabolize a vast array of clinically significant pharmaceutical compounds, CYP3A4 is responsible for the large number of clinical drug–drug interactions.[72–78] Midazolam and erythromycin are commonly used as *in vivo* probes and midazolam, nifedipine, and testosterone are commonly used as *in vitro* probes for drug interaction studies (Schemes 4.8 and 4.9).

Inhibitors of CYP3A4 include, azole antifungal agents (e.g., ketoconazole, itraconazole, clotrimazole),[79,80] macrolide antibiotics (e.g., erythromycin and troleandomycin),[81,82] human immunodeficiency virus (HIV) protease inhibitor ritonavir, and lopinavir and certain flavones, such as those present in grapefruit juice. A comprehensive list of reversible CYP3A4 inhibitor drugs is given by Thummel and Wilkinson.[78] The furanocoumarins in grapefruit juice, dihydroxyberamottin, and bergamottin, cause irreversible, mechanism-based (suicide) inhibition.[83–86] This result presumably involves CYP3A4 mediated formation of a reactive metabolite that covalently binds to the enzyme, leading to its inactivation. Synthetic therapeutic steroids, such as gestodene, which contains an acetylenic moiety, have been shown *in vitro* studies to deactivate CYP3A4 by N-alkylation of the porphyrine ring.

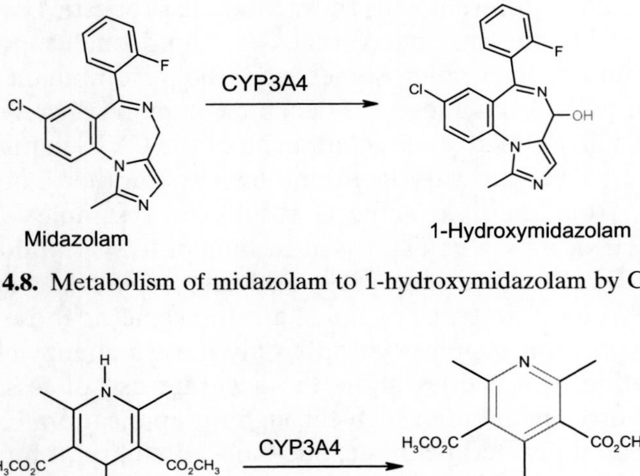

Midazolam   1-Hydroxymidazolam

Scheme 4.8. Metabolism of midazolam to 1-hydroxymidazolam by CYP3A4.

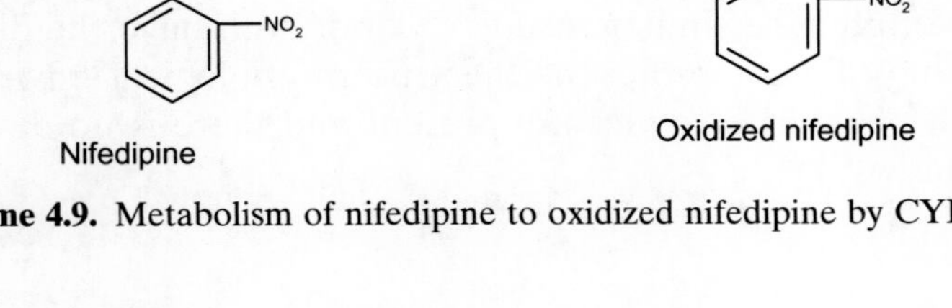

Nifedipine   Oxidized nifedipine

Scheme 4.9. Metabolism of nifedipine to oxidized nifedipine by CYP3A4.

4.1.9 *In vitro* Screening for Inhibition of CYP Enzymes

4.1.9.1 *Rational for High-Throughput CYP Inhibition Screening.*
Significant drug interactions can adversely effect patient safety during
polytherapy and thereby limit the commercial prospects of a drug.
In vitro CYP inhibition screening during the lead optimization phase
enables such attributes to be designed out or sufficiently ameliorated
to minimize likely patient impact. By screening hundreds of compounds
within a chemical, we can develop a structure–inhibition liability relationship. It is important that the *in vitro* inhibition data be able to rank
order compounds sufficiently well to pick or design the winners and
have the throughput to support the medicinal chemistry output.
Typically, this means that only an IC_{50} is determined for a subset of
the most important CYPs (e.g., CYP1A2, CYP2C9, CYP2D6, and
CYP3A4).

4.1.9.2 *Sources of CYPs.* The sources of enzymes available for the
in vitro inhibition screening includes human liver microsomes,[87] human
recombinant enzymes expressed in various cell lines,[88–91] human hepatocytes,[92,93] and liver slices. Although all enzyme systems have pros and
cons, the most commonly used enzyme sources for *in vitro* screening
are human liver microsomes and the human recombinant enzymes that
when expressed in different cells show catalytic properties comparable
with those of human liver microsomes.[89,94] Good quality pooled and
individual human liver microsomes and the recombinant enzymes
expressed in several cell lines have become commercially readily available.[95] Human liver microsomes contain all of the CYPs in human liver,
although their level can vary from one liver to another. Pooling liver
microsomes from multiple subjects results in a sample with more
average levels of all CYPs expressed in human liver. In addition, the
ratio of NADPH cytochrome P450 reductase : P450, the amount of
cytochrome b_5 and the types of lipids are the same as those found in
the liver. Expression systems typically only have one enzyme present
per preparation, which does allow the accurate use of less selective
substrates more amenable to high-throughput application. Expression
systems are an unlimited resource, but the availability of human liver
samples can be limited by availability and ethical concerns. These two
models generally give similar results,[96–102] but both have the disadvantage that they do not represent the true physiological environment
(e.g., not all phase II enzymes are present and there is no directional
transport activity).

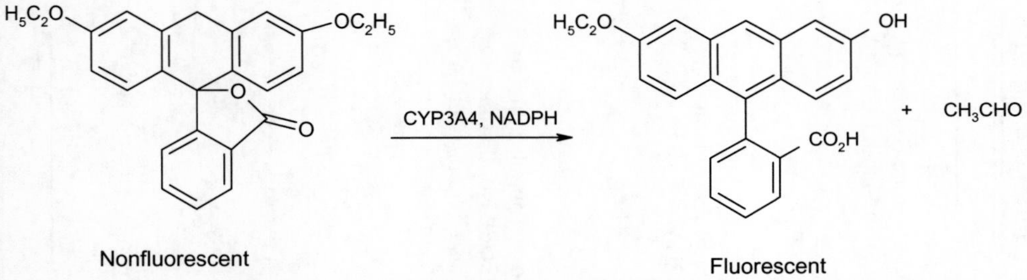

Scheme 4.10. Metabolism of diethoxyfluorescein to ethoxyfluorescein by CYP3A4.

It has been argued that hepatocytes offer advantages over human liver microsomes and recombinant enzymes, because hepatocellular uptake of drugs in isolated hepatocytes are predictable in mimicking the *in vivo* situation.[92] However, the disadvantage in the case of hepatocytes is that the interaction could be based on competition for the uptake mechanism rather than the CYP, making the understanding and extrapolation of any findings more difficult.[103] More significantly supplies of human hepatocytes are more limited and variable than human liver microsomes making them a poor choice for high-throughput applications.

4.1.9.3 *Fluorescence Assay in Human Recombinant Enzymes.*
Fluorescence substrates–products with human recombinant enzymes are commonly used across the pharmaceutical industry for lead optimization and selection in drug discovery. Several groups have described the development of high-throughput inhibition assay in a microtiter plate.[91,99,104–107] These assays have been highly automated.[108] The substrates used in the assays are generally nonfluorescent at the monitored wavelengths, which upon metabolism by the enzyme in the presence of NADPH, generates a fluorescent metabolite. For example, diethoxyfluorescein metabolized by human recombinant CYP3A4 enzyme in the presence of NADPH generates the highly fluorescent ethoxyfluorescein metabolite (Scheme 4.10).[109] For the most part, the use of such substrates has been enabled by single CYP recombinant enzyme sources that obviate the need for highly CYP selective substrates.

4.1.9.4 *The CYP Inhibition Assays in Human Liver Microsomes.*
CYP inhibition assays in human liver microsomes to assess the *in vitro* drug interaction potential is the approach recommended by the regulatory authorities. Enzyme specific substrates are needed due to the

TABLE 4.1. Recommended *In Vitro* Probe Substrates and Inhibitors for P450 Inhibition Assays in Human Liver Microsomes[a]

CYP	Substrate		Inhibitor	
	Preferred	Acceptable	Preferred	Acceptable
1A2	Ethoxyresorufin Phenacetine	Caffeine (low turnover) Theophylline (low turnover) Acetanilide (mostly applied in hepatocytes) Methoxyresorufin	Furafylline	α-naphthoflovone (but can also activate and inhibit CYP3A4)
2A6	Coumarin			Coumarin (but high turnover)
2B6	(S)-Mephenytoin (N-desmethylation)	Bupropion (availability of metabolite standards?)		Sertralin (but also inhibits CYP2D6)
2C8	Paclitaxel (availability of standards?)		"Glitazones" (availability of standards?)	
2C9	(S)-Warfarin	Tolbutamide; Dichlofenac	Sulfaphinazole (low turnover)	
2C19	(S)-Mephenytoin (4-hydroxy metabolite) Omeprezole			Ticlopidine (but also inhibits CYP2D6); Nootkatone (but also inhibits CYP2A6)
2D6	Bufuralol Dextromethorphan	Metoprolol Debrisoquine Codeine (all with no problems, but less commonly used)	Quinidine	
2E1	Chlorzoxazone	4-Nitrophenol Lauric acid		4-Methyl pyrazole
3A4	Midazolam Testosterone (strongly recomended to use at least 2 structurally unrelated substrates)	Nifedipine, Felodipine, Cyclosporine Terfenadine Erythromycin Simavastatin	Ketoconazole (but recent evidence indicates that it is also a potent inhibitor of 2C8) Trolyendomycin	Cyclosporin

[a]See Ref. 57.

presence of multiple CYPs in human liver microsomes. These are generally defined following clinical observations and are therefore mostly clinical drugs. Thus they can be used in clinical drug interaction studies. The selection of substrates listed in Table 4.1 are based on the consensus paper following the conference held in Basel, November 2001.[57] Due to the allosteric nature of the CYP3A4 enzyme and multiple binding sites, it is recommended that at least two to three substrates be used to determine the inhibitory effects of the test compound.

The analytical endpoint for these assays now typically involves liquid chromatography/tandem mass spectrometry (LC-MS/MS), but also can include radiometric or ultraviolet (UV) and fluorescent detection couple with high-performance liquid chromatography (HPLC) and direct radiometric approaches. All of these have much lower throughput than the microtiter approach is capable of, usually due to the relatively long HPLC run time (5–50 min) or other approach necessary to separate the substrate and the metabolite.[87,110–112]

i *Direct Radiometric Assays.* These assays are simple, rapid, and involve radiometric measurement of ^{14}C-acetaldehyde or formaldehyde. These are generated by N- or O-dealkylation of an ethyl and methyl moiety from enzyme-specific substrates, as shown by ^{14}C-phenacetin and ^{14}C-caffeine example in Scheme 4.11. ^{14}C-Acetaldehyde or ^{14}C-fomaldehyde generation is measured by a liquid scintillation analyzer after a simple single-step solid-phase extraction procedure to remove excess substrate. This obviates the need for HPLC and is reasonably amenable for high throughput, although sample preparation by a solid-phase extraction step can be time consuming.

Other enzyme specific radiometric substrates used in human liver microsomes (HLM) include naproxen O-demethylation for CYP2C9,[113,114] diazepam N-demethylation for CYP2C19,[115,116] dextromethorphan O-demethylation for CYP2D6,[117,118] and erythromycin N-demethylation for CYP3A4.[119] Alternatively, tritiated substrates like diclofenac and testosterone, for CYP2C9 and CYP3A4, respectively have been described. The assays are based on the release of tritium as tritiated water that occurs upon hydroxylation of diclofenac and testosterone.[120,121] The radiometric assays are sensitive, flexible, robust, and free from analytical interference. The automated high-throughput screening method using the aforementioned radiolabel substrates has been described.[122]

ii *The LC-MS/MS Based Assays.* Assays in HLM based on liquid chromatography-tandem mass spectrometry (LC-MS/MS) methods of

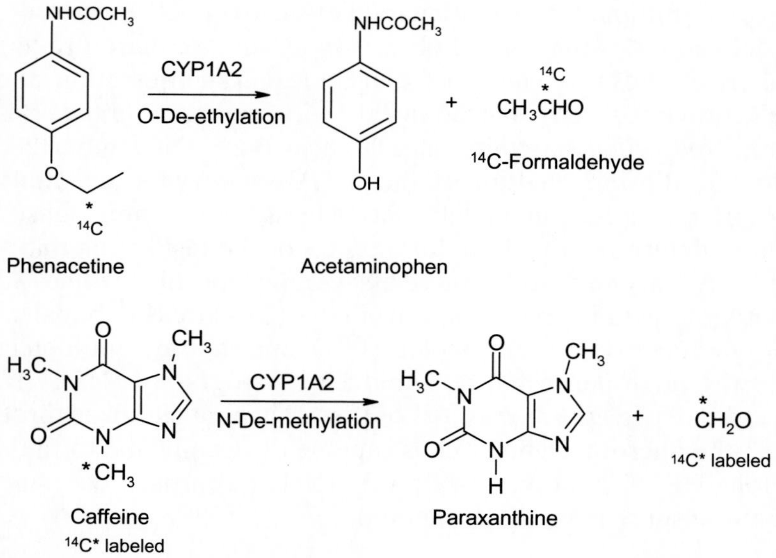

Scheme 4.11. Metabolism of ^{14}C-phenacetin by CYP1A2 and ^{14}C-caffeine by CYP3A4.

detection are now the assays of choice for *in vitro* drug interaction studies for regulatory submission in the pharmaceutical industry. The commonly used substrates for LC-MS/MS assays are shown in Table 4.1. The MS/MS method of detection provides highly selective and sensitive assays with a low limit of quantitation and rapid HPLC run times. Many LC-MS/MS assays have been described.[96,123–128] Incubation approaches using microtiter plates and liquid-handling robots can automate the process sufficiently so that the LC-MS/MS becomes the rate-limiting step. An analytical cocktail approach (i.e., all the incubations at a given concentration of test drug are analyzed for the signal due to each substrate metabolite simultaneously using the specificity of LC-MS/MS) can somewhat address even that limitation.

4.2   THE CYP INHIBITION

4.2.1   Drug–Drug Interactions

A drug interaction occurs when the effectiveness or toxicity of a drug is altered by the administration of another drug or substance.[83] When any two drugs are prescribed together the potential for interaction has been reported as ~6%.[129] The risk of drug interaction significantly increases with the number of drugs the patients takes. Adverse effects of drugs are one of the major causes of hospital admission. As a consequence, interest in mechanisms of drug–drug interactions also has increased.

Drug–drug interaction mediated by CYPs are PK in nature as a result of a change in the metabolism of a drug by the coadministration of another. This result can occur by the induction of new protein synthesis, which accelerates drug metabolism and decrease the magnitude and duration of drug response, or from inhibition, which results in elevated plasma drug concentrations with increased potential for enhanced beneficial or, in most cases, adverse effect. The clinical significance of the enzyme inhibition is measured primarily by the extent to which the plasma level of the drug rises. If the plasma level remains within the therapeutic range, the interaction may not be a problem. If not, the interaction may become adverse as the serum level climbs into the toxic range. For example, felodipine and nifedipine are dihydropyridine calcium antagonists antihypertensive medication, which shows drug interaction with CYP3A4 inhibitor itraconazole. Concomitant use of itraconazole with felodipine and nifedipine can cause a swelling of the ankles and legs within a few days. Ankle swelling is a typical side effect of dihydropyridine calcium antagonist when their plasma concentrations are high.[83]

An example of toxicity due to drug–drug interaction is cisapride—a narrow therapeutic index drug is a gastrointestinal (GI) tract motility agent that was first marketed in the United States in 1993 with a label indication for nocturnal heartburn. Cisapride increases muscle tone in the esophageal sphincter in people with gastroesophageal reflux disease. It also increases gastric emptying in people with diabetic gastroparesis. It has been used to treat bowel constipation. Cisapride caused life-threatening cardiac arrhythmias in patients susceptible either because of concurrent use of medications that interfere with cisapride metabolism or prolong the time between the start of the Q wave and the end of the T wave in the heart's electrical cycle (QT interval) or because of the presence of other diseases that predispose to such arrhythmias. In 1998, the US Food and Drug Administration (FDA) determined that use of cisapride was contraindicated in such patients. In many countries, it has been either withdrawn or has had its indications limited due to reports about long QT syndrome.[130] Cisapride is largely metabolized by CYP3A4 by an N-dealkylation pathway and has been associated with drug–drug interaction during concomitant therapy with antifungal agents, macrolides, or antidepressants.[131–134] The FDA issued a report on 34 patients who had developed proarrhythmias and 23 patients with prolonged QT intervals during medication with cisapride.[135] Four patients died and another 16 survived resuscitation.

Fifty-six percent of the patients were on concomitant treatment with other drugs that affected the metabolism of cisapride through inhibition of the hepatic CYP3A4 enzyme, namely, macrolides antibiotics (e.g., erythromycin), or antifungal (ketoconazole). The FDA issued widespread warnings concerning a drug interaction between cisapride and other drugs known to be metabolized by CYP3A4. Cisapride has a relatively low absolute bioavailability (40–50%) due to significant first pass metabolism. Based on K_m determination, it was unlikely that cisapride would inhibit competitively the metabolism of a coadministered drug.[134] Drugs that are metabolized by CYP3A4 include antifungal agents, (ketoconazole, itraconazole), macrolide antibiotics (erythromycin, clarithromycin), protease inhibitor (ritonavir), and the antidepressive drugs SSRIs, fluoxetine, paroxetine, and nefazodone. When ketoconazole was coadministered with cisapride, the serum ketoconazole levels were increased resulting in an eightfold increase in the area under the curve (AUC) compared with the AUC of ketoconazole alone.[136–140]

Another example of a CYP inhibitor drug with a clinical safety issue is terfenadine (Saldane). Terfenadine was withdrawn from the market in Canada and the United States in 1998. Terfenadine is a nonsedating H1 receptor antagonist formerly used in the treatment of allergic conditions. Terfenadine is a prodrug, which normally undergoes rapid and complete first-pass biotransformation into (by hepatic CYP3A4) a pharmacologically active acid metabolite and inactive desalkyl metabolite. The concentration of terfenadine in the plasma of the patients receiving terfenadine is usually undetectable at the usual dosages of 120 mg/day. However, it is terfenadine that is responsible for the observed QT prolongation. Therefore concurrent administration of the drugs that inhibit CYP3A4 metabolism [macrolide antibacterial (e.g., erythromycin, clarithromycin) and azole antifungal agents (e.g., ketoconazole)] can result in the accumulation of terfenadine and induction of potentially lethal ventricular arrhythmias, such as Torsade de points.[141,142] Patients with 120-mg daily dose of terfenadine and 200-mg twice daily doses of ketoconazole resulted in an excessive concentration of terfenadine in serum causing terfenadine-induced cardiotoxicity previously seen only in cases of overdose.[143] Metabolite terfenadine carboxylate did not inhibit this potassium current even at concentrations 30 times higher than the concentrations of terfenadine producing a half maximal effect. The previous two examples are where the withdrawn drug is the victim of a drug–drug interaction.

If a drug is a significant perpetrator of interactions it is equally, if not more likely, to be a risk to patient safety, the point in case is Posicor

(Mibefradil). Mibefradil was a drug used for treating hypertension and angina, first marketed in 1997. It had significant inhibitory properties against CYP3A4, and there were contraindication and warnings for its use in combination with three specific drugs, astemizole, cisapride, and terfenadine.[144–146] The drug was subsequently available in 38 countries. Therefore, two more drugs (simvastatin and lovastatin) were added to the labeling as drugs that could never be administered with Posicor. Eventually, in 1998, the drug was withdrawn from the market. Withdrawal had come after reports of dangerous; sometimes fatal interactions with at least 25 other drugs, including common antibiotics, antihistamine, and cancer drugs.[147] Because of the number and the diversity of the drugs involved it was not practical to address the problem in standard label warnings.[146,148] Of the 330 cases of statin induced rhabdomyolysis reviewed between 1997–2000 by the FDA, 16% were associated with CYP3A inhibition by mibefradil.[149]

Even if withdrawal is not the outcome, drugs that are CYP inhibitors are at competitive disadvantage to those with less or no interaction with CYP enzymes if they offer no patient benefits, but are with increased risks. Cimetidine was the first H2 receptor antagonist to become commercially available with ranitidine following a few years later.[150,151] The CYP enzymes are inhibited by cimetidine, but not by ranitidine, and cimetidine has several pharmacokinetically significant interaction whereas ranitidine does not. The PKs of many drugs have been shown to be influenced by cimetidine, but only to a small degree by ranitidine or not at all by the newer H2 receptor anatagonist drugs famotidine and nizatidine.[152–155] It has been suggested that nifedipine plasma levels are considerably increased in the presence of cimetidine and that this causes a pharmacodynamic effect in hypertensive patients, with the combination producing a significantly greater reduction in blood pressure than nifedipine alone.[156] Ranitidine, at a dose of 130 mg, taken with nifedipine, does not appear to share this effect or show relatively less interaction.[157]

4.2.2   Prediction of *In Vivo* Drug–Drug Interaction from *In Vitro* Inhibition Data

As a consequence of the significance of CYP mediated drug–drug interactions in patient safety, this issue has generated much interest within the pharmaceutical industry, academia, and the regulatory authorities. Our knowledge of human P450 enzymes and their role in drug metabolism has advanced enormously and in particular there is an increasing interest in developing a quantitative relationship between *in vitro* and *in vivo* data on drug–drug interaction.[158,159] With the technological advancement in the conduct of *in vitro* inhibition studies, and various enzyme system models and sensitive analytical tools now available, the measurement of CYP inhibition liability has been served well for some time. However, the extrapolation of these *in vitro* data to provide a quantitative *in vivo* prediction has been more challenging.

4.2.2.1 *Prediction of In Vivo Drug Interaction from In Vitro Parameters.*

Relating *in vitro* potency for inhibition of drug metabolizing enzymes to *in vivo* concentrations of inhibitors along with other information (plasma protein binding, dose, etc.), can yield satisfactory projections of drug–drug interactions.[160–165] The general approach considered is when the metabolism of a drug (substrate) is reversibly inhibited by another drug (inhibitor), the extent of decrease in the metabolic intrinsic clearance (CL_{int}) of the victim drug is related to the inhibitor concentration [I] available to the enzyme and the inhibition constant, K_i, as shown by Eq. 4.1.

$$CL_{int_1} = \frac{CL_{int}}{1 + [I]/K_i} \tag{4.1}$$

In human *in vivo* interaction studies, drug plasma concentration profiles are determined in the presence and absence of inhibitor (after multiple oral dosing) and the degree of interaction is expressed as the increase in the area under the plasma concentration–time curve (AUC) of substrate. For orally administered drugs, assuming the drug is completely absorbed, the AUC ratio is related to the ratio of the metabolic intrinsic clearance (CL_{int}) as described by Eq. 4.2. The drug concentration *in vivo* is usually much lower than the K_m value and the mechanism of inhibition (competitive or noncompetitive) is not relevant; therefore, Eq. 4.2 is valid for both inhibition types,[159]

$$\frac{AUC_i}{AUC} = \frac{CL_{int}}{CL_{int,i}} = 1 + \frac{[I]}{K_i} \tag{4.2}$$

where [I] is the inhibitor concentration available to the enzyme and subscript i indicates the presence of the inhibitor.

Therefore the ratio of AUCs in the presence and absence of inhibitor is dependent on the [I]/K_i ratio (Eq. 4.3 based on certain assumptions mentioned above.

$$AUC\ ratio = 1 + [I]/K_i \tag{4.3}$$

Equation 4.3 is widely used to describe the degree of *in vivo* interaction between two drugs. The K_i values can be obtained from *in vitro* studies using HLM or recombinant enzyme systems. However, it is not normally possible to measure the inhibitor concentration [I] available to the hepatic enzyme *in vivo* in humans. Several predictions have been made using Eq. 4.3 and inhibitor concentration [I] as based on average systemic total drug plasma concentration ($[I]_{av}$), average systemic unbound drug plasma concentration ($[I]_{av,u}$), maximum systemic plasma concentration ($[I]_{max}$), and maximum hepatic input concentration ($[I]_{in}$). The $[I]_{in}$ concentration represents the theoretical maximum drug concentration entering the liver, which is the sum of the hepatic artery and portal vein concentrations during the absorption process.[166] The uncertainty in assigned [I] is perceived as a major hurdle in realizing the potential of DDI predictions.

According to Eq. 4.3, interactions are regarded to be with low risk if the estimated $[I]/K_i$ ratio is <0.1, and high risk if it is >1. A theoretical plot of AUC ratio against $[I]/K_i$ is shown in Figure 4.4. According to the plot, predictions can be categorized into four zones: true positives ($AUC_{ratio} > 2$, $[I]/K_i > 1$), true negatives ($AUC_{ratio} < 2$, $[I]/K_i < 1$), false positives ($AUC_{ratio} < 2$, $[I]/K_i > 1$), or false negatives ($AUC_{ratio} > 2$, $[I]/K_i < 1$). The threshold of a twofold increase in the AUC was selected based on a consensus report.[57] According to Pharmaceutical Research and Manufacturers of America (PhRMA) recommendations, the clinical drug interaction based on AUC_i/AUC is classified as follows: Potent inhibition $AUC_i/AUC \geq 5$, moderate inhibition $AUC_i/AUC < 5$ to >2; and weak inhibition $AUC_i/AUC \leq 2$.

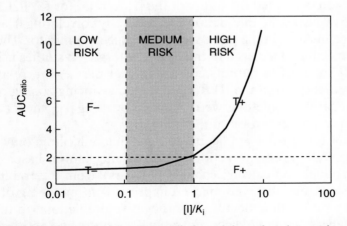

Figure 4.4. Qualitative zoning for the prediction of drug–drug interactions involving CYP inhibition. The curve represents the theoretical curve based on Eq. 4.1. F– = false negative, T– = true negative, F+ = false positive, T+ = true positive. [Reproduced from Ito K. et al., *Br. J. Clin. Pharmacol.*, **2004**, 57, 473–486.]

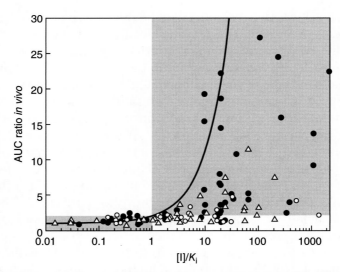

Figure 4.5. Relationship between the observed AUC ratio and the $[I]_{in}/K_i$ ratio for 146 drug–drug interactions involving CYP2C9 (○), CYP2D6 (△), and CYP3A4 (●). The line shown is the theoretical relationship based on Eq. 4.2. The shaded areas represent the regions corresponding to negative and positive drug–drug interactions as defined by the borderlines of an AUC ratio of 2 and an $[I]/K_i$ of 1. [Reproduced from Brown HS, et al. *Br. J. Clin. Pharmacol*, **2005**, 60, 5, 508–518. Ref. 159.]

Qualitative predictions of CYP inhibitions can be achieved from the $[I]/K_i$ ratio using *in vitro* kinetic parameters and the hepatic input concentration of the inhibitor, as shown in Figure 4.5. From the 146 *in vivo* drug–drug interaction studies for the marketed drugs from the literature, Houston evaluated the utility of the $[I]/K_i$ ratio for CYP2C9, 2D6, and 3A4/5 *in vivo* drug interaction prediction by correlating it with the fold change in AUC in the presence and absence of inhibitor. The $[I]/K_i$ ratio was calculated for each of the *in vivo* interaction studies using the various [I] values. The authors concluded that the best correlation of *in vivo* prediction from the $[I]/K_i$ ratio with convincing zoning of positive and negative predictions were obtained by using $[I]_{in}$, the maximum hepatic input concentration of the inhibitor.[159,167]

Equation $1 + [I/K_i]$ is applicable to reversible inhibitors only, therefore, by excluding the interactions based on mechanism-based inhibitors (macrolides and calcium channel blockers), from the training set, these investigators observed marked improvement in zoning of drug–drug interaction with almost no false-negative predictions. In this prediction analysis, the *in vivo* concentration measured as a ratio of AUC or a plasma concentration measured at a single concentration gave similar results.

4.2.2.2 Factors Affecting Prediction of In Vivo Drug Interaction.

The above analysis provides a generic approach for initial assessments from *in vitro* data. There are a number of other factors related to both the substrate and inhibitor that affects the *in vivo* predictions. A refinement in the quantitative prediction of drug–drug interaction can be made by incorporating the fraction of the substrate metabolized by the inhibited CYP pathway (fmCYP) in the analysis, as shown in Eq. 4.4.

$$\frac{AUC(+inhibitor)}{AUC(control)} = \frac{1}{\frac{f_{mCYP}}{1+[I]/K_i}+(1-f_{mCYP})} \tag{4.4}$$

By incorporating the f_{mCYP} values for the victim drug, marked improvement in the prediction of 115 drug–drug interactions have been observed as compared to the use of the $[I]/K_i$ ratio alone. In addition to f_{mCYP}, inclusion of absorption rate constant (k_a) values to refine estimates of $[I]_{in}$ provides the most useful estimate of $[I]$ and results in successful predictions.[166]

In another refinement of drug interaction prediction, the effect of microsomal-protein binding and the plasma-protein binding was evaluated on the accuracy of *in vivo* drug interaction prediction of 8 inhibitors and 18 different 2C9, 2D6, and 3A4 substrates in 45 clinical drug interaction studies using Eq. 4.4. The K_i values were corrected for microsomal protein binding to give $K_{i,u}$. Using the unbound K_i values ($K_{i,u}$), the prediction was significantly improved for CYP3A4 and 2D6, while there was no improvement in CYP2C9 prediction. The impact of plasma protein binding was also considered, for prediction using unbound inhibitor concentration $[I]_{in,u}$ and unbound K_i values, $K_{i,u}$. The use of unbound inhibitor concentration significantly underestimated the extent of the *in vivo* DDI for CYP2D6 and CYP3A4.[166] However, frequently investigators advocate the use of unbound concentration in such predictions.[168-170]

Additional approach for the prediction of drug interactions for reversible inhibitors that are predominantly metabolized by CYP1A2, 2C9, 2C19, and 2D6 include use of free hepatic inlet C_{max}, Figure 4.6.[158]

Drug interaction predictions for CYP3A4 reversible inhibitors can be improved by incorporating contribution from an intestinal metabolism $F_{g,inh}/F_g$ (i.e., a relative contribution of intestinal extraction of victim drug by CYP3A4 in the presence and absence of inhibitor). By using the unbound hepatic inlet C_{max}, $F_{g,inh}/F_g$ and f_{mCYP}, in the Eq. 4.5 seems to improve the drug–drug interaction prediction for the orally

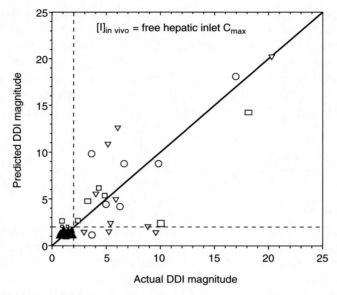

Figure 4.6. Predicted magnitude of DDI versus actual DDI magnitude using the estimated unbound hepatic inlet C_{max} provide the best correlation. Symbols: $\bigcirc$ = reversible inhibitors; $\triangledown$ = known mechanism-based inactivators; $\square$, inhibitors with known inhibitory metabolites. Dashed lines represent the boundaries of twofold interactions and the solid diagonal line is a line of unity. [Reproduced from R. Scott Obach, *J. Pharmacol. Exp. Therap.*, **2006**, 316, 336–348. Ref. 158.]

administered drugs that undergoes considerable intestinal metabolism, such as midazolam, alprazolam, and buspirone.

$$\frac{AUC_{inhibited}}{AUC_{control}} = \frac{F_{g,inh}}{F_g} \times \frac{1}{\left(\dfrac{f_{m(CYP3A)}}{1+\left(\dfrac{[I]_{in\ vivo}}{K_i}\right)}\right) + \left(1 - f_{m(CYP3A)}\right)} \qquad (4.5)$$

4.2.2.3 *Prediction of Irreversible Drug Interaction with CYP.*

Irreversible or metabolism-dependent inhibition (MDI) interaction involves the metabolism of an inhibitor by CYP enzyme to a reactive metabolite that inactivates the catalyzing enzyme in a concentration- and time-dependent manner.[171,172] The interaction between the inactivating species could be covalent or noncovalent involving binding to a protein or heme moiety, respectively.[173] The two major kinetic parameters that characterize MDI interactions are k_{inact} and K_i, the maximal inactivation rate constant and the inhibitor concentration leading to

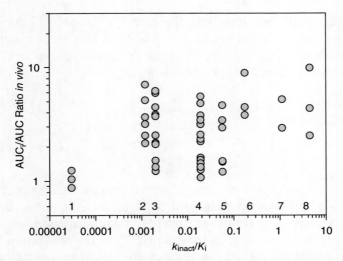

Figure 4.7. Relationship between obtained kinact/K_i ratio and the degree of interaction observed *in vivo* for azithromycin (1), erythromycin (2), clarithromycin (3), diltiazem (4), verapamil (5), mibefradil (6), saquinavir (7), and ritonavir (8) (inhibitors are listed in order of increasing k_{inact}/K_i. [Reproduced from Galetin A. DMD, **2006**, 34, 166–175, Ref. 171.]

50% of k_{inact}, respectively.[172] The k_{inact}/K_I ratio is commonly taken as an indicator of the intrinsic rate of a mechanism-based inhibitor. In contrast to reversible inhibition, the enzyme activity for irreversible inhibition can only be restored by synthesis of a new enzyme. Quantitative *in vitro–in vivo* drug interaction prediction based on the [I]/K_i approach for reversible interactions if applied to irreversible inhibitors, generally gives under prediction of drug-drug interaction (DDI).[167]

A mechanism-based inactivation model based only on K_{inact}/K_i gives a poor prediction of *in vivo* drug interaction. Evaluation based on literature data for macrolides time-dependent inhibitors, namely, erythromycin, clarithromycin, diltiazem, verapamil, mibefradil, saquinavir, and ritonavir, showed no direct relationship between the *in vitro* potency parameters [k_{inact}/K_i] and the *in vivo* AUC$_i$/AUC ratios as shown in Figure 4.7.[171]

These findings are only partially dose related as the same dose of erythromycin (1500 mg/day) results in either no effect (carbamazepine), or a sixfold increase in the AUC ratio (simvastatin), confirming that the k_{inact}/K_i, although good, indicator of potency are not sufficient to predict the extent of MDI. Additional substrate and indicator related parameters are required.[171] Further improvement in the *in vitro* prediction of *in vivo* DDI is achieved by incorporating such parameters as, enzyme degradation rate (k_{deg}), differential contribution of CYP3A4 to the victim drug clearance, and the effect of intestinal inhibition in the *in vitro* model as shown in Eq. 4.6. Thus the mechanism-based inactivation model predicts the extent of drug interactions in CYP3A4 from the *in vitro* data using the following equation:

$$\frac{AUC_i}{AUC} = \frac{F'_G}{F_G} \times \frac{1}{1+\sum_{i=1}^{n} \dfrac{k_{inact,i} \times I_{u,i}}{k_{deg} \times (K_{I,u} + I_u)_i} + (1 - f_{mCYP3A4})} \tag{4.6}$$

In Eq. 4.6, k_{inact} represents the maximal inactivation rate constant, K_I is the inhibitor concentration at 50% of k_{inact}, I_u is the unbound inhibitor concentration (either the average systemic plasma concentration after repeated oral administration ($[I]_{av}$) or the maximum hepatic input concentration ($[I]_{in}$), $f_{mCYP3A4}$ is the fraction of victim drug metabolized by CYP3A4, k_{deg} is the endogenous degradation rate constant of the enzyme, and F'_G and F_G are the intestinal wall availability in the presence and absence of inhibitor, respectively.[171,174] When verapamil was orally coadministered with midazolam, the irreversible inhibition model predicted a two- to fourfold increase in the AUC of a coadministered midazolam that is completely metabolized by hepatic CYP3A.

4.2.2.4 Empirical Guidance for Prediction of In Vivo Drug Interaction Based on In Vitro Data.

The most effective predictions of *in vivo* drug–drug interaction from *in vitro* data require a substantial amount of data beyond that generated in the initial *in vitro* experiment. At early stages of the drug discovery and development processes, such information is not available and would be disproportionately expensive to obtain. As a result there is much interest in empirical guidance, such as that shown in Table 4.2. This is based on a survey of known drug–drug interactions for which both *in vivo* and *in vitro* data are available and enables prediction of *in vivo* interaction. It is estimated that for the drugs with a reversible mechanism, the interaction is highly likely if the ratio of inhibitor $[I]/K_i$ was >1 or an experimentally determined K_i value <1 μM. If K_i is >50 μM and I/K_i is <0.1, the likelihood of an interaction is deemed to be remote. For drugs with a I/K_i ratio between 0.1 and 1, the risk of interaction is medium.[57,175]

In case of irreversible inhibitor, if the reversible K_i parameter is <20 μM, an *in vivo* interaction is highly likely (Table 4.2). If the reversible K_i is >100 μM, the *in vivo* interactions are not seen. It is suggested that a minimum binding affinity is necessary if there is to be sufficient

TABLE 4.2. Empirical Guide to the Likelihood of a Significant Inhibitory Interaction Based on _In Vitro_ K_i Values

	Reversible Mechanism		
K_i, µM	Or	I/K_i	Prediction
<1	Or	>1	Likely
>1, but <50	Or	<1, but >0.1	Possible
>50	And	<0.1	Unlikely
	Slowly Reversible or Irreversible Mechanism		
Reversible K_i, µM		Prediction	
<20		Likely	
>20, but <100		Possible	
>100 µM		Unlikely	

inactivation of the total enzyme pool for which new enzyme synthesis cannot fully compensate. If the reversible K_i is <100 µM, but >20 µM, the interaction is possible.[175]

Alternatively, if the objective is to rank compounds and just ensure that the best candidates progress to the next stage of evaluation, then a different approach to setting empirical guidelines can be considered. Cutoff criteria should eliminate a substantial fraction of compounds, yet not too many either. It is ineffective to run hundreds of compounds through any screen with a high rate of success or failure. With the high rate of success, we will still need to find methods and means to differentiate most compounds for the next level of evaluation. On the other hand, with the high rate of failure there will be insufficient compounds passing the screen for the next level.[176]

From the collection of empirical considerations and more detailed attempts at prediction of drug interactions across the pharmaceutical companies, similar cut-off criteria are used. Generally, for reversible nonmechanism-based inhibitors, the compounds are typically classified as potent ($IC_{50} < 1$ µM), moderate (IC_{50} 1–10 µM), or weak inhibitors ($IC_{50} > 10$ µM). Similar guidance has evolved for mechanism-based inhibition. A large decrease (>10-fold) in the apparent IC_{50} after preincubation with NADPH and the test compound is evidence of metabolism/mechanism-based inhibition and usually terminates interest in the compound.[176]

There is good data to support these arbitrary "rules". Researchers in Pfizer studied _in vitro_ inhibition of 69 drugs for CYP inhibition in human liver microsomes and correlated with the _in vivo_ clinical drug interaction data from the literature (Fig. 4.8).[158] With two exceptions

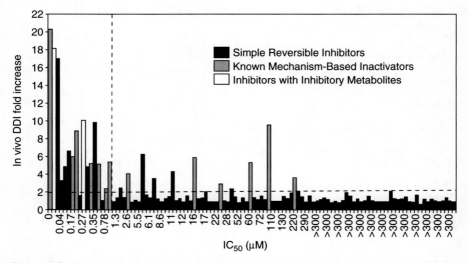

Figure 4.8. Bar graph of the magnitude of drug interactions versus *in vitro* inhibitory potency. [Reproduced from R. Scott Obach, *J. Pharmacol. Exp. Therap*, **2006**, 316, 336–348. Ref. 158.]

(disulfiram and dicumarol), all inhibitors possessing *in vitro* potency values (IC$_{50}$) <1 µM demonstrated drug interactions of at least twofold. The major exceptions of unexpected interactions included several CYP3A inhibitors known to cause irreversible inactivation (e.g., clarithromycin, erythromycin, and diltiazem).

4.3   THE CYP INDUCTION

Induction is defined as the increase in the amount and activity of a drug metabolizing enzyme that generally requires more than acute exposure to the inducing agent.[177] Induction of CYPs and other ADME enzymes may cause reduction in therapeutic concentration, and thereby the efficacy of comedications. For example, by this mechanism rifampicin caused acute transplant rejection in patients treated with cyclosporine, presumably because of induction of the clearance of cyclosporine.[178,179] Also, induction may create an undesirable imbalance between detoxification and activation as a result of increased formation of reactive metabolite leading to an increase in risk of metabolite induced toxicity.[180,181] Unlike CYP inhibition, which is almost immediate, CYP induction is a less immediate process. It takes time to reach a higher steady-state enzyme level as a result of a new balance between

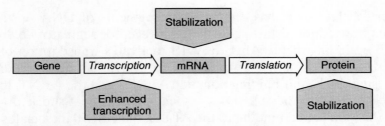

Figure 4.9. Mechanism by which enzyme may be induced. [Reproduced from Park B. K., *Br. J. Clin. Pharmacol*, **1996**, 41, 477–491. Ref. 189.]

a rate of biosynthesis and degradation.[182] Similarly, it takes time to return the enzyme basal level after discontinuing the treatment with inducer.[183]

Because CYP induction is a metabolic liability in drug therapy, it is highly desirable to develop new drug candidates that are not potent CYP inducers. Ideally, this liability should be identified and designed out of a series before the drug candidate is progressed to clinical development. Several *in vitro* models have been established to asses the potential of CYP induction including liver slices, immortalized cell lines, and primary hepatocytes.[184–187] Perhaps as a consequence it has been estimated that up to the year 2000, clinical induction as a reason for development failure was on the order of <2%.[188]

4.3.1 Mechanism of Enzyme Induction

Enzymes levels can be controlled at pretranslational, translational, and post-translational level, as shown in Figure 4.9.[189]

4.3.2 The CYP Induction by Nuclear Receptor

4.3.2.1 Aryl Hydrocarbon Receptor (AhR). Polycyclic aromatic hydrocarbons (PAH) typified by 2,3,7,8-tetrachlorodibenzo-*p*-dioxine (TCDD) are effective inducers of CYP1A1 and CYP1A2 that are under similar regulatory control.[189] Induction of CYP1A1 involves interaction of the inducer with a hydrophobic cytosolic receptor termed aromatic hydrocarbon receptor (AhR), and translocation of the ligand receptor complex to the nucleus followed by *de novo* protein synthesis. Studies in the mouse hepatoma cell line led to the identification of a second regulatory protein, AhR nuclear transporter (ARNT), in CYP1A induction.[190] Both AhR and ARNT receptors are required for CYP1A induction.

The CYP1A1 gene has one or more segments of DNA upstream from its transcription start site called Ah-receptor regulatory element (AhRE). Binding of the AhR to AhRE activates transcription of the *CYP1A1* gene. The AhR in its active form consists of heterodimer comprising the ligand-binding domain (ALBD) and the ARNT. In the absence of ligand, the ALBD is associated with heat-shock protein HSP-90. Upon ligand binding to the ALBD, the HSL90 dissociates and ARNT binds yielding the receptor complex capable of interacting with AhRE, as shown in Figure 4.10.

4.3.2.2 Constitutive Androstane Receptor. The functional role of constitutive androstane receptor (CAR) in CYP2B6 induction has been demonstrated in transgenic mice. The endogenous steroids androstanol and androstenol are the natural ligands for CAR receptor.

The CAR/RXR heterodiamer transcriptionally activates the *CYP2B* genes by interacting with the PB responsive enhancer module (PBREM). Sequence comparison of rat CYP2B2 PBREM, mouse CYP2b10 PBREM, and human CYP2B6 PBREM revealed that PBREM is a conserved arrangement of two nuclear-binding sites (NR1 and NR2) and a nuclear factor 1 (NF1) binding site between NR1 and NR2.[191–193] Only the NR binding sites are essential for the PB response activity, although the NF1 binding site may be required to confer full PBREM activity. The responsive elements that confer induction by PB also have been identified for *CYP2C* and *CYP3A* genes. In contrast to the highly conserved CYP2B PBREM, there are marked species differences in the amino acid sequence of PBREM of *CYP2C* and *CYP3A* genes.[194]

Constitutive androstane receptor is predominantly expressed in liver and to a lesser extent in the intestine.[195] Phenobarbital has not been shown to bind directly to either human or mouse CAR. Therefore ligand binding dose not seem to be critical for CAR nuclear translocation.

4.3.2.3 Pregnane X Receptor. The major CYP enzyme in humans, CYP3A4 along with many other ADME proteins are inducible by Pregnane X Receptor (PXR) ligands, making it perhaps the most significant induction mechanism. Kliewer[196] in 1998 discovered mouse PXR receptor, which was soon followed by the discovery of the Human PXR receptor by Bertilsson.[197] These nuclear receptors were first defined by their activation by pregnanes, hence they are named as

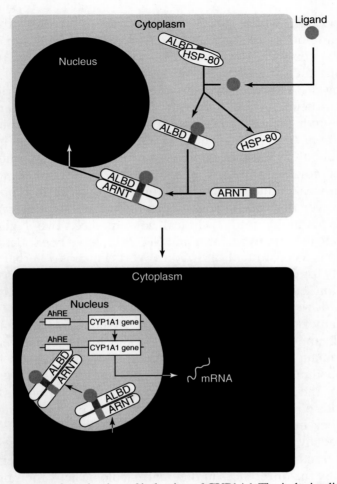

Figure 4.10. Proposed mechanism of induction of CYP1A1. The inducing ligand enters the cell cytoplasm and displaces the heat-shock protein, HSP-91 from its binding site on the ligand-binding domain (ALBD) of the Ah receptor. This allows the nuclear transporter ARNT to associate with ALBD to form the receptor–ligand complex. Translocation of this complex into the nucleus allows it to bind to the Ah receptor response element (AhRE) upstream of the CYP1A1 gene leading to enhanced transcription of the gene. [Reproduced from Park B. K. et al. *Br. J. Clin. Pharmacol,* **1996,** 41, 477–491, Ref 189.]

pregnane X receptors. The PXR ligand is expressed predominantly in human liver and to a lesser extent in small intestine. It mediates the induction of CYP3A4, 2B6, and CYP2C enzymes, as well as many other non-CYP ADME processes. The PXR gene is a promiscuous nuclear receptor, which can be activated by numerous structurally diverse xenobiotics and drugs, and is referred to as the "master" regulator of CYP enzymes. The number of compounds identified as PXR ligands continues to grow.

By using a PXR reporter gene assay, compounds have been rank ordered for their CYP3A4 induction potential based on binding affinity. Compounds are ranked as follows: lovastatin, simvastatin, troglitazone, rifampicin, pioglitazone, dexamethasone as potent inducers; fexofenadine, PCN, carbamazepine clothrimazole, and spironolactone as medium inducers; and CPA, phenobarbital, metyropone, and sulfinpyrazole as weak inducers; and phenytoin and pravastatin as noninducers.[198] However, dose and exposure is an important factor in translating this *in vitro* affinity into a clinical consequence. Two high-affinity human PXR ligands, hyperforin and SR12813, have been identified.[199] Hyperforin is a constituent of St. Jon's Wort, which is a herbal remedy used widely for depression and is the hyperforin that is responsible for the induction seen with its use. The SR12813 ligand is an investigational cholesterol-lowering drug.

Like many other nuclear receptors, PXR contains two functional domains: ligand-binding domain (LBD) and highly conserved DNA binding domain (DBD).[200] Crystal structure analyses suggest that the LBD of the human PXR is highly hydrophobic and flexible. The unique structure of the ligand pocket not only allows PXR to bind a diverse set of ligands of different molecular size, but also permits a single molecule to dock in multiple orientations.[201] This explains why PXR can be activated by various structurally diverse ligands. Although these diverse interactions imply promiscuity, PXR also exhibits specificity, as evidenced by the differences in the pharmacologic activation profile of PXR across species. For example, human PXR is activated by rifampicin and the cholesterol-lowering drug SR12813,[202,203] whereas mouse PXR is not;[204] mouse PXR is activated by the synthetic steroid 5-pregnen-3β-ol-20-one-16α-carbonitrile (PCN), whereas the human receptor is not.

Accumulating evidence from *in vitro* studies indicates that there is a redundancy between CAR and PXR with regard to the overlapping ligand spectrum. In addition, there is also a significant overlapping affinity between the binding of CAR and PXR to the DNA response elements of many genes. Each of the *CYP* genes contains multiple xenobiotic response elements, and each of the response elements can be recognized by more than one nuclear receptor. The process that an individual gene can be activated by more than one nuclear receptor is often referred to as "cross-talk".

The cross-talk between CAR and PXR is best illustrated by the use of CAR and PXR null mice. For example, both *Cyp2b10* and *Cyp3a11* genes were significantly induced by PB and 1,4-bis-[2-(3,5,-dichloropyridyloxy)]benzene (TCPOBOP) in $CAR^{(+/+)}$ mice, whereas the inducers failed to induce *Cyp2b10* and *Cyp3a11* genes in $CAR^{(-/-)}$ mice.[205] In contrast, dieldrin and clotrimazole (PXR activators) greatly increased *Cyp3a11* gene, but not *Cyp2b10* gene in both $CAR^{(+/+)}$ and $CAR^{(-/-)}$ mice. These results suggest that the *Cyp3a11* gene can be activated not only by PXR, but also CAR. The CAR mediated induction of *Cyp3a11* gene is further supported by the study with $PXR^{(-/-)}$ mice. In the PXR null mice, *Cyp3a11* was efficaciously induced by clotrimazole and PB.[206] Collectively, these results strongly suggest that *CYP3A* genes can be induced by both PXR and CAR through a cross-talk.

4.3.3 *In Vitro* Assays for CYP Induction

Both mammalian cell-based functional assays and PXR ligand-binding assays have been developed for rapid *in vitro* screening for induction of compounds. In a cell-based functional assay, full length PXR is cotransfected with a reporter plasmid driven by multiple copies of the DR-3 type PXR response element motif of the mouse CYP3A1 promotor. Such cell-based PXR reporter gene assays have been established for some time. Such assays use inexpensive human-derived cell lines, such as the hepatocellular carcinoma HepG2 and are amenable to automated high-throughput formats.[207]

Also frequently applied in assessing induction is the treatment of primary culture of human hepatocytes with test compound and then measuring mRNA, protein, or enzyme activity. One of the most significant disadvantages of human hepatocytes culture model continues to be the availability and quality of the donor tissue.

Luo et al. compared induction of 14 compounds in the PXR reporter gene assay with those from the conventional cultured human hepatocytes assay for their ability to induce CYP3A4 and activate PXR. In general, PXR activation correlated with the induction potential observed in human hepatocyte cultures.

4.3.4 Relationship between CYP Inhibition and Induction

Some drugs, such as drugs used for antiviral, antiepileptic, antifungal, and antimicrobial drugs, are inducers of multiple ADME process, as well as inhibitors of specific processes, such as CYPs. In these cases, the effect of induction can be offset by inhibition properties of the

TABLE 4.3. Inhibition in Human Recombinant (hr) CYP Enzymes and the EC50 Values for hPXR[a]

| | IC50, μM | | | | | |
Compound	CYP3A4 (DEF)[b]	CYP3A4 (7-BQ)[b]	CYP1A2 (ER)[b]	CYP2C9 (FCA)[b]	CYP2D6 (MMC)[b]	PXR EC50 (μM)[b]
Cyproterone	87	100	100	11	100	1.6 ± 0.2[c]
Fexofenidine	100	100	100	100	100	2.4 ± 0.3[c]
Lovastatin	11	11	100	28	64	0.5 ± 0.2[c]
Simvastatin	4.7	16	100	24	39	0.8 ± 0.6[c]
Rifampicin	28	57	100	76	100	1.7 ± 0.8[c]
Carbamazepine	100	100	100	100	100	0.9 ± 0.2[c]
Clotrimazole	<0.1	ND	0.2	0.1	14	1.1 ± 0.1[c]
Spironolactone	62	A[g]	100	100	100	1.1 ± 0.4[c]
Mifepristone RU486	6.5	19	100	2.4	25	5.5[c]
Sulfinpyrazone	100	100	100	100	100	7.9 ± 6.1[c]
PCN	100	A[g]	100	100	100	2.5 ± 0.8[c]
Dexamethasone	100	A[g]	A[g]	100	100	2.6 ± 0.6[c]
SR12813	1.6	2.0	100	3.4	100	0.12[d]
Phenytoin	100	100	100	100	100	25.1 ± 18.4[c]
Troglitazone	4.7	14	73	2.4	100	0.2 ± 0.1[c]
Phenobarbital	100	100	100	100	100	9.7 ± 12.7[c]
Pioglitazone	100	57	100	14	100	1.1 ± 0.2[c]
Pravastatin	100	57	100	100	100	NI[e]
Trans-nonachlor	0.3	1.9	16	22	26	5.5[f]

[a]The CYP inhibition IC50s, μM were determined using fluorescence probe substrates shown in parentheses.

[b]Diethoxyfluorescein = DEF, 7-BQ = 7-benzyloxyquinoline, ER = ethoxy resorufin, FCA = 7-methoxy-4-trifluoromethylcoumarin-3-acetic acid, MMC = 7-methoxy-4-methyl amino methyl coumarin.

[c]Ayrton, DMD, 2001, 29, 1499–1504.

[d]Ekins, DMD, 2002, 30, 96–99.

[e]No statistically significant induction occurred at any dose = NI.

[f]Catalyst predicted, Ekins, DMD, 2002, 30, 96–99.

[g]Stimulation of Enzyme Activity.

drugs and vice versa resulting in difficult to explain clinical interactions. For example, ritonavir, a protease inhibitor, is a PXR ligand and induces CYP3A4 and several other ADME processes. It shows some evidence of autoinduction of its own metabolism[208] and induction of the clearance of other drugs depending on dose and period of administration (e.g., methadone). However, it is also a potent inhibitor of CYP3A4 and on single and multiple doses causes significant elevation of the levels of many CYP3A4 substrates.

Such overlap between inhibition and induction was investigated by Pichard and co-workers who tested 58 drugs as inducers or inhibitors of cyclosporine activity in human hepatocytes culture and microsomes. These drugs could be classified into three categories: inducers, inhibitor, and drugs that do not affect the CsA activity. Rifampicin, sulfadimidine, phenobarbital, phenytoin, phenylbutazone, dexamethasone, sulfinpyrazone, and carbamazepine induced CsA activity in human hepatocytes culture. Several macrolides, antifungals, calcium cannel blockers, and corticosteroids were classified as inhibitors. Whereas, several antibiotics, sulfamides, quinolone antibiotics, antiarrhythmic, H2 antagonists, antipyretic and anti-inflammatory, and antidiuretics were classified as drugs that are neither inducers nor inhibitors. Corticosteroids, such as prednisone and prednisolones, were both moderate inducers, as well as inhibitors of CsA activity. This work suggests that except for few corticosteroids, there was no structural overlap of drugs that could be classified as inducers and inibitors–substates for CYP3A4 and that the structural features of inducers and substrates for CYP3A4 are likely different.[209]

Similarly, we tested several structurally diverse PXR ligands to evaluate the overlap between CYP inhibition and induction (Table 4.3). The CYP inhibition of ligands were estimated using fluorescence probe substrates in human recombinant (hr) CYP enzyme expressed in bactosomes.

Clotrimazole, mifepristone, SR12813, troglitazone, and *trans*-nonachlor showed potent inhibition of either CYP3A4, CYP2C9, CYP2D6, or CYP1A2, and also were potent ligands for PXR, as shown by low EC50 values. Drugs, such as cyproterone, fexofenadine, carbamazepine, spironolactone, PCN, dexamethasone, and pioglitazone, showed a very low potential for CYP inhibition, but were potent PXR ligands. Lovastatin, simvastatin, and rifampicin were moderate inhibitors of CYP3A4, but potent PXR ligands. Phenytoin, which is a known inducer of several CYP enzymes, showed a low potential for CYP inhibition and was also a weak PXR ligand. Thus while examples of overlap exist, it is by no means a significant correlationship.

4.3.5   Clinical Consequences of CYP Induction

4.3.5.1   The CYP1A1 and CYP1A2 Enzymes.   Omeprazole has been shown to induce CYP1A1 and CYP1A2 in humans in a dose-dependent manner. At a dose of 20 mg/day for 7 consecutive days to six human volunteers, there was an average sixfold induction in the *CYP1A1* gene in the alimentary tract. At a higher dose of 60 mg/day, a dramatic increase in CYP1A1 induction was observed. Following a daily dose of 120-mg omeprazole for 7 days to extensive metabolizers, the average increase in plasma clearance of caffeine N-demethylation amounted to 31.6 ± 20.7%. Caffeine N-demethylation is used as an indicator of CYP1A2 activity in humans. Clinically relevant drug interaction based on CYP1A2 induction is not expected with common therapeutic doses in extensive metabolizers, but cannot be ruled out after unusually higher doses or in poor metabolizers.[210,211] Cigarette smoking is known to induce the CYP1A2 enzyme. In a patients smoking 20 cigarettes or more per day, sudden cessation of smoking caused a nearly 36% decrease in caffeine clearance from 2.47- to 1.53-mL/min/kg body weight.[212] The CYP1A2 enzyme is induced by consumption of broccoli, which contains 3-methylindole. Daily consumption of 500 g of broccoli by human volunteers for 12 days increased metabolism of caffeine by 19% as determined by the urinary caffeine metabolic ratio.[213] The CYP1A2 enzyme is also induced by consumption of charbroiled meat that contains polycyclic aromatic amines.[214] Based on a study of 75 colorectal cancer patients or with polyps and 205 control subjects, people with rapid *N*-acetyl transferase (NAT) and rapid CYP1A2 activity were shown to be at a greater risk of developing colorectal cancer when exposed to high dietary levels of heterocyclic amines, such as charbroiled meat. In colorectal cancer patients or with polyps, combined rapid CYP1A2 and rapid NAT phenotypes were twice as prevalent as compared to the control humans.

4.3.5.2   The CYP2C8 and CYP2C9 Enzymes.   Rifampicin is known to induce CYP2C8 and CYP2C9, however, the effect of rifampicin on the drugs that are predominantly metabolized by CYP2C8 and CYP2C9 seems to be less significant compared to that on drugs metabolized by CYP3A4.[215,216] For example, 600-mg daily dose of nifedipine for 4–6 days gives two to threefold induction in low-clearance drugs, such as rosiglitazone, glimepride, glicazide, glyburide, glipizide, and warfarin.[177] It has been shown that barbiturate also induces CYP2C9 enzyme in humans.[217]

Phenobarbital is an archetypical inducer of drug metabolism.[218] Phenobarbital is used in the therapy of epilepsy and has long been known to be a strong and broad spectrum *in vivo* inducer of drug metabolism. The dose of warfarin required for the anticoagulant effect can be increased up to 10-fold during phenobarbital treatment.[219] In another case, the maximum tolerated dose (MTD) of paclitaxel was higher in cancer patients receiving anticonvulsants (phenytoin, carbamazepine, and phenobarbital) than in cancer patient receiving no anticonvulsants ($140 mg/m^2$ vs $200 mg/m^2$). This suggests that patients receiving concurrent anticonvulsants might experience enhance hepatic clearance of paclitaxel that could result in reduced antitumor efficacy.[220,221]

4.3.5.3 The CYP3A4 Enzyme.

Rifampicin is one of the most effective inducers of human CYP3A4 enzyme in clinical use. A 600-mg daily dose of rifampicin for 5–12 days is know to cause 3 to 52-fold induction in CYP3A4 activity and a decrease in AUC of low-clearance drugs, such as cyclosporine, tacrolimus, methadone, alprazolam, diazepam, zolpidem, zopiclone; moderate-clearance drugs, such as quinidine, midazolam, trazolam; and high-clearance drugs, such as nifedipine, indinavir, and verapamil. In addition, an increased dose of oral contraceptive is recommended for women treated over an extended time with rifampin, because the drug produces a 40% decrease in bioavailability of both ethinyl estradiol and norethisterone as a consequence of induction of both oxidation and glucuronidation.[177] Time- and dose-dependent induction of CYP3A4 has been demonstrated in humans during verapamil treatment.[222] Anticonvulsant agents phenobarbital, phenytoin, and carabamazepine has been shown to induce CYP3A4 in humans after prolonged treatment. The CYP3A4 induction may play a role in toxicity due to anticonvulsant agents.[189] Many CYP3A4 inducers, such as rifampin, phenobarbital, clotrimazole, and reserpine, are also P-glycoprotein (Pgp) substrates and may modulate their own CYP3A inductive properties by stimulating their rapid removal from the intracellular environment.

4.3.5.4 The CYP2E1 Enzyme.

There are several examples of enhanced toxic effects of drug as a consequence of induced metabolism. The most well know is the enhanced risk of liver damage produced by consumption of acetaminophen as a consequence of induction of CYP2E1. Another risk of hepatotoxicity and other effects are observed on drinkers with exposure of anesthetic halothane, enfurane, and isofluorane that are metabolized by CYP2E1.[223] Ethanol is known to induce CYP2E1 *in vivo* and *in vitro*[224] and may metabolize 10% of the ingested alcohol. Ethanol intake causes up to threefold elevation

TABLE 4.4.   Dose, Total (C_p), and Free Plasma Concentrations (C_p free) of Clinically Used CYP3A4 Inducers[a]

	Dose (mg/kg)	C_p (μM)	C_p free (μM)
Carbamazepine	400–1200	12	3.6
Phenytoin	350–1000	54	5.0
Rifampicin	450–600	12	4.0
Phenobarbitone	70–400	64	32.0
Troglitazone	200–600	7	0.01
Efavirenz	600	29	0.3
Nevirapine	400	31	12.0
Moricizine	100–400	3	0.5
Probenicid	1000–2000	350	35.0
Felbamate	1200–3600	125	95.0

[a]See Ref. 188, Smith DA, Eur. J. Pharm. Sci., 2000, 11, 185–189.

in the amount of both CYP2E1 protein and mRNA in the human liver.[225–228]

4.3.6   Identifying Clinical Risk of Enzyme Induction

In addition to measurement of the affinity of an agent for nuclear hormone receptors or other mechanisms of induction, the major factor in identifying risk of significant induction is the dose. The drugs that cause clinical drug–drug interactions are generally given at high doses and prolonged treatment often in the range of 500–1000 mg/day. This results in a total drug concentration with 10–100-μM range. For example: rifampicin, which is a most effective inducer, is generally given orally as 600-mg daily dose for 4–11 days.[177] Troglitazone is given in daily doses of 200–600 mg, which lowers the plasma concentration of known CYP3A4 substrates, such as cyclosporine, terfenadine, atorvastatin, and ethinylestradiol.[229] In contrast, structurally related rosiglitazone is used as 2–12 mg and shows no evidence of enzyme induction. Table 4.4 shows the dose and the total or free plasma concentration of clinically used CYP3A4 inducers.[188] Thus even a simple empirical assessment (i.e., dose) would be a start in identifying the clinical risk of enzyme induction.

4.4   CONCLUSIONS

This chapter briefly has covered many of the main structural, functional aspects of cytochrome P450, and illustrated the many roles it has that are relevant to the discovery and development of new pharmaceutical agents. To properly do justice to this intensively studied enzyme would require a whole book or even several. This topic interest also of great as a research topic from biophysicists to clinical pharmacologists and many in between. This interest is driven at one end by its complex mechanism of action and wide-ranging biochemical capabilities to the impact it can have on the safety and efficacy of drugs and other xenobiotics, and therefore human health. It is easy to forget that even in this latter context other drug metabolizing enzymes, the action of transporters, and perhaps other processes yet to be discovered, that cytochrome P450 only accounts for perhaps 40% of drug clearance.[6] Even then it must be remembered that this is a superfamily of enzymes that although having very much in common from a patient perspective, are really often very different from one another. If all transporters were similarly treated as one in the short-hand way cytochrome P450 is, then they would surely be equally significant. Additionally, at present ADME research is arguably most vibrant in the transporter area; however, it is unlikely that cytochrome P450 would relinquish its pre-eminence any time soon. In addition to their role in so many drugs' clearance and their sensitivity to inhibition and induction, which confers so much pharmacokinetic significance, cytochrome P450 biotransforms changing the chemical nature of its substrates. It is these wide-ranging properties that makes an understanding of cytochrome P450 required reading for anyone involved in drug discovery and development.

REFERENCES

1. Nelson, D. R.; Koymans, L.; Kamataki, T.; Stegeman, J. J.; Feyereisen, R.; Waxman, D. J.; Waterman, M. R.; Gotoh, O.; Coon, M. J.; Estabrook, R. W.; Gunsalus, I. C.; Nebert, D. W. *Pharmacogenetics* **1996**, 6, 1–42.
2. Emoto, C.; Murase, S.; Iwasaki, K. *Xenobiotica* **2006**, 36, 671–683.
3. Loew, G. *Int. J. Quantum Chem.* **2000**, 77, 54–70.
4. Negishi, M.; Uno, T.; Darden, T. A.; Sueyoshi, T.; Pedersen, L. G. *FASEB, J.* **1996**, 10, 683–689.
5. Parkinson, A. in *Biotransformation of Xenobiotics* Ed., Klassen, C. D. **2001**, 133–224, McGrow-Hill.
6. Clarke, S. E.; Jones, B. in *Drug–Drug Interactions* Ed., Rodrigues, A. D. **2002**, 116, 55–88, Taylor & Francis.
7. Thummel, K. E.; Wilkinson, G. R. *Annu. Rev Pharmacol. Toxicol.* **1998**, 38, 389–430.
8. Spatzenegger, M.; Jaeger, W. *Drug Metab. Rev.* **1995**, 27, 397–417.

9. McGinnity, D. F.; Parker, A. J.; Soars, M.; Riley, R. J. *Drug Metab. Dispos.* **2000**, 28, 1327–1334.

10. Guengerich, F. P. *J. Biol. Chem.* **1991**, 266, 10019–10022.

11. Schenkman, J. B.; Jansson, I. *Pharmacol. Ther.* **2003**, 97, 139–152.

12. Sergeev, G. V.; Gilep, A. A.; Estabrook, R. W.; Usanov, S. A. *Biochem. (Moscow)*, **2006**, 71, 790–799.

13. Ito, A.; Hayshi, S.; Yoshida, T. *Biochem. Biophys. Res. Commun.* **1981**, 101, 591–598.

14. Gonzalez, F. J. *Pharmacol. Rev.* **1988**, 40, 243–288.

15. Nelson, D. R.; Kamataki, T.; Waxman, D. J.; Guengerich, F. P.; Estabrook, R. W.; Feyeceisen, R.; Gonzalez, F. J.; Coon, M. J.; Gunsalus, I. C.; Gotoch, O.; Okuda, K.; Nelbert, D. W. *DNA Cell Biol.* **1993**, 12, 1–51.

16. Nebert, D. W.; Nelson, D. R. *Methods Enzymol.* **1991**, 206, 3–11.

17. Testa, B. in *The Metabolism of Drugs and Other Xernobiotics*, Eds. Testa, B.; Caldwell, J. **1995**, 70–121, Academic Press.

18. Shimada, T.; Yamazaki, H.; Mimura, M.; Inui, Y.; Guengerich, F. P. *J. Pharmacol. Exp. Ther.* **1994**, 270, 414–423.

19. Rowland, Y. K. *Br. J. Clin. Pharmacol.* **2004**, 57, 678–679.

20. Jones, D. *Nature Rev. Drug Discov.* **2003**, 2, 685.

21. Williams, P. A.; Cosme, J.; Ward, A.; Angove, H. C.; Vinkovi, D. M.; Jhoti, H. *Nature (London)* **2003**, 424, 464–468.

22. Rowland, P.; Blaney, F. E.; Smyth, M. G.; Jones, J. J.; Leydon, V. R.; Oxbrow, A. K.; Lewis, C. J.; Tennant, M. G.; Modi, S.; Eggleston, D. S.; Chenery, R. J.; Angela, M.; Bridges, A. M. *J. Biol. Chem.* **2006**, 281, 7614–7622.

23. Williams, P. A.; Cosme, J.; Vinkovic, D. M.; Ward, A.; Hayley, C.; Angove, P. J.; Day, P. J.; Vonrhein, C.; Tickle, I. J.; Jhoti, H. *Science* **2004**, 305, 683–686.

24. Schoch, G. A.; Jason, K.; Yano, M. R.; Wester, K. J.; Griffin, C.; Stout, D.; Johnson, E. F. *J. Biol. Chem.* **2004**, 279, 9497–9503.

25. Yano, J. K.; Hsu, M. H.; Griffin, K. J.; Stout, C. D.; Johnson, E. F. *Nature Structural Molec. Biol.* **2005**, 12, 822–823.

26. Tucker, G., T. *J. Pharmacy Pharmacol.* **1994**, 46, 417–424.

27. Meyer, U. A. *J. Pharmacy Pharmacol.* **1994**, 46, 409–415.

28. Smith, G. *Xenobiotica* **1998**, 28, 1129–1165.

29. Bertilsson, L. *Clin. Pharmacokinet.* **1995**, 29, 192–209.

30. Wilkinson, G. R.; Guengerich, F.; Peter, R. A.; Branch, R. A. *Pharmacol. Ther.* **1989**, 43, 53–76.

31. Westlind, A.; Löfberg, L.; Tindberg, N.; Andersson, T. B.; Ingelman-Sundberg, M. *Biochem. Biophys. Res. Commun.* **1999**, 259, 201–205.

32. Daly, A. K.; Brockmoller, J.; Broly, F.; Eichelbaum, M.; Evans, W. E.; Gonzalez, F. J.; Huang, J. D.; Idle, J. R.; Ingelmansundberg, M.;

Ishizaki, T.; Jacqzaigrain, E.; Meyer, U. A.; Nebert, D. W.; Steen, V. M.; Wolf, C. R.; Zanger, U. M. *Pharmacogenet.* **1996**, 6, 193–201.

33. Pelkonen, O. *Xenobiotica* **1998**, 28, 1203–1253.

34. Krauser, J. A.; Guengerich, F. P. *J. Biol. Chem.* **2005**, 280, 19496–19506.

35. Thierry, C. T.; Monsarrat, B.; Dubois, J.; Sonnier, M.; Alvinerie, P.; Gueritte, F. *Drug Metab. Dispos.* **2002**, 30, 438–445.

36. Gorski, J. C.; Hall, S. D.; Jones, D. R.; VandenBranden, M. *Biochem. Pharmacol.* **1994**, 47, 1643–1653.

37. Yu, A.; Haining, R. L. *Drug Metab. Dispos.* **2001**, 29, 1514–1520.

38. Kato, R.; Yamazoe, Y. *Drug Metab. Rev.* **1994**, 26, 413–429.

39. Schweikl, H.; Taylor, J. A.; Kitareewan, S.; Linko, P.; Nagorney, D.; Goldstein, J. A. *Pharmacogenet.* **1993**, 3, 239–249.

40. Shimada, T.; Yun, C. H.; Yamazaki, H.; Gautier, J. C.; Beaune, P. H.; Guengerich, F. P. *Mol. Pharmacol.* **1992**, 41, 856–864.

41. Shimada, T.; Martin, M. V.; Pruess-Schwartz, D.; Marnett, L. J.; Guengerich, F. P. *Cancer Res.* **1989**, 49, 6304–6312.

42. MacLeod, S.; Sinha, R.; Kadlubar, F. F.; Lang, N. P. *Mutation Res.* **1997**, 376, 135–142.

43. Lang, N. P.; Butler, M. A.; Massengill, L. M.; Stotts, R. C.; Hauer-Jensen, M.; Kadlubar, F. F. *Cancer Epidemiol. Biomarkers Prev.* **1994**, 3, 675–682.

44. Rost, K. L.; Roots, I. *Clin. Pharmacol. Ther.* **1994**, 55, 402–411.

45. Hanne, M. H.; Rasmussen, B. B.; Brøsen, K. *Clin. Pharmacol. Ther.* **1997**, 61, 319–324.

46. Patten, C. *Chem. Res. Toxicol.* **1993**, 6, 511–518.

47. Brøsen, K.; Skjelbo, E.; Rasmussen, B. B.; Poulsen, H. E.; Loft, S. *Biochem. Pharmacol.* **1993**, 45, 1211–1214.

48. Clarke, S. E.; Ayrton, A. D.; Chenery, R. J. *Xenobiotica* **1994**, 24, 517–526.

49. Kunze, K. L. *Chem. Res. Toxicol.* **1993**, 6, 649–656.

50. Brian, W. R. *Biochemistry* **1989**, 28, 4993–4999,

51. Zilly, W.; Breimer, D. D.; Richter, E. *Eur. J. Clin. Pharmacol.* **1977**, 11, 287–293.

52. Leemann, T.; Transon, C.; Dayer, P. *Life Sci.* **1993**, 52, 29–34.

53. Leeman, T. D.; Transon, C.; Bonnabry, P.; Dayer, P. *Drug Exp. Clin. Res.* **1993**, 19, 189–195.

54. Veronese, M. E.; Mackenzie, P. I.; Doecke, C. J.; McManus, M. E.; Miners, J. O.; Birkett, D. J. *Biochem, Biophys. Res. Commun.* **1991**, 175, 1112–1118.

55. Relling, M. V.; Aoyama, T.; Gonzalez, F. J.; Meyer, U. A. *J. Pharmacol. Exp. Ther.* **1990**, 252, 442–447.

56. Mayumi, N.; Einosuke, T.; Shogo, M.; Tsutomu, S.; Susumu, I.; Yoshihiko, F. *Biochem. Pharmacol.* **1994**, 47, 247–251.

57. Tucker, G. T.; Houston, J. B.; Huang, S. M. *Br. J. Clin. Pharmacol.* **2001**, 52, 107–117.

58. Baldwin, S. J.; Bloomer, J. C.; Smith, G. J.; Ayrton, A. D.; Clarke, S. E.; Chenery, R. J. *Xenobiotica* **1995**, 25, 261–270.

59. Koenigs, L. L.; Peter, R. M.; Hunter, A. P.; Haining, R. L.; Rettie, A. E.; Friedberg, T.; Pritchard, M. P.; Shou, M.; Rushmore, T. H.; Trager, W. F. *Biochemistry* **1999**, 38, 2312–2319.

60. Yasumori, T.; Murayama, N.; Yamazoe, Y.; Kato, R. *Clin. Pharmacol. Therp.* **1990**, 47, 313–322.

61. Koymans, L.; Vermeulen, N. P.; van Acker, S. A.; te Koppele, J. M.; Heykants, J. J.; Lavrijsen, K.; Meuldermans, W.; Donné-Op den Kelder, G. M. *Chem. Res. Toxicol.* **1992**, 5, 211–219.

62. de Groot, M. J.; Ackland, M. J.; Horne, V. A.; Alex, A. A.; Jones, B. C. *J. Med. Chem.* **1999**, 42, 1515–1524.

63. Rowland, P.; Blaney, F. E.; Smyth, M. G.; Jones, J. J.; Leydon, V. R.; Oxbrow, A. K.; Lewis, C. J.; Tennant, M. G.; Modi, S.; Eggleston, D. S.; Chenery, R. J.; Bridges, A. M. *J. Biol. Chem.* **2006**, 281, 7614–7622.

64. Pelkonen, O.; Maenpaa, J.; Taavitsainen, P.; Rautio, A.; Raunio, H. *Xenobiotica* **1998**, 28, 1203–1253.

65. Baker, G. B.; Fang, J.; Sinha, S.; Coutts, R. T. *Neurosci. Biobehav. Rev.* **1998**, 22, 325–333.

66. Caccia, S. *Clin. Pharmacokinet.* **1998**, 34, 281–302.

67. Sproule, B. A.; Naranjo, C. A.; Brenmer, K. E.; Hassan, P. C. *Clin. Pharmacokinet.* **1997**, 33, 454–471.

68. Wrighton, S. A.; Ring, B. J. *Drug Metab. Rev.* **1999**, 31, 15–28.

69. Benet, L. Z. in *Goodman, Gilman's the Pharmacological Basis of the Therapeutics*, 9th ed, Ed. Hardman, J. H.; Molinoff, P. B.; Gilman, A. G. **1996**, 3–28, McGraw-Hill.

70. Lewis, D. V. *Curr. Med. Chem.* **2003**, 10, 1955–1972.

71. Guengerich, F. P. *Annu. Rev. Pharmacol. Toxicol.* **1999**, 39, 1–17.

72. Venkatesan, K, *Clin. Pharmacokinet.* **1992**, 22, 47–65.

73. Wilkinson, G. R. *Pharmacokinet. Biopharmacol.* **1996**, 24, 475–490.

74. Ameer, B.; Weintraub, R. A, *Clin. Pharmacokinet.* **1997**, 33, 103–121.

75. Bertz, R. J.; Granneman, G. R. *Clin. Pharmacokinet.* **1997**, 32 210–258.

76. Lin, J. H. *Annu. Rev. Med. Chem.* **1997**, 32, 295–304.

77. Lin, J. H.; Lu, A. Y. *Pharmacol. Rev.* **1997**, 49, 403–449.

78. Thummel, K. E.; Wilkinson, G. R. *Annu. Rev. Pharmacol. Toxicol.* **1998**, 38, 389–430.

79. Lomaestro, B. M.; Piatek, M. A. *Ann. Pharmacother.* **1998**, 32, 915–928.

80. Albengres, E.; Le Louët, H.; Tillement, J. P. *Drug Safety* **1998**, 18, 83–97.
81. Ludden, T. M. *Clin. Pharmacokinet.* **1985**, 10, 63–79.
82. Nahata, M. *J. Antimicrob. Chemother.* **1996**, 37 (Suppl C), 133–142.
83. Dresser, G. K.; Spence, J. D.; Bailey, D. G. *Clin. Pharmacokinet.* **2000**, 38, 41–57.
84. Edwards, D. J.; Bellevue, F. H. 3rd; Woster, P. M. *Drug Metab. Dispos.* **1996**, 24, 1287–1290.
85. Schmiedlin-Ren, P.; Edwards, D. J.; Fitzsimmons, M. E.; He, K.; Lown, K. S.; Woster, P. M.; Rahman, A.; Thummel, K. E.; Fisher, J. M.; Hollenberg, P. F.; Watkins, P. B. *Drug Metab. Dispos.* **1997**, 25, 1228–1233.
86. Guengerich, F. P. *Chem. Res. Toxicol.* **1990**, 3, 363–371.
87. Ed. Ian, P.; Shephard, A. E. *Methods in Molecular Biology*, **1998**, 107, 123, and 129, Human Press, Totawa.
88. Rodrigues, A. D. *Biochem. Pharmacol.* **1999**, 57, 465–480.
89. Masimirembwa, C. M.; Otter, C.; Berg, M.; Jönsson, M.; Leidvik, B.; Jonsson, E.; Johansson, T.; Bäckman, A.; Edlund, A.; Andersson, B. *Drug Metab. Dispos.* **1999** 27, 1117–1122.
90. Yoshitomi, S.; Ikemoto, K.; Takahashi, J.; Miki, H.; Namba, M.; Asahi, S. *Toxicol. In Vitro* **2001**, 15, 245–256.
91. Crespi, C. L.; Miller, V. P.; Penman, B. W. *Anal. Biochem.* **1997**, 24, 188–190.
92. Li, A. P. *IDrugs* **1998**, 1, 311–314.
93. Donato, M. T.; Jiménez, N.; Castell, J. V.; Gómez-Lechón, M. J. *Drug Metab. Dispos.* **2004**, 32, 699–706.
94. Gonzalez, F. J.; Korzekwa, K. R. *Annu. Rev. Pharmacol. Toxicol.* **1995**, 35, 369–390.
95. Rodrigues, A. D. *Med. Chem. Res.* **1998**, 8, 422–433.
96. Li, D.; Kerns, E. H.; Li, S. Q.; Carter, G. T. *Int. J. Pharma.* **2007**, 335, 1–11.
97. Zlokarnik, G.; Grootenhuis, P. D.; Watson, J. B. *Drug Disc. Today* **2005**, 10, 1443–1450.
98. Favreau, L. V.; Palamanda, J. R.; Lin, C. C.; Nomeir, A. A. *Drug Metab. Dispos.* **1999**, 27, 436–439.
99. Bapiro, T. E.; Egnell, A. C.; Hasler, J. A.; Masimirembwa, C. M. *Drug Metab. Dispos.* **2001**, 29, 30–35.
100. Nomeir, A. A.; Ruegg, C.; Shoemaker, M.; Favreau, L. V.; Palamanda, J. R.; Silber, P.; Lin, C. C. *Drug Metab. Dispos.* **2001**, 29, 748–753.
101. Cohen, L. H.; Remley, M. J.; Raunig, D.; Vaz, A. D. N. *Drug Metab. Dispos.* **2003**, 31, 1005–1015.

102. Weaver, R.; Graham, K. S.; Beattie, I. G.; Riley, R. J. *Drug Metab. Dispos.* **2003**, 31, 955–966.

103. Madan, A.; Usuki, E. L.; Burton, A.; Ogilve, B. W.; Parkinson, A. in *Drug–Drug Interactions* Ed. Rodrigues, A. D. Drugs and the Pharmaceutical Sciences **2002**, vol. 116, 217–294, Marcel-Dekker.

104. Stresser, D. M.; Turner, S. D.; Blanchard, A. P.; Miller, V. P.; Crespi, C. L. *Drug Metab. Dispos.* **2002**, 30, 845–852.

105. Bloomer, J.; Ramesh, B.; Stephen, E. C. Characterization of novel CYP2C9 and CYP2D6 substrates for fluorescence P450 assays. *13th International Symposium on Microsomes and Drug Oxidations* Stressa, Italy, 10–14 July **2000**.

106. Yamamoto, T.; Suzuki, A.; Kohno, Y. *Drug Metab. Pharmacokinet.* **2002**, 17, 437–448.

107. Venhorst, J.; Onderwater, R. C. A.; Meerman, J. H. N.; Nico, P. E.; Vermeulen, N. P. E.; Jan, N. M.; Commandeur, J. N. M. *Eur. J. Pharma. Sci.* **2002**, 12, 151–158.

108. Jenkins, K. M.; Angeles, R.; Quintos, M. T.; Xu, R.; Kassel, D. B.; Rourick, R. A. *J. Pharma. Biomed. Anal.* **2002**, 34, 989–1004.

109. Bambal, R.; Bloomer, J. C.; Clarke, S. E.; Chenery, R.; Characterization of diethoxyfluorescein as a novel fluorescence substrate for CYP3A4 and CYP2C8. *Patent* P32490, **2000**.

110. Rasmussen, B. B.; Nielsen, K. K.; Brosen, K. *Anal. Biochem.* **1994**, 222, 9–13.

111. Bourrie, M.; Meunier, V.; Berger, Y.; Fabre, G. *J. Pharmacol. Exp. Ther.* **1996**, 277, 321–332.

112. Butler, M. A.; Iwasaki, M.; Guengerich, F. P.; Kadlubar, F. F. *Proc. Natl. Acad. Sci. USA* **1989**, 86, 7696–7700.

113. Rodrigues, A. D.; Kukulka, M. J.; Roberts, E. M.; Ouellet, D.; Rodgers, T. R. *Drug Metab. Dispos.* **1996**, 24, 126–136.

114. Rodrigues, A. D.; Surber, B. W.; Yao, Y.; Wong, S. L.; Roberts, E. M. *Drug Metab. Dispos.* **1997**, 25, 1097–1100.

115. Ono, S.; Hatanaka, T.; Miyazawa, S.; Tsutsui, M.; Aoyama, T.; Gonzalez, F. J.; Satoh, T. *Xenobiotica* **1996**, 26, 1155–1166.

116. Jung, F.; Richardson, T. H.; Raucy, J. L.; Johnson, E. F. *Drug Metab. Dispos.* **1997**, 25, 133–139.

117. Bloomer, J. C.; Woods, F. R.; Haddock, R. E.; Lennard, M. S.; Tucker, G. T. *Br. J. Clin. Pharmacol.* **1992**, 33, 521–523.

118. Rodrigues, A. D.; Kukulka, M. J.; Surber, B. W.; Thomas, S. B.; Uchic, J. T.; Rotert, G. A.; Michel, G.; Thome-Kromer, B.; Machinist, J. M. *Anal. Biochem.* **1994**, 219, 309–320.

119. Riley, R. J.; Howbrook, D. *J. Pharmacol. Toxicol. Methods* **1997**, 38, 189–193.

120. Di Marco, A.; Marcucci, I.; Verdirame, M.; Pérez, J.; Sanchez, M.; Fernando, F.; Chaudhary, A.; Laufer, R. *Drug Metab. Dispos.* **2005**, 33, 349–358.

121. Di Marco, A.; Marcucci, I.; Chaudhary, A.; Taliani, M.; Laufer, R. *Drug Metab. Dispos.* **2005**, 33, 359–364.

122. Moody, G. C. *Xenobiotica* **1999**, 29, 53–75.

123. Obach, R. S. *Drug Metab. Dispos.* **1997**, 25, 1359–1369.

124. Margolis, J. M.; Obach, R. S. *Drug Metab. Dispos.* **2003**, 31, 606–611.

125. Walsky, R. L.; Obach, R. S. *Drug Metab. Dispos.* **2004**, 32, 647–660.

126. Wu, J.; Hughes, C. S.; Picard, P.; Letarte, S.; Gaudreault, M.; Lévesque, J.-F.; Nicoll-Griffith, D. A.; Bateman, K. P. *Anal. Chem.* **2007**, 79, 4657–4665.

127. Ayrton, J.; Plumb, R.; Leavens, W. J.; Mallett, D.; Dickins, M.; Dear, G. J. *Rapid Commun. Mass Spectrue* **1998**, 12, 217–224.

128. Dierks, E. A.; Stams, K. R.; Lim, H. K.; Cornelius, G.; Zhang, H.; Ball, S. E. *Drug Metab. Dispos.* **2001**, 29, 23–29.

129. Kuhlmann, J.; Wolfgang, M. *Drug Safety* **2001**, 24, 715–725.

130. Williams, C. N. *Can. J. Gastroentorol.* **1998**, 12, 535.

131. Furutaa, S.; Kamadaa, E.; Omataa, T.; Sugimotoa, T.; Kawabataa, Y.; Yonezawab, K.; Wuc, X. C.; Kurimotoa, T. *Eur. J. Pharmacol.* **2004**, 497, 223–231,

132. Bedford, T. A.; Rowbotham, D. J. *Drug Safety* **1996**, 15, 167–175,

133. Michalets, E. L.; Williams, C. R. *Clin. Pharmacokinet.* **2000**, 39, 49–75,

134. Simard, C.; O'Hara, G. E.; Prévost, J.; Guilbaud, R.; Massé, R.; Turgeon, J. *Eur. J. Clin. Pharmacol.* **2001**, 57, 229–234,

135. Darpö, B. *Eur. Heart, J. Suppl.* **2001**, 3, K70–K80.

136. Alderman, J. *Clin. Ther.* **2005**, 27, 1050–1062.

137. Laine, K.; Forsstrom, J.; Gronroos, P.; Irjala, K.; Kailajarvi, M.; Scheinin, M. *Ther. Drug Monit.* **2000**, 20, 503–509.

138. Furutaa, S.; Kamadaa, E.; Omataa, T.; Sugimotoa, T.; Kawabataa, Y.; Yonezawab, K.; Wuc, X. C.; Kurimoto, T. *Eur. J. Pharmacol.* **2004**, 497, 223–231.

139. McMullin, S. T.; Reichley, R. M.; Watson, L. A.; Steib, S. A.; Frisse, M. E.; Bailey, T. *Arch. Int. Med.* **1999**, 159, 2077–2082.

140. Anderson, T.; Hassan-Alin, M.; Hasselgren, G.; Rohss, K. *Clin. Pharmacokinet.* **2001**, 40, 523–537.

141. Kivisto, K. T.; Neuvonen, P. J.; Klotz, U. *Clin. Pharmacokinet.* **1994**, 27, 1–5.

142. Honig, P. K.; Woosley, R. L.; Zamani, K.; Conner, D. P.; Cantilena, L. R. Jr. *Clin. Pharmacol. Ther.* **1992**, 52, 231–238.

143. Honig, P. K.; Wortham, D. C.; Zamani, K.; Conner, D. P.; Mullin, J. C.; Cantilena, L. R. *JAMA* **1993**, 269, 1513–1518.

144. Bradbury, J. *Lancet* **1998**, 351, 1791.
145. Editorial news, Posicor warning issued, *Geriatric Nursing* **1998**, 19, 118–119.
146. Sorelle, R. *Circulaltion* **1998**, 98, 831–832.
147. Available at http://www.fda.gov/opacom/hpnews.html.
148. Jacobson, T. A. *Am. J. Cardiol.* **2004**, 94, 1140–1146.
149. Van der Vring, J. A.; Cleophas, T. J.; Van der Wall, E. E.; Niemeyer, M. G. *Curr. Ther. Res.* **1998**, 59, 754–761.
150. Smith, S. R.; Kendall, M. J. *Clin. Pharmacokinet.* **1988**, 15, 44–54.
151. Baciewicz, A. M.; Baciewicz, F. A. Jr. *Am. Heart, J.* **1989**, 118, 144–154.
152. Reynolds, J. C. *J. Clin. Gastroenterol.* **1990**, 12, S54–S63.
153. Lauritsen, K.; Laursen, Laurits, S.; Rask-Madsen, J. *Clin. Pharmacokinet.* **1990**, 19, 11–31.
154. Shinn, A. F. *Drug Safety* **1992**, 7, 245–267.
155. Klotz, U.; Kroemer, H. K. *Pharmacol. Ther.* **1991**, 50, 233–244
156. Smith, S. R. *Br. J. Clin. Pharmacol.* **1987**, 23, 311–315.
157. Cross, D. *J. Biopharmaceut. Sci.* **1991**, 2, 339–377.
158. Obach, R. S.; Walsky, R. L.; Venkatakrishnan, K.; Gaman, E. A.; Houston, J. B.; Tremaine, L. M. *J. Pharmacol. Exp. Ther.* **2006**, 316, 336–348.
159. Brown, H. S.; Ito, K.; Galetin, A.; J. Houston, B. J. *Br. J. Clin. Pharmcol.* **2005**, 60, 508–518.
160. Yao, C.; Levy, R. H. *J. Pharm. Sci.* **2002**, 91, 1923–1935.
161. Houston, J. B.; Galetin, A. *Drug Metab. Rev.* **2003**, 35, 393–415
162. Neal, J. M.; Kunze, K. L.; Levy, R. H.; O'Reilly, R. A; Trager, W. F. *Drug Metab. Dispos.* **2003**, 31, 1043–1048.
163. Venkatakrishnan, K.; von Moltke, L. L.; Obach, R. S.; Greenblatt, D. J. *Curr. Drug Metab.* **2003**, 4, 423–459.
164. Blanchard, N.; Richert, L.; Coassolo, P.; Lave, T. *Curr. Drug Metab.* **2004**, 5, 147–156.
165. Shou, M. *Curr. Opin. Drug Disc. Dev.* **2005**, 8, 66–77.
166. Brown, H. S.; Galetin, A.; Hallifax, D.; Houston, J. B. *Clin. Pharmacokinet.* **2006**, 45, 1035–1050.
167. Ito, K.; Brown, H. S.; Houston, J. B. *Br. J. Clin. Pharmacol.* **2004**, 57, 473–486.
168. Blanchard, N.; Richert, L.; Coassolo, P.; Lave, T. *Curr. Drug Metab.* **2004**, 5, 147–156,
169. McGinnity, D. F.; Tucker, J.; Trigg, S.; Riley, R. J. *Drug Metab. Dispos.* **2005**, 33, 1700–1707.
170. Grime, K.; Riley, R. J. *Curr. Drug Metab.* **2006**, 7, 251–264.
171. Galetin, A.; Burt, H.; Gibbons, L.; Houston, J. B. *Drug Metab. Dispos.* **2006**, 34, 166–175.

172. Silverman, R. B. *Methods Enzymol.* **1995**, 249, 240–283.

173. Zhou, S.; Yung Chan, S.; Cher Goh, B.; Chan, E.; Duan, W.; Huang, M.; McLeod, H. L. *Clin. Pharmacokinet.* **2005**, 44, 279–304.

174. Wang, Y. H.; Jones, D. R.; Hall, S. D. *Drug Metab. Dispos.* **2004**, 32, 259–266.

175. Wrighton, S. A.; Schuetz, E. G.; Thummel, K. E.; Shen, D. D.; Korzekwa, K. R.; Watkins, P. B. *Drug Metab. Rev.* **2000**, 32, 339–361.

176. White, R. *Annu. Rev. Pharmacol. Toxicol.* **2000**, 40, 133–157.

177. Lin, J. H. *Pharm. Res.* **2006**, 23, 1089–1116.

178. Modry, D. L.; Stinson, E. B.; Oyer, P. E. *Transplantation* **1985**, 39, 313–314.

179. Hebert, M. F.; Roberts, J. P.; Prueksaritanont, T.; Benet, L. Z. *Clin. Pharmacol. Ther.* **1992**, 52, 453–457.

180. Lin, J. H.; Lu, A. Y. H. *Clin. Pharmacokinet.* **1998**, 35, 361–390.

181. Beresford, A. P. *Drug Metab. Rev.* **1993**, 25, 503–517.

182. Pelkonen, O.; Manenpaa, J.; Taavitsainen, P.; Rautio, A.; Rautio, H. *Xenobiotics* **1998**, 28, 1203–1253.

183. Fromm, M. F.; Busse, D.; Kroemer, H. K.; Eichelbaum, M. *Hepatology* **1996**, 24, 796–801.

184. Silva, J. M.; Morin, P. E.; Day, S. H.; Kennedy, B. P.; Payette, P.; Rushmore, T.; Yergey, J. A.; Nicoll-Griffith, D. A. *Drug Metab. Dispos.* **1998**, 26, 490–496.

185. Kostrubsky, V. E.; Ramachandran, V.; Venkataramanan, R.; Dorko, K.; Esplen, J. E.; Zhang, S.; Sinclair, J. F.; Wrighton, S. A.; Strom, S. C. *Drug Metab. Dispos.* **1999**, 27, 887–894.

186. Maurel, P. *Adv. Drug Deliv. Rev.* **1996**, 22, 105–132.

187. LeCluyse, E. L. *Eur. J. Pharm. Sci.* **2001**, 13, 343–368.

188. Smith, D. A. *Eur. J. Pharm. Sci.* **2000**, 11, 185–189.

189. Park, B. K.; Kitteringham, N. R.; Pirmohammad, M.; Tucker, G. T. *Br. J. Clin. Pharmacol.* **1996**, 41, 477–491.

190. Miller, A. G.; Israel, D. I.; Whitlock, J. P. Jr. *J. Biol. Chem.* **1983**, 258, 3523–3527.

191. Trottier, E.; Belzil, A.; C. Stoltz, C.; Anderson, A. *Gene* **1995**, 158, 263–268.

192. Honkakoski, P.; Moore, R.; Gynther, J.; Negeshi, M. *J. Biol. Chem.* **1996**, 271, 9746–9753.

193. Sueyoshi, T.; Kawamato, T.; Zelko, I.; Honkakoshi, P.; Negeshi, M. *J. Biol. Chem.* **1996**, 274, 6043–6046.

194. Handschin, C.; Meyers, U. A. *Pharmacol. Rev.* **2003**, 55, 649–673.

195. Baes, M.; Gulick, T.; Choi, H. S.; Martinoli, M. G.; Simha, D.; Moore, D. D. *Mol. Cell Biol.* **2003**, 14, 1544–1555.

196. Kliewer, S. A.; Moore, J. T.; Wade, L.; Staudinger, J. L.; Watson, M. A.; Jones, S. A.; McKee, D. D.; Oliver, B. B.; Wiltson, T. M.; Zetterstrom, R. H.; Pellerman, T.; Lehmann, J. M. *Cell* **1998**, 92, 73–82.

197. Bertilsson, G.; Heidrich, J.; Svensson, K.; Asman, M.; Jendeberg, L.; Sydow-Backman, M.; Ohlsson, R.; Postlind, H.; Blomquist, P.; Berkenstam, A. *Proc. Natl. Acad. Sci. USA* **1998**, 95, 12208–12213.

198. El-Sankary, W.; Gibson, G. G.; Ayrton, A.; Plant, N. *Drug Metab. Dispos.* **2001**, 29, 1499–1504.

199. Moore, L. B.; Goodwin, B.; Jones, S. A.; Wisely, G. B.; Serabjit-Singh, C. J.; Wilson, T. M.; Coliins, J. L.; Kliewer, S. A. *Proc. Natl. Acad. Sci. USA* **2000**, 97, 7500–7502.

200. Wang, H.; LeCluyse, E. L. *Clin. Pharmacokinet.* **2003**, 42, 1331–1357.

201. Watkins, R. E.; Wisely, G. B.; Moore, L. B.; Collins, J. L.; Lambert, M. H.; Williams, S. P.; Willson, T. M.; Kliewer, S. A.; Redinbo, M. R. *Science* **2001**, 292, 2329–2333.

202. Berkhout, T. A.; Simon, H. M.; Patel, D. D.; Bentzen, C.; Niesor, E.; Jackson, B.; Suckling, K. E. *J. Biol. Chem.* **1996**, 271, 14376–14382.

203. Berkhout, T. A.; Simon, H. M.; Jackson, B.; Yates, J.; Pearce, N.; Groot, P. H.; Bentzen, C.; Niesor, E.; Kerns, W. D.; Suckling, K. E. *Atherosclerosis* **1997**, 139, 203–212.

204. Jones, S. A.; Moore, L. B.; Shenk, J. L.; Wisely, G. B.; Hamilton, G. A.; McKee, D. D.; Tomkinson, N. C. O.; LeCluyse, E. L.; Lambert, M. H.; Willson, T. M.; Kliewer, S. A.; Moore, J. T. *Mol. Endocrinol.* **2000**, 14, 27–39.

205. Wei, P.; Zhang, J.; Dowhan, D. H.; Han, Y.; Moore, D. D. *Pharmacogenomics, J.* **2002**, 2, 117–126.

206. Xie, W.; Barwick, J. L.; Simon, C. M.; Pierce, A. M.; Safe, S.; Blumberg, B.; Guzelian, P. S.; Evans, R. M. *Genes Dev.* **2000**, 14, 3014–3023.

207. Luo, G.; Cunningham, M.; Kim, S.; Burn, T.; Lin, J.; Sinz, M.; Hamilton, G.; Rizzo, C.; Jolley, S.; Gilbert, D.; Downey, A.; Mudra, D.; Graham, R.; Carroll, K.; Xie, J.; Ajay Madan, A.; Parkinson, A.; Christ, D.; Selling, B.; LeCluyse, E.; Gan, L. S. *Drug. Metab. Dispos.* **2002**, 30, 795–804.

208. Hsu, A.; Grammemain, G. R.; Bertz, R. J.; *Clin. Pharmacokinet.* **1998**, 35, 275–291.

209. Pichard, L.; Fabre, I.; Fabre, G.; Domergue, J.; Aubert, S. B.; Mourad, G.; Maurel, P. *Drug Metab. Dispos.* **1990**, 18, 595–606.

210. Rost, K. L.; Brösicke, H.; Heinemeyer, G.; Roots, I. *Hepatology* **1994**, 20, 1204–1212.

211. McDonnell, W. M.; Scheiman, J. M.; Traber, P. G. *Gastroenterology* **1992**, 103, 1509–1516.

212. Faber, M. S.; Fuhr, U. *Clin. Pharmacol. Ther.* **2004**, 76, 178–184.

213. Kall, M. A.; Vang, O.; Clausen, J. *Carcinogenesis* **1996**, 17, 793–799.

214. Lang, N. P.; Butler, M. A.; Massengill, J.; Lawson, M.; Stotts, R. C.; Hauer-Jensen, M.; Kadlubar, F. F. *Cancer Epidemiol. Biomark. Preve.* **1994**, 3, 675–682.

215. Synold, T. W.; Dussault, I.; Forman, B. M. *Nature Med.* **2001**, 7, 584–590.

216. Gerbal-Chaloin, S.; Pascussi, J. M.; Pichard-Garcia, L.; Martine Daujat, M.; Waechter, F.; Fabre, J. M.; Carrère, N.; Maurel, P. *Drug Metab. Dispos.* **2001**, 29, 242–251.

217. Zilly, W.; Breimer, D. D.; Richter, E. *Eur. J. Clin. Pharmacol.* **1977**, 11, 287–293.

218. Waxman, D. J.; Azaroff, L. *Biochem. J.* **1992**, 281, 577–592.

219. Patsalos, P. N.; Duncan, J. S. *Drug Safety* **1993**, 9, 156–184.

220. Fetell, M. R.; Grossman, S. A.; Fisher, J. D.; Erlanger, B.; Rowinsky, E.; Stockel, J.; Piantadosi, S. *J. Clin. Oncol.* **1997**, 15, 3121–3128.

221. Baker, A. F.; Dorr, R. T. *Cancer Treat. Rev.* **2001**, 27, 221–233.

222. Fromm, M. F.; Busse, D.; Kroemer, H. K.; Eichelbaum, M. *Hepatology* **1996**, 24, 796–801.

223. Silva, J. M.; Nicoli-Griffith, D. A. in *Drug–Drug Interactions* Ed. Rodrigues, A. D. **2002**, 116, Taylor & Francis.

224. Sotaniemi, E. A.; Pelkonen, R. O. Eds. *Enzyme Induction in Man* **1987**, Taylor & Francis.

225. Perrot, N.; Nalpas, B.; Yang, C. S.; Beaune, P. H. *Eur. J. Clin. Invest.* **1989**, 19, 549–555.

226. Takahashi, T.; Lasker, J. M.; Rosman, A. S.; Lieber, C. S. *Hepatology* **1993**, 17, 236–245.

227. Pelkonen, O. *Xenobiotica* **1998**, 28, 1203–1253.

228. Ronis, M. J. J.; Ingelman-Sunberg, M. in *Hand Book of Drug Metabolism*, Ed. Woolf, T. F. **1999**, 239–262, Marcel Dekker.

229. Loi, C. M.; Young, M.; Randinitis, E.; Vassos, A.; Koup, J. R. Clinical pharmacokinetics of troglitazone, *Clin. Pharmacokinet.* **1999**, 37, 91–104.

CHAPTER 5

THE ROLE OF DRUG METABOLISM AND METABOLITE IDENTIFICATION IN DRUG DISCOVERY

XIANGMING GUAN

South Dakota State University, Department of Pharmaceutical Sciences, College of Pharmacy, Brookings, SD

Evaluation of Drug Candidates for Preclinical Development: Pharmacokinetics, Metabolism, Pharmaceutics, and Toxicology, Edited by Chao Han, Charles B. Davis, and Binghe Wang
Copyright © 2010 John Wiley & Sons, Inc.

5.1 INTRODUCTION

Drug discovery is a costly, slow, and high-risk process. Only 1 in 10 chemical entities that enter clinical development could be successful. The average cost for one marketed product has been estimated to be >$1 billion[1] with a typical time scale of 14.8 years from preclinical discovery research to regulatory approval.[2] The staggering cost of drug development may partially be due to difficulties in identifying undesirable compounds at an early enough stage of development. The undesirable compounds include those with inappropriate pharmaceutical, pharmacokinetic (PK), and unacceptable toxicological properties. It has been reported that 63% of all preclinical compounds nominated for clinical development failed due to poor PKs [absorption, distribution, metabolism, and excretion (ADME)] and/or drug induced toxicity (Tox).[3] It is now well recognized that selection of a robust candidate requires a balance of potency, safety, and PKs. Maximizing potency against a biological target is no longer a primary driving force in developing a drug candidate. It is, therefore, no surprise that the pharmaceutical industry is making all efforts possible to eliminate compounds with poor "developability" at an early stage to minimize attrition in late development stages, which is more costly and time consuming. Consequently, determination of pharmaceutical, PK, and toxicological properties of a drug candidate has been shifted from its traditional supporting role to a more proactive guiding role, and from being conducted in the drug development stage [from a clinical candidate to final US Food and Drug Administration (FDA) approval] to being integrated throughout the drug discovery (hit generation, lead selection and optimization, and candidate selection) and development processes.

Drug metabolism properties constitute the most important component of the PK properties and play a significant role in the toxicological properties. Drug metabolism describes the biotransformation of a chemical entity. Research in this area involves identification, structural characterization, quantitation of metabolites, and examination of responsible enzyme systems. From the drug metabolism viewpoint, the rate of metabolism, the nature of the metabolites, and the corresponding metabolizing enzymes are important information for evaluating whether a chemical entity is "developable". The rate of metabolism largely affects the eventual drug concentration, which determines the biological effects and whether the response is desirable or not. Although most compounds lose their biological activities after metabolism, some could be converted to reactive intermediates leading to adverse effects. On the other hand, plenty of examples have been reported that some metabolites could possess better developability than the parent compound and can be served as a new lead or be developed into a better drug. Additionally, knowledge of a given chemical entity is a substrate, inhibitor, or inducer of a given metabolizing enzyme is extremely valuable for understanding potential toxicity, drug–drug interactions, and dosage related issues of the drug candidate. Integration of drug metabolism at the drug discovery stage makes metabolism information available early enough to help the evaluation of whether or not a drug candidate merits further development. Further, such information also provides medicinal chemists guidance, from a drug metabolism perspective, in conducting further structural modification by blocking, enhancing, or switching metabolism to optimize the PK and safety profiles.[4]

5.2 THE PROCESSES OF DRUG DISCOVERY AND DEVELOPMENT

To fully understand the role of drug metabolism in drug discovery and development, it is beneficial to briefly discuss the process of discovery and development. Figure 5.1 provides a flow diagram describing the traditional and current drug discovery and development processes, as well as the role of drug metabolism in each stage.[5–7] The discovery phase involves hit identification, lead identification and optimization, and clinical candidate selection. In a traditional linear approach, discovery and development departments play two independent functions. The drug discovery department primarily has the responsibility of synthesizing milligram quantities of compounds exhibiting desired biological activities. The preclinical department has the responsibility of characterizing the PKs, toxicity, initial formulation, and physicochemical properties (solubility, pK_a, $\log P$, etc.) of the candidate. By using a current parallel approach, the two organizations would have a significant preclinical collaboration between them, as illustrated in Figure 5.1. The integrated approach makes the best use of experimental and *in silico* ADME–Tox evaluation and enables them to complement each other well. The earlier use of *in silico* ADME–Tox evaluation on a large number of compounds serves as a filter for obtaining a manageable number of compounds with improved candidates entering *in vitro* ADME–Tox testing. The availability of *in vitro* results on the sets of

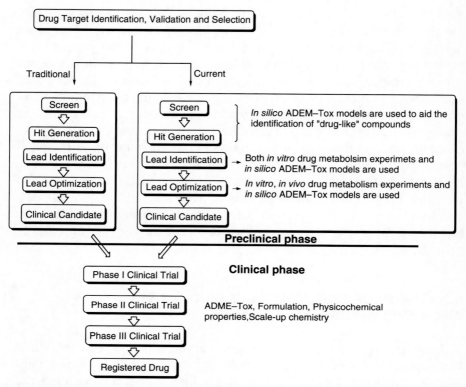

Figure 5.1. A flow diagram of traditional and current drug discovery and development processes and integration of ADME–Tox evaluation.

compounds predicted to have desirable properties provides valuable feedbacks to assess the predictability of *in silico* ADME–Tox models and, more importantly, helps to adjust the parameters and refine the models in the continuous improvement of predictability.[7]

5.3 DRUG METABOLISM AND THE FATE OF A COMPOUND AS A DRUG CANDIDATE

Drug metabolism related to the fate of a compound as a drug candidate primarily involves metabolic stability, drug or drug metabolite related toxicities, and metabolizing enzyme inhibition or induction. Of these properties, drug or drug metabolite related toxicities and metabolizing enzyme inhibition are the major causes leading to a termination of drug candidacy.

5.3.1 Issues Related to Toxicity

Drug-induced toxicity has been reported as the major cause of attrition in drug discovery and development.[8] It is also a major cause of post-market withdrawal and usage modification of medications,[8] as exemplified by the recall of diethyaminoethoxyhexestrol,[8] terfenadine,[9] and vioxx,[10] the abrupt termination of clinical trials with fialuridine, and essential abandonment of perhexiline, and issuance of new guidelines for tetracycline and valproic acid.[8] Further, toxicity study is the foundation of an investigational new drug application.

The severity of chemical-induced toxicity is a function of three major determinants: (1) the intrinsic toxic property of a chemical; (2) its local concentration at a particular organ; and (3) the ability of the host defense systems to detoxify the chemical and cope with chemical injuries. The first determinant is embedded in the chemical structure and considered as an intrinsic toxic property of a chemical.[8]

Depending on the therapeutic applications of a potential drug, the scope of the toxicity investigation can vary. In general, toxicity evaluation can include the study of genetic toxicity, hepatic toxicity (steatosis, intrahepatic cholestasis, phospholipidosis) and cardiotoxicity,[8] severe cutaneous reactions, anaphylaxis, and blood dyscrasias.[11] In most cases, reactive drug metabolites or reactive drugs appear to be the major contribution to drug related toxicity.[12,13] Reactive metabolites are also considered to be the primary cause of idiosyncratic drug reactions.[13–15] Therefore, identifying reactive metabolites is an important part of drug discovery and development.

5.3.1.1 Reactive Metabolites

5.3.1.1a Functional Groups That Can Be Bioactivated to a Reactive Species. There are many different types of reactive metabolites that can be formed. A detailed description of which can be found elsewhere.[16,17] In general, reactive metabolites are electrophiles (electron-deficient species), free radicals, peroxides, or other oxidizing agents. Electrophiles react with nucleophilic functional groups of biological molecules like the sulfhydryl or amino group of proteins resulting in toxicity. Free radicals can cause cleavage of biological molecules, while oxidizing agents would lead to cellular oxidative stress. Some functional groups can be converted to reactive toxic species through metabolic conversion. Table 5.1 lists representative types of reactive functional groups resulting from bioactivation of various drugs or chemicals. A detailed discussion on the generation of these reactive

TABLE 5.1. Different Types of Reactive Intermediates Generated from Drugs or Chemicals[a]

Compounds	Toxicity	Compounds	Toxicity
Aryl oxidation to either an epoxide or a quinone		**Formation of quinone imines**	
Benzo[a]pyrene	Lung toxicity	Acetaminophen	Hepatotoxicity
Bromobenzene	Hepatotoxicity	Amodiaquine	Hepatotoxicity
Carbamazepine	Teratogenicity	Diclofenac	Hepatotoxicity
Phenytoin drug-induced hypersensitivity	Teratogenic	Phenacetin	Kidney toxicity
Naphthalene	Lung, but covalent binding higher in liver and kidney	**Formation of an acyl glucuronide conjugate**	
Estrogens	Carcinogenicity (breast, liver, endometrial, kidney)	Bromofenac	Hepatotoxicity; withdrawn in 1998; six deaths
Tamoxifen	Endometrial cancer	Benoxaprofen	Hepatotoxicity; withdrawn from market
Raloxifene	Jaundice accompanied by elevated liver enzymes	Ibufenac	Hepatotoxicity; withdrawn from market
Practolol	Skin and eye lesions	Zomepirac	Hepatotoxicity; withdrawn from market
Furan epoxidation, ring opening to yield an aldehyde		**Formation of isocyanate**	
4-Ipomeanol	Lung	Troglitazone	Hepatotoxicity
Furosemide	Teratogenicity	**Formation of imine methide**	
L-739010	Hepatotoxicity in dogs	3-Methylindole	Pneumotoxicity (in ruminant)
Pulegone	Hepatotoxicity	**Miscellaneous**	
L-754394	Bone marrow toxicity in dogs	Halothane	Idiosyncratic hepatoxicity
		Isoniazid	Hepatotoxic in humans following N-acetylation and liberation of acetylhydrazine
Formation of a Michael acceptor			
Valproic acid	Hepatotoxicity	Clozapine	Agranulocytosiss nitrenium ion implicated
		Tienillic acid	Immunogenic, hepatitis

[a]See Ref. 17.

functional groups is presented in Figures 5.2–5.9. It should be recognized that despite the rather extensive literature on the mechanisms by which drugs and other foreign compounds undergo metabolic activation, it is likely that numerous functional groups that have not hitherto been recognized as precursors to reactive intermediates also can undergo bioactivation.

1. *Formation of Quinones and Related Structures.* A common type of reactive metabolite is quinones and related quinone imines and quinone methides. These can be formed by oxidation whenever there are –OH groups para or ortho to one another on an aromatic ring (Fig. 5.2). The quinone imine and quinone methide are formed when one of the –OH groups is replaced by an amino or methylene group, respectively (Fig. 5.2).[18,19] These quniones and related structures can serve as Michael acceptor-like electrophiles.

2. *Reactive Species from Aromatic Amines, Aromatic Nitro Compounds, Hydrazines, and Hydrazides.* Aromatic amines are less

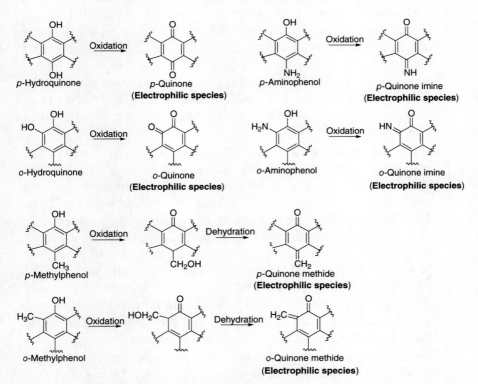

Figure 5.2. Formation of reactive electrophilic species related to quinones and their derivatives.

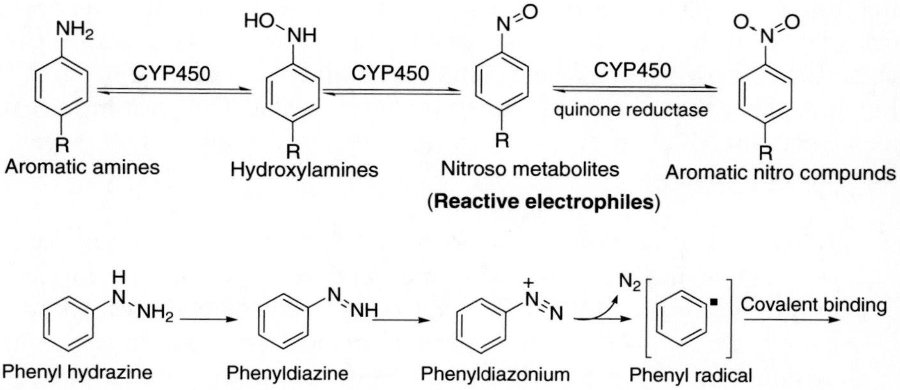

Figure 5.3. Metabolic activation of aromatic amines, nitro compounds, and hydrazines.

commonly present in drugs, but they are usually associated with significant side effects. Aromatic amines are often oxidized to reactive nitroso groups (Fig. 5.3). The same reactive metabolites can also form by reduction of a nitro group (Fig. 5.3).[17,20,21]

Monosubstituted hydrazines are readily oxidized through several steps to reactive intermediates, probably including diazines and possibly diazonium ions (Fig. 5.3).[17,20,21] Loss of molecular nitrogen leads to an alkyl free radical or carbocation. The chemistry is complex and in many cases it is unclear what the identity of the reactive intermediates is. Hydrazides [RC(O)–NHNH$_2$] can be hydrolyzed to hydrazines or they may be directly oxidized to acylonium ions.[17,20,21]

3. *Acyl Glucuronides as Reactive Species.* Some carboxylic acid containing drugs have been implicated in rare but serious adverse reactions. These compounds can be bioactivated via two distinct pathways: by uridine 5′-diphosphate (UDP)-glucuronosyltransferase catalyzed conjugation with glucuronic acid, resulting in the formation of acyl glucuronides, or by acyl-coenzyme A (CoA) synthetase catalyzed formation of acyl-CoA thioesters (Fig. 5.4).[17,22] Conversion of a carboxylic acid to acyl glucornides and/or CoA thioester activates the carboxylic acid and makes acyl transfer possible. It should be recognized that in most cases, acyl glucuronide formation is a common and nontoxic phase-II metabolic pathway for carboxylic acids.

4. *Formation of Epoxides.* Epoxide is a common intermediate in the metabolism of alkenes and aromatic rings (Fig. 5.5) and is a reactive electrophile. If the formed epoxide exists long enough, it can

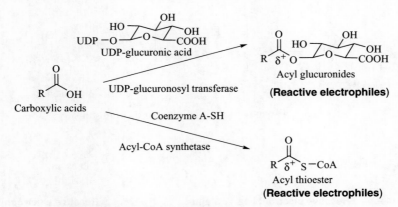

Figure 5.4. Mechanism of carboxylic acid bioactivation.

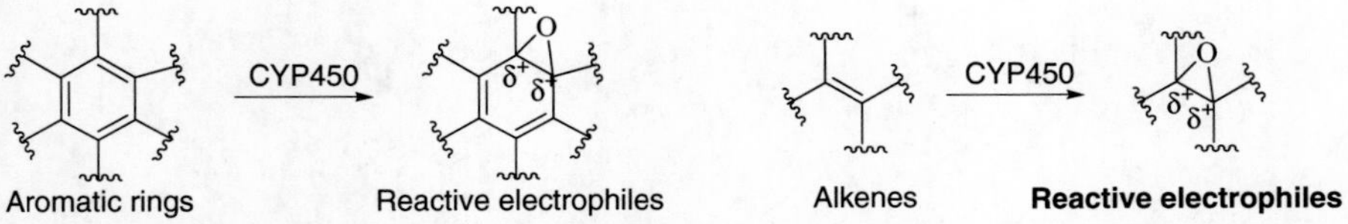

Figure 5.5. Formation of epoxides from aromatic systems or alkenes.

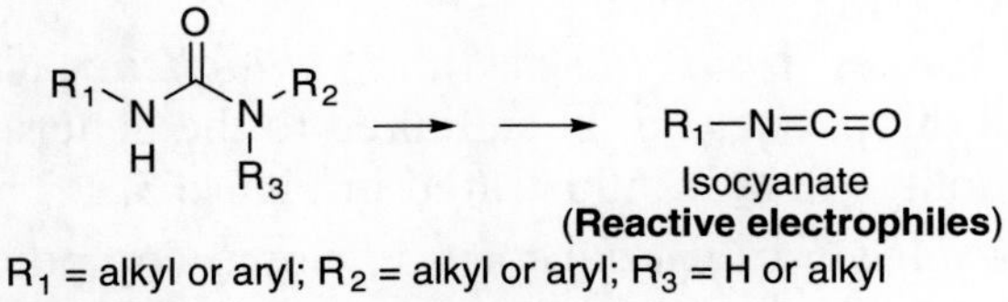

Figure 5.6. Bioactivation of N,N′-substituted ureas.

react with nucleophilic functional groups of biological systems resulting in toxicity.[18]

5. *Formation of Carbamoylating Species.* N,N′-Substituted urea structures can undergo metabolic activation to generate a carbamoylating species. The process has been reported to involve a reactive isocyanate (Fig. 5.6).[17]

6. *Bioactivation of Halogenated Carbons.* The halogenated carbons are known to be bioactivated to reactive species by P450 mediated oxidation reactions. The formed reactive species are usually an acid halide (Fig. 5.7). A representative example is the hepatotoxicity of inhalation anesthetic halothane. Halothane is metabolized to an acid chloride resulting in toxicity.[17,23]

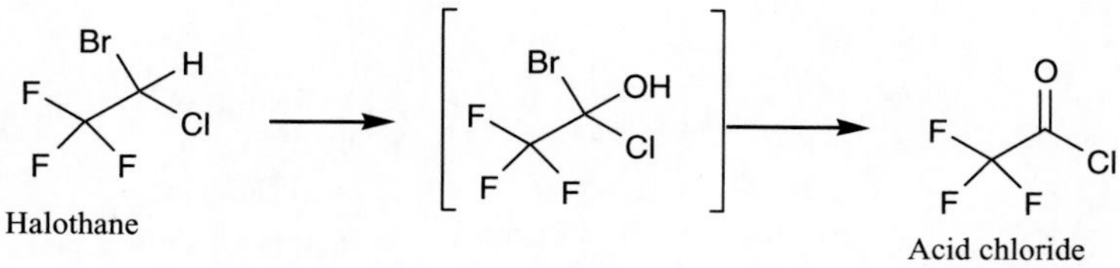

Figure 5.7. Bioactivation of halogenated compounds.

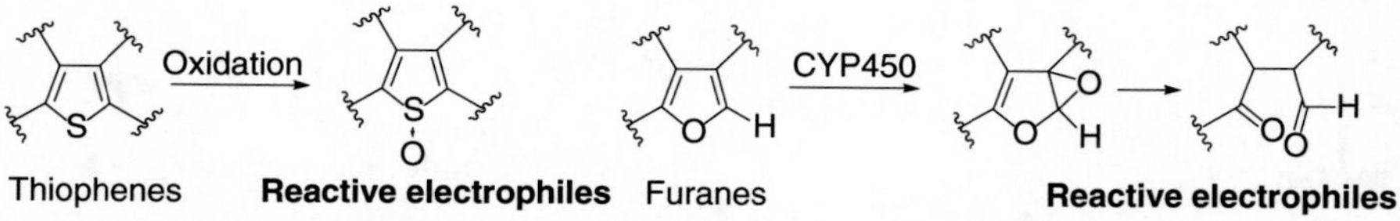

Figure 5.8. Bioactivation of thiophenes and furans.

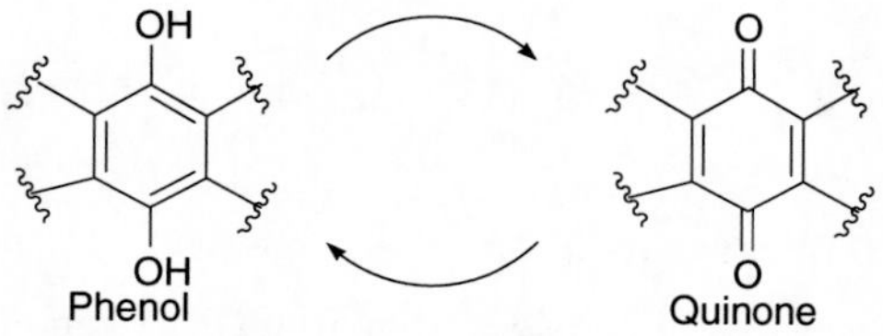

Figure 5.9. Redoxy cycline of quinines.

7. *Reactive Species from Furans and Thiophenes.* Oxidation of furans and thiophenes has been linked to the generation of reactive metabolites that are illustrated in Figure 5.8.[12,13,17]

8. *Redox Cycling and Oxidative Stress.* Some compounds, such as aryl amines and quinones, can also undergo redox cycling that eventually depletes intracellular reducing agents [e.g., glutathione (GSH)] resulting in oxidative stress (Fig. 5.9).[20]

5.3.1.1b   Detection of Reactive Intermediates. Due to the impact of reactive intermediate formation on the drug candidacy of a new chemical entity, detection of reactive metabolites is an important part of drug discovery and development. High-throughput methods to screen for reactive intermediates have been reported[13] and methods for probing the mechanistic aspects of metabolite-mediated toxic reactions using deuterium isotope effects have been developed.[13] In addition, significant advances have also been made in identifying the nature of the protein adducts formed with reactive intermediates.[13] Two major approaches have been adopted in identifying reactive intermediates: use of radiolabeld analogs and use of reactive intermediate trapping agents.

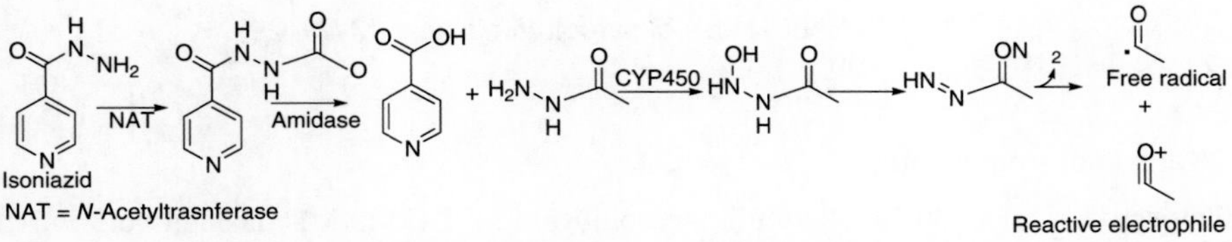

Figure 5.10. Formation of reactive species (free radical and reactive electrophile) from isoniazid.

1. *Use of Radiolabeled Analogs.* An important method for detecting, as well as quantifying, a reactive intermediate is the use of radiolabeling to measure irreversible binding. Radiolabeld analogs of lead candidates can facilitate the assessment of reactive intermediates in rats and human microsomes, hepatocytes, and *in vivo* experiments in rats.[13] Radiolabeling is obviously limited by the availability of the radiolabeled compound and, therefore, is not often used in the initial screen. Another practical issue that needs to be considered is the appropriate location of the radiolabeled atom. This is best exemplified in the case of isoniazid, where, had the primary metabolite acetylisoniazid been labeled in the pyridine moiety, as opposed to the acetyl group, for covalent-binding studies, no radioactivity would have become associated irreversibly with liver proteins (Fig. 5.10).[18,21]

   One challenging issue in assessing protein-reactive intermediate adducts with a radiolabeling technique is variability caused by different experimental conditions. It is imperative that data derived be standardized and comparable in order to conduct an appropriate assessment. To solve this issue, Merck has developed a system to assess radiolabeld protein adducts under standardized conditions for studies involving microsoms, hepatocytes as well *in vivo* experiments in rats.[18]

2. *Use of Reactive Intermediate Trapping Agents.* Formation of reactive intermediates can also be assessed by use of a trapping agent. The most commonly used trapping agent is GSH, which can react with most reactive electrophiles to form glutathione conjugates. Detection of a glutathione conjugate indirectly reflects the formation of a reactive metabolite. Other trapping agents include cyanide anion (CN^-), methoxylamine and semicarbazide.

   Detection of glutathione conjugates can be achieved by liquid chromatography/tandem mass spectrometry (LC/MS/MS) because glutathione conjugates have a characteristic fragment ion

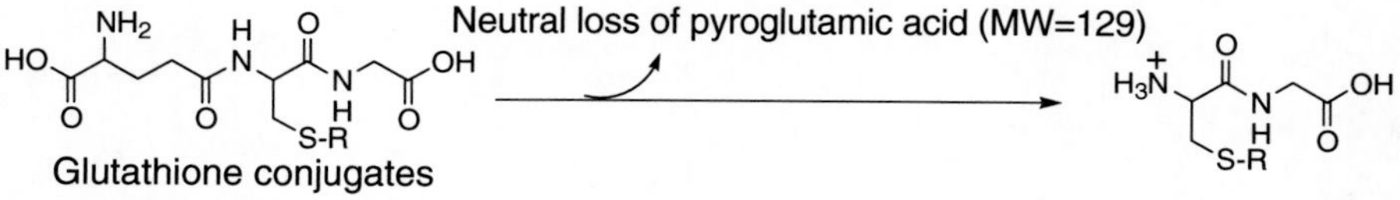

Figure 5.11. Detection of a glutathione conjugate by LC/MS/MS through collision-induced neutral loss of pyroglutamic acid (MW = 129).

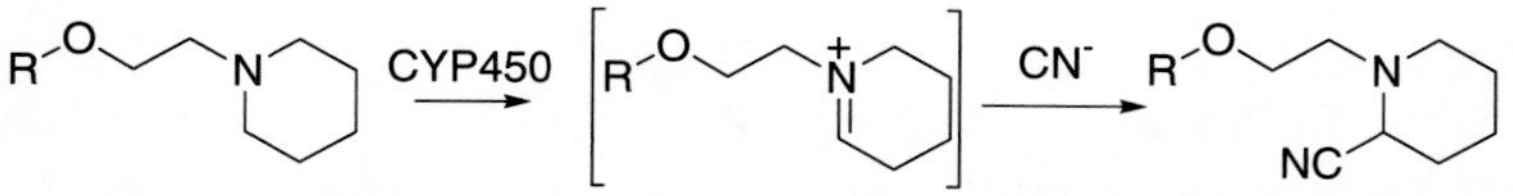

Figure 5.12. Trapping of iminium by cyanide ion (CN⁻).

that can be detected by a neutral loss of 129 resulted from the loss of pyroglutamic acid (Fig. 5.11).[12] Studies of glutathione conjugate formation are best done *in vitro* (e.g., in hepatic microsomes or hepatocytes) because the conjugates are often further metabolized *in vivo*.[15] Typically, *in vitro* experiments are conducted at 0.2–5-mM GSH concentration. Unfortunately, this method does not detect all reactive metabolites, mainly because some of the conjugates are not sufficiently stable, (as in the case of glutathione conjugates derived from acylglucuronides/or CoA esters), or the conjugates react with other nucleophils, usually nitrogen nucleophiles. Further, glutathione conjugates can be converted to cysteine conjugates or mercapturic acids. Therefore, detection of cysteine conjugates or mercapuric acids is an alternative way of revealing the formation of a reactive electrophile.

The cyanide anion (CN⁻) can be used to trap certain electrophilic drug metabolites, for example, iminium (Fig. 5.12). Typically, 1-mM KCN (a mixture of CN and ^{13}C ^{15}N at 1:1 ratio) is used as the trapping agent. The detection of cyano adducts by LC/MS is facilitated by the presence of prominent isotopic "doublets" that differed in mass by 2 (monoadducts) or 4 Da (bisadducts). Furthermore, the MS/MS spectra of these adducts are characterized by a neutral loss of 27–29 Da (HCN/H ^{13}C ^{15}N).[18]

Both methoxylamine and semicarbazide can form Schiff base with an aldehyde (Fig. 5.13), a process mimicking reactions between aldehyde metabolites with lysine residues on proteins. Typical conditions require the addition of 5 mM of either trapping agent to the incubation mixture followed by LC/MS/MS analysis.[18]

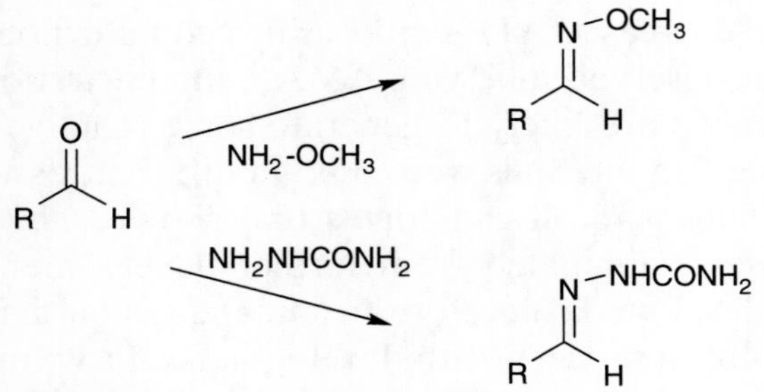

Figure 5.13. Trapping of an aldehyde by methoxylamine (NH_2OCH_3) or semicarbazide ($NH_2NHCONH_2$).

5.3.1.1c Reactive Metabolites and Drug Developability.

Although there is plenty of evidence linking reactive metabolites to toxicity, not all compounds that generate reactive metabolites will cause clinically significant toxicity. There are ample examples of drugs that produce reactive metabolites but are still used as effective and safe therapeutic agents, as demonstrated in Table 5.1. An important factor in determining whether or not a reactive metabolite-generating compound will produce clinically significant toxic effects is dosage. It is generally accepted that drugs producing reactive metabolites might be considered safe if the dose does not exceed 10 mg/day.[11,15] Clozapine and olanzepine serve as good examples to illustrate the importance of dosage in generating toxicity. Clozapine, an antipsychotic drug, is bioactivated to a nitrenium metabolite leading to agranulocytosis while olanzepine, a neuroleptic with a similar structure to clozapine, also exhibits the potential to undergo nitrenium ion formation, has not been associated with a significant incidence of agranulocytosis. The difference in toxicity between the two compounds with a potentially similar mechanism of bioactivation is the maximum daily dose. Olanzepine is given at ~10 mg/day, whereas clozapine is given up to ~900 mg/day.[11] Another factor in determining whether a reactive metabolite would produce clinically significant toxicity obviously is the nature of the biomolecule on which the reactive metabolite affects, which is difficult to identify.[14] Timenstein and Nelson[24] found that although the reactive metabolite of 3'-hydroxyacetanilide (AMAP), a regioisomer of acetaminophen (APAP) produced similar covalent binding compared to the reactive metabolite of acetaminophen, it is not hepatotoxic. The difference was explained by the observation that APAP treated mice displayed decreased plasma membrane calcium–adenosine triphosphate (ATP)ase activity and impaired mitochondrial calcium sequestration characterized by oxidative stress, increased hydrogen peroxide production, and decreased ATP synthesis by cell mitochondria. Similar effects were not observed following AMAP administration.[24]

Most compounds are likely to generate some reactive metabolites. If different screening methods were used in different tissues to screen all drug candidates, and all candidates that showed any evidence of bioactivation were eliminated from further development, few drugs would ever be developed. Therefore, in a final decision-making process on whether or not to proceed with development of a compound, other factors should also be considered, such as the availability of existing treatments, the nature of the disease, the duration of the therapy, the intended population, and the possibility of chemical structural modification to minimize or remove the metabolic pathway leading to the reactive species, and so on.[18]

By considering the potential of a wide array of functional groups that can produce reactive intermediates, it would be impractical for medicinal chemists to avoid the use of reactive metabolite generating functionalities in the design of new chemical entities. Nevertheless, their presence should be considered as a "structural alert" for electrophilic and potentially toxic intermediates.

5.3.2   Issues Related to Drug–Drug Interactions

Drug–drug interactions can be pharmaceutical, pharmacokinetic, or pharmacodynamic. The discussion presented here will be limited to drug–drug interactions related to drug metabolism (pharmacokinetic). It is well recognized that metabolizing enzyme inhibition and induction are serious problems in medication. One of the objectives of drug metabolism studies is to identify the enzyme(s) responsible for the metabolism of the chemical entity, as well as to identify chemical entities that inhibit or induce metabolizing enzymes. Although all metabolizing enzymes are potentially inhibitable and inducible, it is the P450 enzyme system that is the most clinically relevant source of drug–drug interactions.[6,25] Perturbation of CYP450 activities can have profound effects on therapeutic efficacy and in extreme cases may lead to life-threatening toxicities. Among all CYP450 isoforms, five major metabolizing CYPs: CYP1A2, CYP2C9, CYP2C19, CYP2D6, and CYP3A4 isoforms, have been selected for investigation due to their clinical relevance.[8]

5.3.2.1   *Identification of Metabolizing CYP450 Isoforms.* It is important to identify metabolizing enzymes involved in the major metabolic pathways of a chemical entity. The identification helps predicting probable drug–drug interactions. In general, compounds with more

than one metabolic pathway have a lower likelihood of clinically significant drug–drug interactions. A red flag should be raised if a compound is (1) exclusively metabolized by one CYP450 isoform; (2) rapidly metabolized by one CYP450 isoform and; (3) metabolized by polymorphically expressed isoforms (i.e., 2C9, 2C19, and 2D6).[8] Early investigation and identification of the metabolites of a drug candidate related to these potential red flags could help address the issue early at low cost.

In vitro assays designed to identify the particular CYP450 enzyme(s) that mediate the major pathways of metabolism are more likely to be carried out later in the development of promising drug candidates. The identification can be achieved through the use of selective inhibitory antibodies, recombinant CYP isoforms, and specific chemical inhibitors. Correlation with substrates known to be metabolized by specific pathways is considered to be nonselective and less commonly used. These assays can provide valuable information on the potential for variability in drug exposure due to metabolism by polymorphically expressed enzymes, the comparative metabolic fate in preclinical species to that in humans, and as a predictor of clinical interactions due to inhibition or induction of metabolizing enzymes.[8,26]

5.3.2.2 The CYP450 Inhibition and Induction.
Inhibition of CYP450 dependent metabolism is the most frequently encountered form of metabolism-based drug–drug interactions. From among all the CYP450s, CYP3A4 is the most abundant isoform in humans. Agents that are clinically important CYP3A4 inhibitors include ketoconazole, itraconazole, erythromycin, clarithromycin, and nefazodone. These inhibitors can cause marked increases in the plasma concentrations of drugs that are CYP3A4 substrates. For example, ketoconazole has been shown to produce 16-, 22-, and 73-fold increases in serum concentrations of midazolam,[27] triazolam,[28] and terfenadine,[29] respectively. When the antihistamine drug terfenadine was administered simultaneously with ketoconazole, the combination produced serious and, in some cases, fatal cardiac arrhythmias.[30] Inhibitory drug–drug interactions have led to issues with many marketed drugs and the withdrawal of some.[31] Therefore, screening for inhibition should be an essential part of the discovery process.

The CYP450 inhibition studies have typically been conducted using liver microsomes from humans and various other animal species as well as recombinant CYP450 with analysis of samples using high-performance liquid chromatography (HPLC) with ultraviolet (UV), fluorescence, or mass spectrometry detection. The methods and theory are discussed in more details in Chapter 4.

An issue related to CYP450 inhibition screening is whether the observed inhibition is direct (reversible or irreversible), metabolism-based (reversible), or mechanism-based (metabolism-based irreversible).[6] Metabolism–mechanism-based inhibition increases with time while direct inhibition is constant or decreases with time so they can be distinguished experimentally in a high-throughput mode by determining the apparent IC_{50} of the test compound toward a standard substrate with or without a preincubation period of the enzyme with the test compound. A large decrease in the apparent IC_{50} after preincubation is evidence of metabolism–mechanism-based inhibition. Typically, a compound is classified as a potent inhibitor if the IC_{50} is <1 μM.[6]

Hepatic enzyme induction may be viewed as a general homeostatic adaptive mechanism whereby an organism responds to exposure to potentially harmful chemicals via upregulation of detoxifying enzymes, which may be specific (CYP) proteins (monofunctional inducers) or a combination of CYP450 and detoxifying phase-II enzymes (multifunctional inducers). There is a general consensus that drug–drug interactions arising through enzyme induction have less of a clinical impact compared to enzyme inhibition.[6,32] However, CYP3A4 inducers, such as rifampicin and rifabutin, can reduce plasma concentrations of certain drugs up to 40-fold, effectively abolishing their efficacy.[33,34] Induction of CYP3A4 can also produce enhanced metabolic activation of substrates catalyzed by this P450, resulting in toxicity. For example, autoinduction of CYP3A4 by troglitazone produces enhanced bioactivation and toxicity in HepG2 cells and human hepatocytes.[35,36] In clinical studies, troglitazone was implicated in severe and fatal hepatotoxicity in patients receiving this antidiabetic in the absence of other therapeutics.[37,38] Thus, screening new drugs for their ability to induce CYP enzymes should be considered as important as identifying inhibitors of metabolizing enzymes.[39] Early screening and investigation of these potentially unwanted properties of chemical entities with metabolism information, such as metabolite and/or reactive metabolite search and identification can help decision making.

5.3.3 Issues Related to Pharmacokinetic Properties

Two important PK parameters: oral bioavailability and half-life, which define the pharmacological and toxicological profile of drugs as well as patient compliance, are affected by drug metabolism. Although a number of other factors, such as drug solubility, dissolution, drug efflux pumps, transporters, physiological conditions of the gastrointestinal

(GI) system, and so on, can affect oral bioavailability, drug metabolism in the liver and GI system is, in most cases, the major determinant. Conceivably, a drug that is quickly metabolized would exhibit low oral bioavailability and a short half-life. On the other hand, it should also be recognized, that a chemical entity that does not undergo quick metabolism may not necessarily exhibit a long half-life. This finding is especially true for a hydrophilic compound that experiences extensive renal filtration. Another conceivable impact of drug metabolism on oral bioavailability and half-life is related to inhibition and induction of drug metabolizing enzymes, which can affect the half-life of the drug itself or other drugs. Therefore, prediction of pharmacokinetic parameters from *in vivo* animal, *in vitro* cellular–subcellular, and computational systems in their early stages would help to assess their developability as drug candidates. Metabolic stability studies represent some of the earliest *in vitro* studies used in the pharmaceutical industry in an effort to predict *in vivo* PK parameters. In retrospective studies however, quantitative predictions of *in vivo* clearance from *in vitro* metabolism data for many compounds, have been shown to be poor. Several excellent reviews have been published describing the *in vitro* methods and their application in early screening.[40]

5.4 BASIC TECHNIQUES FOR DRUG METABOLISM STUDIES IN DRUG DISCOVERY

Metabolism studies in the drug development stage have been well established. However, metabolism studies in drug discovery, especially in their early stages, are still evolving. One of the challenges is how to meet the high-throughput demand of drug discovery.[5,6,40] With major advances in combinatorial library production and increased automation in chemical synthesis and purification, the number of high-quality compounds generated by medicinal chemists has far surpassed the capacity for traditional drug metabolism studies.[8] The limited throughput of drug metabolism study does not enable every compound to be evaluated. Consequently, as indicated in Figure 5.1, *in silico* drug metabolism studies play a significant role especially in the hit generation, lead identification and optimization stages. Experimental metabolism studies in the early drug discovery stage primarily involve *in vitro* studies. Integration of *in silico* and experimental metabolism studies in a complementary and synergistic manner is crucial to the decision-making process. Due to page limitation, this chapter will not cover techniques employed for metabolite identification, characterization, and quantification. Readers are referred to other sources for these topics.[41–50] The main focus of the following will be on biological systems and *in silico* methods employed in drug metabolism studies in the drug discovery phase.

5.4.1   *In Vitro* Biological Systems

Various biological systems have been developed to examine the metabolic stability,[6] enzyme induction and inhibition,[5,6,8] and toxicity[8] of compounds. These systems include tissue slices, hepatocyte cultures, and subcellular fractions.

As always, each biological system has its advantages and disadvantages. The most commonly employed biological system is liver microsomes due to its simplicity and suitability to high-throughput screening.[6] However, hepatic microsomes may not always be appropriate for metabolism screening if cytosolic or other nonmicrosomal enzymes are important in the clearance of the compound.[6] Hepatocyte cultures, on the other hand, provide the complete range of enzymes operating in the cell, including conjugating enzymes, esterases, and the amidases in addition to the CYP enzymes. Cofactor supplies should also resemble the *in vivo* situation instead of adding unphysiologically high amounts, which is the case in microsomal incubations. The substances also have to cross the membrane as *in vivo*. The role of plasma protein binding, which is not dealt with when using subcellular systems, may also be solved by incubating liver cells in serum.[40] Recently, several laboratories have described cryopreserved hepatocytes.[40] The use of cryopreserved material considerably improves flexibility and access to the systems, especially since cryopreserved hepatocytes are now offered by several commercial companies. It is obvious that whole cell systems should be more reliable for predicting *in vivo* metabolic clearance than subcellular systems.[40]

Although cells offer technical simplicity and thus higher throughput, they may lack physiologic characteristics of the organ cell types. Primary cultures and tissue slices have been employed in order to have a better representation of the cell characteristics *in vivo*. Because these systems require animals to derive cultures and can be more technically demanding than continuous cell lines, these models are used most often for mechanistic research or comparing a small number of lead compounds. Primary cultures and slices can be obtained from a variety of species including mouse, rat, rabbit, pig, dog, monkey, and humans. This provides the opportunity to assess species differences. Despite the large number of variables that come into play with these systems, they have proven to be valuable tools in early screening programs.[51] However, tissue slices have not been characterized to the same extent as microsomes and hepatocyte suspensions. Poor diffusion of substrate to the inner layer of the tissue slice has been discussed and associated with lower clearance values than from microsomes or hepatocyte suspensions.[40]

Another biological system, which has been adopted in a high-throughput manner, is recombinant human CYP450.[6] This system offers the possibility to mix exact proportions of enzymes or incubate with single enzymes. This can be advantageous over liver microsomes, especially when studying human metabolism, because of the great variations in enzyme levels in human liver microsomes. However, the major disadvantage is that the studies are restricted to the enzymes available. There is also concern that we might not reproduce the coenzyme requirement for the different isoenzymes of CYP450 and for different test compounds, as this has been shown to be important for some CYPs (e.g., CYP1A2 and 3A4) and for some compounds.[40] In drug discovery, studies using expressed enzymes are mainly used to identify enzymes responsible for the metabolism of drug candidates.[40]

5.4.2 *In Silico* ADME–Tox Models

Computational models are widely available for predicting ADME–Tox properties.[52,53] The followings are sources that provide software to predict ADME–Tox properties: http://www.accelrys.com (Cerius^{2TM} ADME, http://www.bio-rad.com (knowItAll^{TM}), http://www.compudrug.com (MetabolExpert^{TM}), http://www.multicase.com (META^{TM}), http://www.genego.com (MetaDrug^{TM}), http://www.compudrug.com (Hazard Expert^{TM}), http://www.leadscope.com (LeadScope^{TM}), MultiCase^{TM}, and http://www.multicase.com (MultiCase^{TM}).

5.5 CONTRIBUTION OF DRUG METABOLISM TO RATIONAL STRUCTURAL MODIFICATION OF DRUG CANDIDATES

It is conceivable that information related to metabolic stability, reactive intermediates, inhibition, and induction of metabolizing enzymes can serve as a valuable guidance to medicinal chemists in the selection and structural modification of drug candidates.[54] Structural modifications can be made to change metabolic stability (blocking, accelerating, or switching metabolic pathways) to produce compounds with better developability. In addition, although in most cases metabolism of drugs leads to pharmacological inactivation, there are plenty of cases where a metabolite exhibits a better "drug-like" property than the parent compound and eventually is developed into a marketable drug or served as a new lead.[55] Presented below are a few examples highlighting the guiding role of drug metabolism in drug discovery.

5.5.1 Blocking a Metabolic Pathway

Extensive metabolism is generally considered a liability as it limits the systemic exposure and shortens the half-life of a compound. Several strategies, such as reduction of lipophilicity to reduce its affinity for CYP enzymes, modification, and/or blocking of metabolically soft spots, have been developed to combat metabolism. Among these, modification and/or blocking metabolically soft spots with a metabolic resistant structure are the most commonly adopted practices.

Metoprolol (Fig. 5.14) is a cardioselective beta-adrenoceptor antagonist. The *p*-methoxylethyl substituent is a major site of metabolism resulting in a low bioavailability (38%) and a short half-life (3.2h). Replacement of the methyl with a cyclopropyl group sterically hinders the metabolism. The resulting betaxolol exhibits an excellent oral bioavailability (96%) and a longer half-life.[54]

The nitro group of chloramphenicol (Fig. 5.14) was thought by many to be responsible for the aplastic anemia associated with the drug. This led to the replacement of the nitro group with a methyl sulfone group in thiamphenicol, a drug that has similar antibacterial activities to that of chloramphenicol. Although this drug was first believed to be safe, it

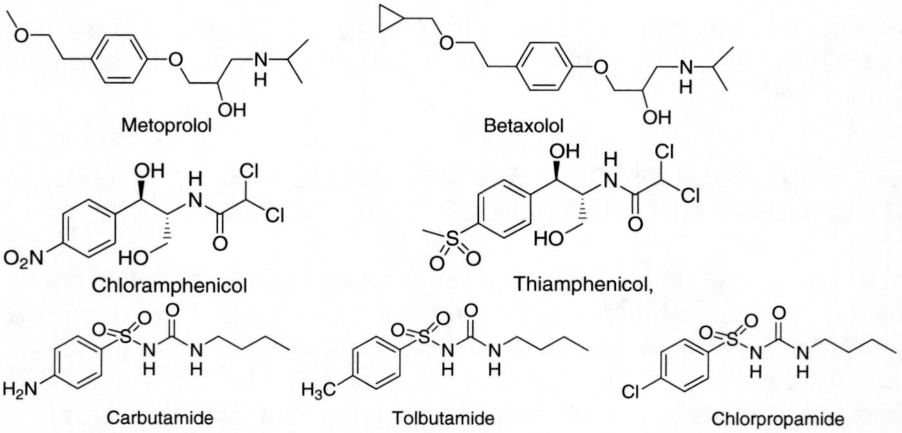

Figure 5.14. Structures of metabolic labile and resistant compounds discussed in this section.

now appears that it may also cause aplastic anemia, which might be caused by the dichloroacetamide present in both drugs.[54]

Carbutamide (Fig. 5.14) was the first clinically useful sulfonylurea for the treatment of diabetics. This compound was found to cause adverse effects on the bone marrow due to the aromatic amine structure. Replacement of the amino group with a methyl led to tolbutamide, which maintained the hypoglycemic activities, but had no side effect to bone marrow. However, tolbutamide exhibits a moderate half-life (7 h) due to the metabolism of the metabolically labile benzylic methyl group. To improve its metabolic stability, the benzylic methyl group was replaced by a chloro group. The resulting chlorpropamide significantly increases its half-life (36 h).

5.5.2 Accelerating Metabolism

In case a chemical entity exhibits a half-life that is too long, structural modification can be made to shorten the half-life through incorporation of a metabolically labile functional group (e.g., a sterically easily accessible benzylic methyl group or an ester group). Such structural modification is exemplified by the initial structural lead for celecoxib. The initial lead exhibited half-lives (in male rats) up to 220 h (Fig. 5.15). To reduce the long half-life, a benzylic methyl group, which is a metabolically labile functional group, was employed to replace the metabolically resistant fluoro group. The resulting compound celecoxib had a half-life in rats of 3.5 h.[54]

5.5.3 Metabolic Switching

Structural modification can also be made to achieve the objective of switching away from an undesired metabolic pathway by incorporating a more metabolically labile function group. Ticlopidine (Ticlid) is an antithrombotic agent (Fig. 5.16). Its clinical use has been limited by a 1–2% incidence of agranulocytosis and several reports of aplastic anemia. Ticlopidine has been reported to generate a GSH adduct of

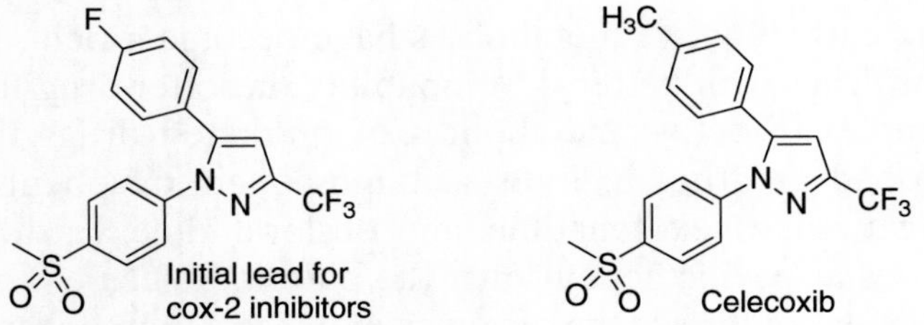

Figure 5.15. Structures of celecoxib and its initial lead.

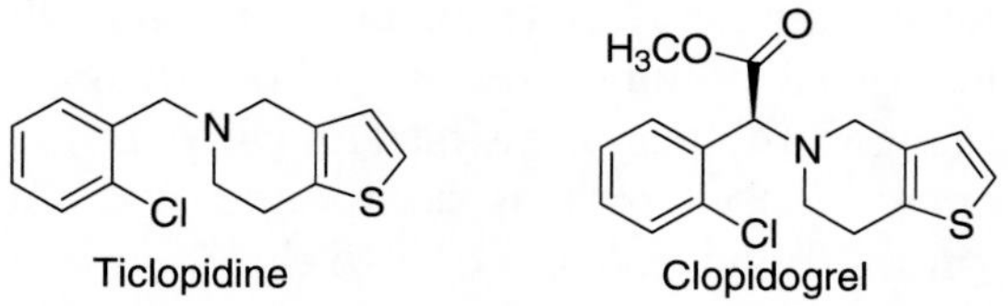

Figure 5.16. Structures of ticlopidine and clopidogrel.

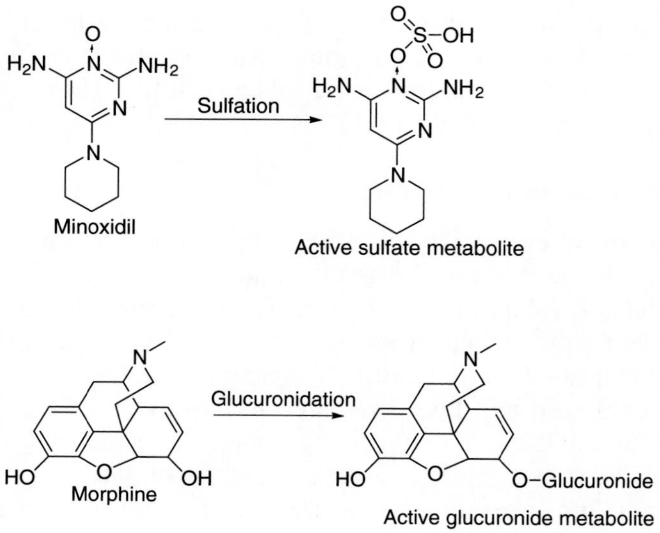

Figure 5.17. Representative examples of active metabolites generated from phase-II metabolism.

the thiophene moiety in activated neutrophils *in vitro*. Incorporation of a methyl ester into the structure switches the metabolic pathway to methyl ester cleavage. The resulting clopidogrel (Fig. 5.16) does not have comparable toxicity as ticlopidine.[13]

5.5.4   Active Metabolites

As indicated earlier, active metabolites have become a rich source for new leads or drugs with better developability or better drug-like properties. Examples of active metabolites of marketed drugs that have been developed as drugs include acetaminophen, oxyphenbutazone, oxazepam, cetirizine, fexofenadine, and desloratadine. Each of these drugs provides a specific benefit over the parent molecule.[55] Although most active metabolites are the products of phase-I metabolism, phase-II metabolism can also yield active metabolites (Fig. 5.17).[55]

5.6 CONCLUSIONS

Integration of drug metabolism studies into the drug discovery phase reflects the effort of the pharmaceutical industry to terminate "undesirable" drug candidates at the early stage to reduce attrition rates in the late and costly development stage. One of the challenges of this effort is to develop high-throughput assays to meet the demand of the explosive number of new hits and leads generated from various high-throughput technologies. Due to the fact that the evaluation of compounds in early discovery is not likely to require the details and depth of data provided by traditional drug metabolism studies, *in silico* studies play a significant role in the early screening of hits and leads for its high speed. A proper use of experimental and computational technologies in drug discovery will help the decision-making process in candidate evaluation. Decision-making is a complex process, which needs to take into consideration factors other than PK properties. One should also keep in mind that a number of currently marketed drugs might not have been developed if current candidate selection standards were used. The example provided by Smith et al.[54] illustrate this scenario. Omeprazole, a prototype proton-pump inhibitor and one of the world's best selling drugs, is acid labile and has a short PK half-life and variable PKs due to metabolism by the polymorphically expressed CYP2C19. Omeprazole never would have been discovered in today's modern paradigm based on its "undesirable" PK features.

Another advantage of integrating drug metabolism into drug discovery is its guiding role in aiding medicinal chemists to conduct rational structural modification to improve PK properties. It is strongly believed that with a close working relationship between medicinal chemists and drug metabolism research scientists, not only undesirable drug candidates can be dropped in the early enough stage to reduce cost but also the structural modifications would be conducted in a more rational and effective fashion.

REFERENCES

1. DiMasi, J. A.; Hansen, R. W.; Grabowski, H. G. *J. Health Econ.* **2003**, 22, 151–185.
2. Frank, R. G. *J. Health Econ.* **2003**, 22, 325–330.
3. Kassel, D. B. *Curr. Opin. Chem. Biol.* **2004**, 8, 339–345.
4. Nassar, A. E.; Talaat, R. E. *Drug Discov. Today.* **2004**, 9, 317–327.

5. Caldwell, G. W.; Ritchie, D. M.; Masucci, J. A.; Hageman, W.; Van, Z. *Curr. Top. Med. Chem.* **2001**, 1, 353–366.

6. Roberts, S. A. *Xenobiotica.* **2001**, 31, 557–589.

7. Yu, H.; Adedovin, A. *Drug Discov. Today.* **2003**, 8, 852–861.

8. Lin, J.; Sahakian, D. C.; de Morais, S. M.; Xu, J. J.; Polzer, R. J.; Winter, S. M. *Curr. Top. Med. Chem.* **2003**, 3, 1125–1154.

9. Ashworth, L. *Home Care Provid.* **1997**, 2, 117–120.

10. Sooriakumaran, P. *Postgrad. Med. J.* **2006**, 82, 242–245.

11. Williams, D. P.; Park, B. K. *Drug Discov. Today.* **2003**, 8, 1044–1050.

12. Bailie, T. A.; Kassahun, K. *Adv. Exp. Med. Biol.* **2001**, 500, 45–51.

13. Evan, D. C.; Bailie, T. A. *Curr. Opin. Drug Discov. Devel.* **2005**, 8, 44–50.

14. Uetrech, J. P. *Curr. Drug Metab.* **2000**, 1, 133–141.

15. Uetrecht, J. *Drug Discov. Today.* **2003**, 8, 832–837.

16. Uetrecht, J. Bioactivation. in Lee, J. S.; Obach, S.; Fisher, M. B. Eds. *Drug Metabolizing Enzymes.* **2003**, 87–145; Lausanne. Fontis Media. Switzerland.

17. Evans, D. C.; Watt, A. P.; Nicoll-Griffith, D. A.; Baillie, T. A. *Chem. Res. Toxicol.* **2004**, 17, 3–16.

18. Kalgutkar, A. S.; Gardner, I.; Obach, R. S.; Shaffer, C. L.; Callegari, E.; Henne, K. R.; Mutlib, A. E.; Dalvie, D. K.; Lee, J. S.; Nakai, Y.; O'Donnell, J. P.; Boer, J.; Harriman, S. P. *Curr. Drug Metab.* **2005**, 6, 161–225.

19. Monk, T. J.; Jones, D. C. *Curr. Drug. Metab.* **2002**, 3, 425–438.

20. Uetrech, J. N. *Drug Metab. Rev.* **2002**, 34, 651–665.

21. Kalgutkar, A. S.; Dalvie, D. K.; O'Donnell, J. P.; Taylor, T. J.; Sahakian, D. C. *Curr. Drug Metab.* **2002**, 3, 379–424.

22. Sidenius, U.; Skonberg, C.; Olsen, J.; Hansen, S. H. *Chem. Res. Toxicol.* **2004**, 17, 75–81.

23. Satoh, H.; Martin, B. M.; Schulick, A. H.; Christ, D. D.; Kenna J. G.; Pohl, L. R. *Proc. Nat. Acad. Sci. USA.* **1989**, 86, 322–326.

24. Tirmenstein, M. A.; Nelson, S. D. *J. Biol. Chem.* **1989**, 264, 9814–9819.

25. Weaver, R. J. *Xenobiotica.* **2001**, 31, 499–538.

26. Baipai, M.; Esmay, J. D. *Drug Metab. Rev.* **2002**, 34, 679–689.

27. Tsunoda, S. M.; Velez, R. L.; von Moltke, L. L.; Greenblatt, D. J. *Clin. Pharmacol. Ther.* **1999**, 66, 461–471.

28. Varhe, A.; Olkkola, K. T.; Neuvonen, P. J. *Clin. Pharmacol. Ther.* **1994**, 56, 601–607.

29. Honig, P. K.; Worham, D. C.; Zamani, K.; Conner, D. P.; Mullin, J. C.; Cantilena, L. R. *J. Am. Med. Assoc.* **1993**, 269, 1513–1518.

30. Wilkinson, G. R. *J. Pharmacokinet. Biopharm.* **1996**, 24, 475–490.

31. Mullins, M. E.; Horowitz, B. Z.; Linden, D. H.; Smith, G. W.; Norton, R. L.; Stump, J. *J. Am. Med. Assoc.* **1998**, 280, 157–158.

32. Worboys, P. D.; Carlile, D. J. *Xenobiotica.* **2001**, 1, 539–556.

33. Gillum, J. G.; Israel, D. S.; Polk, R. E. *Clin. Pharmacokinet.* **1993**, 25, 450–482.

34. Grange, J. M.; Winstanley, P. A.; Davies, P. D. *Drug Safety.* **1994**, 11, 242–251.

35. Kostrubsky, V. E.; Sinclair, J. F.; Ramachandran, V.; Venkataramanan, R.; Wen, Y. H.; Kindt, E.; Galchev, V.; Rose, K.; Sinz, M.; Strom, S. C. *Drug Metab. Dispos.* **2000**, 28, 1192–1197.

36. Tettey, J. N.; Maggs, J. L.; Rapeport, W. G.; Pirmohamed, M.; Park, B. K. *Chem. Res. Toxicol.* **2001**, 14, 965–974.

37. Gitline, N.; Julie, N. L.; Spurr, C. L.; Lim, K. N.; Juarbe, H. M. *Ann. Intern. Med.* **1998**, 129, 36–38.

38. Herrine, S. K.; Choudhary, C. *Ann. Intern. Med.* **1999**, 130, 163–164.

39. Dayna, C.; Mankowski, A.; Sean Ekins, B. *Curr. Drug Metab.* **2003**, 4, 381–391.

40. Masimirembwa, C. M.; Bredberg, U.; Andersson, T. B. *Clin. Pharmacokinet.* **2003**, 42, 515–528.

41. Clarke, N. J.; Rindgen, D.; Korfmacher, W. A.; Cox, K. A. *Anal. Chem.* **2001**, 73, 430A–439A.

42. Pochapsky, S. S.; Pochapsky, T. C. *Curr. Top. Med. Chem.* **2001**, 1, 427–441.

43. Watt, A. P.; Mortishire-Smith, R. J.; Gerhard, U.; Thomas, S. R. *Curr. Opin. Drug. Discov. Devel.* **2003**, 6, 57–65.

44. King, R.; Fernandez-Metzler, C. *Curr. Drug Metab.* **2006**, 7, 541–545.

45. Ma, S.; Chowdhury, S. K.; Alton, K. B. *Curr. Drug Metab.* **2006**, 7, 503–523.

46. Jemal, M.; Xia, Y. Q. *Curr. Drug Metab.* **2006**, 7, 491–450.

47. Hsieh, Y.; Korfmacher, W. A. *Curr. Drug Metab.* **2006**, 7, 479–489.

48. Yang, Z. *J Pharm. Biomed. Anal.* **2006**, 40, 516–527.

49. Liu, D. Q.; Hop, C. E. *J. Pharm. Biomed. Anal.* **2005**, 37, 1–18.

50. Hop, C. E. *Curr. Drug Metab.* **2006**, 7, 557–563.

51. Johnson, D. E.; Wolfgang, G. H. *Curr. Top. Med. Chem.* **2001**, 1, 233–245.

52. Ekins, S.; Nikolsky, Y.; Nikolskaya, T. *Trends Pharmacol. Sci.* **2005**, 26, 202–209.

53. Kulkami, S. A.; Zhu, J.; Blechinger, S. *Xenobiotica.* **2005**, 35, 955–973.

54. Smith, D.; Schmid, E.; Jones, B. *Clin. Pharmacokinet.* **2002**, 41, 1005–1019.

55. Fura, A.; Shu, Y. Z.; Zhu, M.; Hanson, R. L.; Roongta, V.; Humphreys, W. G. *J. Med. Chem.* **2004**, 47, 4339–4351.

CHAPTER 6

PROTEIN BINDING IN DRUG DISCOVERY AND DEVELOPMENT

VIKRAM RAMANATHAN and NIMISH VACHHARAJANI
Drug Metabolism and Pharmacokinetics and Clinical Pharmacology,
Advinus Therapeutics Pvt. Ltd., Bangalore, India

Evaluation of Drug Candidates for Preclinical Development: Pharmacokinetics, Metabolism, Pharmaceutics, and Toxicology, Edited by Chao Han, Charles B. Davis, and Binghe Wang
Copyright © 2010 John Wiley & Sons, Inc.

6.1   INTRODUCTION

It is generally believed that only unbound or free-drug mediates efficacy and toxicity[1] (Fig. 6.1). Most drugs, with a few exceptions (e.g., anticoagulant heparin), exert their effects in tissues not within plasma. Direct measurement of drug concentrations at receptor sites is seldom possible due to inaccessibility of tissues. For this reason, pharmacokinetics (PKs) of drugs is characterized by measuring drug concentration in plasma; consequently, protein-binding measurements are typically performed in the plasma. While the relevance of free-drug levels to drug effect is well accepted, it is important to understand the circumstances under which protein binding affects drug dispositional characteristics sufficiently to be clinically relevant. For example, it is generally perceived that higher protein binding could result in slower elimination

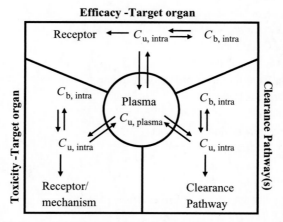

Figure 6.1. Free-drug hypothesis: Free-drug crosses membranes, mediates efficacy and toxicity, and is cleared. Drug exists in both bound and unbound forms in all tissues including plasma. Unbound drug levels in plasma are assumed too equilibrate with intracellular levels in tissue. The binding process can exhibit nonlinearity. Experimental determinations of plasma–protein binding are typically made across a therapeutic–toxicologically relevant concentration range to provide mechanistic explanations for the results. The parameters C_u and C_b are concentrations of unbound and bound drug, respectively; subscript intra refers to intracellular.

of a drug. This is, however, an oversimplification and in many cases other factors can predominate. Similarly, displacement of protein-bound drug has previously been implicated as a mechanism for various clinical drug–drug and disease–drug interactions; however, only in a few instances does it affect PKs sufficiently to become pharmacologically relevant.

In this chapter, the theoretical basis for drug–protein binding and its effects on PK parameters are described. Various experimental methodologies to measure protein binding are presented along with practical considerations, with a view to enable the reader to judiciously select an appropriate approach depending on the stage of drug development. Finally, examples of the effects of protein binding in drug discovery and development are provided. As described in earlier chapters, one of the key factors for early termination of drugs from development is inadequate PK characteristics. We hope that the information provided here will enable a nonpharmacokineticist to better appreciate the role and implications (or lack thereof) of protein binding.

6.2 THEORETICAL CONSIDERATIONS

The unbound (f_u) or bound fraction (f_b; $f_b = 1 - f_u$) are the commonly determined experimental measures of plasma protein binding and are typically expressed as a percentage:

$$\% f_u = 100 \times C_u / C_{total} \tag{6.1}$$

$$\% f_b = 100 \times C_b / C_{total} \tag{6.2}$$

where C_u, C_b, and C_{total} are concentrations of unbound, bound, and total drug in plasma, respectively. The reversible equilibrium between a protein and binding drug obeys the law of mass action and can be written as:

$$[D]+[P] \underset{k_{-1}}{\overset{k_1}{\rightleftharpoons}} [DP] \tag{6.3}$$

where [D], [P], and [DP] are the molar concentrations of the unbound drug, unoccupied protein, and the drug–protein complex, respectively, and k_1 and k_{-1} are the rate constants for association and dissociation. The thermodynamic binding affinity constant (K_A) for the equilibrium is thus given by

$$K_A = \frac{[DP]}{[D][P]} = \frac{k_1}{k_{-1}} \tag{6.4}$$

The dissociation constant K_D is simply the inverse of the affinity constant, or $1/K_A$.

The unbound fraction, f_u, is an equilibrium or thermodynamic measurement that is inversely proportional to the binding affinity (K_A) as shown below:

$$f_u = \frac{C_u}{C_{total}} = \frac{[D]}{[D]+[DP]} = \frac{1}{1+K_A[P]} \tag{6.5}$$

Equation 6.5 shows (1) that f_u reflects the binding affinity and (2) when the molar concentrations of the drug and binding protein are similar, a decrease in concentration of the protein (e.g., due to disease) results in an increase in the free fraction of the drug. Equation 6.5 assumes the simple case of a single site in the binding protein; albumin has several binding sites and more complex derivations have been described for these cases. For some compounds, the equilibrium binding value of f_u does not predict *in vivo* efficacy and PKs in a manner consistent with the free-drug hypothesis. Therefore recently there has been a renewed interest in kinetics of drug–protein binding (in particular the off-rate k_{-1}; discussed in Sections 6.4.2, 6.4.3, and 6.5.5).

6.3   MAJOR PLASMA-BINDING PROTEINS

Plasma contains >60 different soluble proteins. Among these, the major proteins that bind drug are albumin, alpha-1 acid glycoprotein (AAG), and to a smaller extent lipoproteins.[2] Although albumin and AAG can both bind acidic and basic drugs, albumin generally binds acidic drugs better while AAG preferentially binds to basic drugs. Table 6.1 summarizes the major circulating plasma proteins relevant to drug development.

6.3.1   Albumin

Albumin is a heart-shaped protein[16] of 585 amino acids. It is the most abundant plasma protein and accounts for >50% of the total plasma proteins.[4] Structurally, albumin has three homologous domains, each comprising subdomains (A and B) with common structural elements.

TABLE 6.1. Major Plasma Proteins that Bind Drugs

	Albumin[a]	Alpha-1 Acid Glycoprotein[b]	Lipoprotein[c]
Molecular mass (Da)	67,000	38,000–48,000	200,000–2,400,000
Normal circulating plasma concentration	35–50 mg/mL (500–700 μM)	0.4–1 mg/mL (12–31 μM)	Variable (<5 mg/mL)
Plasma half-life	19 day[d]	5 days[e]	
Site of biosynthesis	Hepatocytes	Liver parenchymal cells, hepatocytes, granulocytes, monocytes	Intestine, liver
Attributes of ligands	Acidic, basic	Weak bases	Neutral, lipophilic
Prototype ligands	Warfarin Diazepam Ibuprofen Nonesterified fatty acids Bilirubin Thyroxine	Propranolol Saquinivir Ritonivir Nelfinavir Imatinib	Amphotericin B Cyclosporin Halofantrine Nicardipine Propofol Quinidine Tacrolimus
Biochemical–structural features	No carbohydrate; 17 disulfide bonds rich in Lys, Arg, Glu, Asp; Size: 80 × 30 Å	$pK_a = 2.7$ 59% protein 41% carbohydrate	Nonpolar lipid core surrounded by surface amphipathic lipids and protein
Chromosomal location	4q11-13	9q31-34.1	
Genetic variants	Lys372Glu[f] Asp550Gly[f] Glu501Lys[g] Lys573Glu[h]		

[a]References 2–6.
[b]References 2, 4, and 6–9.
[c]References 2, 6, 7, and 10.
[d]Reference 5.
[e]References 11 and 12.
[f]Reference 13.
[g]Reference 14.
[h]Reference 15.

Early work by Sudlow et al.[17] identified two primary drug binding sites in albumin: the first in subdomain IIA for warfarin, sulfonamides, phenytoin, valproic acid, and phenylbutazone, and a second in subdomain IIIA (benzodiazepine site) for penicillins and probenecid. Recently, Curry and co-workers[16,18,19] have elucidated crystal structures of human serum albumin (HSA) bound to 17 ligands including diazepam, indomethacin, warfarin, phenylbutazone, and fatty acids. Their work has identified key residues involved in binding; moreover, it shows that the two primary sites are highly adaptable, and that there are several secondary binding sites across the protein (Fig. 6.2). In a study of 14 structurally diverse compounds,[20] ionization and lipophilicity were major determinants of binding to bovine albumin; in this study, acids bound more strongly than neutral compounds, which in turn bound more strongly than bases.

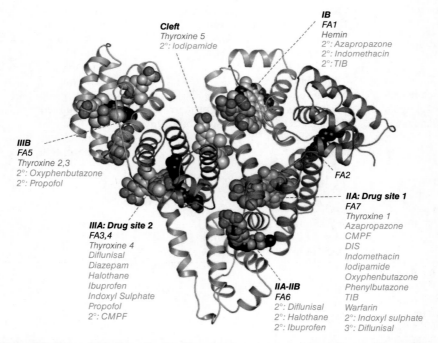

Figure 6.2. Ligand binding sites in albumin: A summary of crystallographic studies of ligand-binding capacity of albumin is depicted. Ligands are shown in space-filling representation. Oxygen atoms are colored red in all cases; other atoms in fatty acid (myristic acid), endogenous ligands (hemin, thyroxin), and drugs are colored dark gray, light gray, and orange, respectively. [From Ghuman, J, Zunszain, P.A., Petitpas, I., Bhattacharya, A.A., Otagiri, M. and Curry, S. Structural basis of the drug-binding specificity of human serum albumin. *J. Mol. Biol.*, 353: 38–52, **2005**. Reproduced with permission from S. Curry and the copyright holder Ref. 16.]

Despite the ability of HSA to accommodate structurally diverse ligands in its binding site, human HSA polymorphisms,[15,21,22] as well as binding differences between species, suggest that subtle differences in albumin structure can affect binding significantly. Human familial dis-albuminemic hyperthyroxinemia results from genetic variants of HSA. Studies with these variant HSA proteins produced recombinantly shows that their affinities for thyroxine and warfarin are increased 10-fold and fivefold, respectively, over wild-type HSA.[22] Also, different species orthologs of albumin share structural and functional homology; however, important specie differences in protein binding have been described.[23,24]

The flexibility of drug-binding sites on HSA, and their number, may mean that a 1:1 drug–protein binding stoichiometry as assumed in Eq. 6.5 is simplistic. Plasma albumin levels $(500–700\,\mu M)^6$ are higher than those of most drugs, making saturation effects unlikely for albumin binding drugs, except in rare cases.[25] It is plausible that higher drug-binding stoichiometric ratios (i.e., multiple drug-binding sites on the protein) may also reduce the likelihood of binding saturation with drugs that bind albumin, relative to those that bind the less abundant AAG.

6.3.2 Alpha-1 Acid Glycoprotein

Alpha-1 acid glycoprotein (AAG; also known as orosomucoid) is ~40% carbohydrate in composition. The normal concentration of AAG in plasma is lower than that of albumin, thus making saturation effects with AAG binding drugs more likely. The AAG is an acute-phase reactant produced in the liver and immune cells in response to stress, inflammatory cytokines, and host neoplasms. Thus, its levels in immu-nocompromised individuals infected by the human immunodeficiency virus (HIV), and in cancer patients are a matter of therapeutic inter-est.[26,27] Alpha-1 acid glycoprotein with its numerous sialyl residues and sialyl-galactosyl linkages shows considerable microheterogeneity,[28] a characteristic of the sugar residues in glycosylated proteins, where addition of simple and complex sugars to the individual protein mol-ecules is a stochastic process; this results in a heterogenous population of post-translationally modified AAG proteins rather than a uniform one. The AAG has a highly acidic isoelectric point (pH between is 1.0 and 2.7) due to a large number of negatively charged acidic residues. The AAG shows characteristic tight-binding affinities for several basic drugs, which likely results from strong ionic interactions between the drug and the binding-site residues and/or the negatively charged sialic acid residues in the glycosylated part of the protein. In humans, there are two AAG genes (AGP1 and AGP2), thought to have arisen by duplication;[29] in some individuals a third gene is also present. Genetic variants of AAG have been reported to show differences in their binding affinities for antimalarials.[30] The AAG may be thought of as a high-affinity, low-capacity binding protein; in contrast, albumin is a low affinity, high-capacity binding protein. In addition to basic drugs, AAG can bind with high affinity to a variety of neutral and even acidic drugs.[31] A comprehensive review of AAG is available.[8]

6.3.3 Lipoproteins

Lipoproteins include high-density lipoproteins (HDL), low-density lipoproteins (LDL), and very low density lipoproteins (VLDL).[10] Ligands that significantly bind lipoproteins appear to be largely lipophilic and neutral molecules, and include the immunosupresant cyclosporin, the systemic antifungal amphotericin B, the oral polyene antibiotic nystatin, and the antimalarial halofantrine.[10,32] In contrast to drugs that bind albumin and AAG, drugs that bind lipoproteins appear to do so primarily by partitioning nonspecifically into the lipid core rather than to a specific binding site.[2,10] This also means that saturation phenomena are relatively unlikely for drug–lipoprotein binding. Studies of binding of nicardipine, binedaline, and darodipine with lipoproteins suggest that, in addition to lipophilic interactions, ligand protonation may also affect binding, possibly through charge–charge interactions with phosphate headgroups of the phospholipids.[33] The observed postprandial correlation between elevated levels of the binding lipoprotein and the drug halofantrine levels *in vivo* were suggested to be causally related and also responsible for the QT prolongation. Direct studies in an anesthetized rabbit model using intravenous (IV) infusion of lipoprotein and halofantrine, however, suggested that this was not the case.[34]

6.4 EFFECTS ON PHARMACOKINETICS

The primary PK parameters, volume of distribution and clearance, can be affected by binding to plasma proteins. Protein binding has the potential to be a significant factor if the compound in question is highly or very highly bound. Compounds that are >99% bound to plasma protein are generally classified as very highly bound, those between 95 and 99% bound as highly bound, those between 85 and 95% bound as moderately highly bound, and those <80% as poorly bound.

6.4.1 Volume of Distribution

The volume of distribution (V_D) is a proportionality constant between amount of drug in the body and its concentration in the plasma (V_D = amount of drug in the body/concentration in plasma); it can also be expressed as:

$$V_D = \frac{f_u}{f_{uT}} \cdot V_T + V_P \qquad (6.6)$$

where f_u and f_{uT} are unbound fractions in plasma and tissue, respectively, and V_P is the volume of plasma. Extensive binding of drug-to-plasma proteins (small f_u) will reduce the volume while extensive binding to tissues (large f_{uT}) will increase it. Propranolol provides an interesting example of a drug with marked specie differences in the apparent volume of distribution. Fichtl et al.[35] showed that this difference lies in differences in the f_u.

Ensuring a large volume of distribution in humans is one way to increase the half-life ($t_{1/2} = 0.693 \cdot V_D/CL$ in the simplest case of a one-compartment model) and make possible once-a-day dosing. The azalide antibiotic azithromycin[36] is poorly bound to plasma proteins (f_u = 50–97% in a concentration-dependent manner), has a very a large V_D (31 L/kg) and a long $t_{1/2}$ = 40 h). The experimental difficulty in determining f_{uT} has made predictions of human volume of distribution difficult; f_u, on the other hand, is readily measured. Animal data have been used to estimate human f_{uT} for predictive exercises for a volume of distribution.[37,38] In an alternative approach, Lombardo et al. used only the routinely measured log D, pK_a, and unbound fractions, and achieved predictability of human V_D within a twofold margin for neutral and basic compounds.[39,40]

Most drugs do not exert their effects in the plasma compartment with exceptions (e.g., heparin). Tissue penetration is thought to be especially important for antibiotics.[41,42] In an elegant study, Woodnutt et al.[43] showed for a series of β-lactam antibiotics that compounds with low plasma protein binding penetrated well into peripheral lymph (a measure of extravascular diffusion), and vice versa. Note, however, that a high plasma protein binding does not necessarily imply sequestration of drug in plasma and unavailability for distribution.

Physiologically, V_T greatly exceeds V_P (~3 L for a 70-kg human). This factor itself can counter the sequestration effect; moreover, the magnitude of f_{uT} can be a significant factor.[44] This may explain why paradoxically some drugs, including the antifungals itraconazole and ketoconazole, are successful despite being very highly protein bound.[45] Telethromycin and cithromycin are also >90% bound in plasma, but show excellent tissue penetration with volumes of distribution of ~500 L and high intracellular concentration.[46] On the other hand, gentamycin shows very low plasma protein binding (<10%),[47] and its dose limiting nephrotoxicity results from its extensive tissue distribution.[48,49]

6.4.2 Hepatic Clearance

Liver is the major organ for metabolic clearance of drugs. The well-known well-stirred venous equilibrium model of hepatic clearance[50,51] is

$$CL_H = Q_H \cdot E = \frac{Q_H \cdot f_{u,Bld} \cdot CL_{int}}{Q_H + f_{u,Bld} \cdot CL_{int}} \qquad (6.7)$$

in which CL_H is the hepatic blood clearance, Q_H is hepatic blood flow, E is the extraction ratio, $f_{u,Bld}$ is the unbound fraction in blood, and CL_{int} is the intrinsic clearance. Equation 6.7 uses blood flow and binding to blood proteins instead of plasma. Note that though fraction unbound in blood ($f_{u,Bld}$) and in plasma (f_u) may differ, the unbound drug concentrations are the same in the two fluids ($f_{u,Bld} \cdot C_{Bld} = f_u \cdot C_P$). The model assumes that only free-drug in blood crosses the sinusoidal membrane of the hepatocyte and enters it prior to being metabolized. Thus, when intrinsic clearance is very small relative to hepatic blood flow, CL_H approximates to $f_{u,Bld} \cdot CL_{int}$, and when it is very high relative to liver flood flow it approximates to Q_H.

Gillette[52] coined the terms "restrictive clearance" and "nonrestrictive clearance"; they relate hepatic clearance and blood flow with the extent of protein binding. Restrictive clearance applies to low-clearance compounds, where $CL_H = f_{u,Bld} \cdot CL_{int}$, in which either the bound fraction or intrinsic clearance determine overall hepatic clearance. On the other hand, high-clearance compounds are those where nonrestrictive clearance applies, and where clearance of drug is equal to its rate of presentation to the liver $CL_H = Q_H$. For such compounds, the intrinsic clearance will be very high and dissociation rate of drug–protein complex must exceed the organ transit time.

Two other scenarios also exist. First, if drug enters the liver via an active transporter, then its affinity for the transporter may exceed that for the binding plasma protein. If the off-rate from plasma protein (k_{-1} in Eq. 6.3 is sufficiently large, it can de-bind and get transported into the hepatocyte during its transit through the perfusing capillary (see also Sections 4.3 and 5.5). Here, binding kinetics rather than the equilibrium bound fraction would be important. Second, for some drugs, uptake of drug-bound albumin complex into the liver can occur via an albumin receptor.[53] Apparently, a drug–albumin complex can bind at the cell surface where a conformational change is triggered by the membrane or its microenvironment following which the ligand dissociates and is taken up into the hepatocyte.[54] Baker and Parton[55] have developed a kinetic model with variables describing the kinetic effects of plasma protein binding, sinusoidal uptake, passive permeability, and cellular disposition in hepatic clearance and disposition.

6.4.3 Renal Clearance

Renal clearance can be subject to restrictive binding and similar principles apply here as described earlier for the liver. In 1980, Levy[56] described two models for the relationship between the unbound fraction and the renal clearance for low renal extraction drugs:

$$CL_R = f_u \cdot [GFR \cdot (1-F) + K_S \cdot (1-F)] \tag{6.8}$$

and

$$CL_R = f_u \cdot GFR \cdot (1-F) + K'_S \cdot (1-F) \tag{6.9}$$

where CL_R is renal clearance, GFR is glomerular filtration rate, K_S is the intrinsic secretion clearance, and F is the fraction of drug that is reabsorbed. Equation 6.8 describes the case where protein binding governs the net secretion clearance, and Eq. 6.9 describes the case where it does not.

Theoretically, the kinetics of dissociation are relevant in determining the extent to which protein binding can be restrictive. (see also Section 6.5.5)[57] The lifetime of the albumin-bound complex of acetrizoate, a highly bound but actively secreted renal contrast agent, was estimated from nuclear magnetic resonance (NMR) measurements of the dissociation rate constants as between 0.03 and 0.012 s.[58] The renal cortical transit time is substantially higher (0.3–3 s); hence, there is potentially substantial opportunity for the active transport mechanism to strip the drug off from the protein as it traverses the capillary, thus explaining its net secretion. The same authors have also shown[59] mathematically that (1) the system is most sensitive to changes in the dissociation rate when the lifetime of albumin–drug complex is close to the cortical transit time and (2) the extent of protein binding decreases the net secretion capacity so long as the system is not operating at saturating conditions.

6.4.4 Oral Bioavailability

Assuming negligible intestinal metabolism, the maximum oral bioavailability is equal to $1 - E$, where E is the hepatic extraction ratio. Thus,

$$F = F_H = 1 - E \tag{6.10}$$

$$= 1 - [CL_{int} \cdot f_{u,Bld} / (Q_H + CL_{int} \cdot f_{u,Bld})] \tag{6.11}$$

$$= 1 - [Q_H / (Q_H + CL_{int} \cdot f_{u,Bld})] \tag{6.12}$$

where F is the bioavailability, F_H is the fraction that passes through the liver and enters the general circulation, E is the extraction ratio, CL_{int} is the intrinsic clearance, $f_{u,Bld}$ is the unbound fraction in blood, and Q_H is the liver blood flow. During discovery for a chemical series exhibiting high liver clearance, oral bioavailability is generally small because of the liver first-pass effect. It might be expected in such a series that, all other things being equal, compounds with higher protein binding would have higher bioavailability.

6.5 EXPERIMENTAL DETERMINATION OF PROTEIN BINDING

Protein-binding studies are typically done with either plasma or serum. Equilibrium dialysis and ultrafiltration are commonly used experimental techniques for protein-binding measurements. A third method, ultracentrifugation, is less widely employed. In an elegant comparative study,[60] valproic acid binding was investigated by all three methods and the conclusion reached was that each has its limitations (discussed below).

Equilibrium dialysis is often considered the gold standard method although there is no conclusive evidence to suggest that this indeed is the case. The ultrafiltration and ultracentrifugation techniques physically separate free and bound drug by external force whose effect on the binding equilibrium is a subject of potential concern.[60] This is not the case for equilibrium dialysis, which is probably the reason why the method is assumed to be the benchmark method. A common misconception about the meaning of the word "equilibrium" in equilibrium dialysis should also be clarified: In all three methods (equilibrium dialysis, ultrafiltration, and ultracentrifugation), the binding equilibrium between drug and plasma is rapidly achieved; it is only the technique that separates bound from free-drug that differs. The use of "equilibrium" in equilibrium dialysis simply refers to allowing attainment of equilibrium between the drug concentrations in plasma and those in a dialyzing medium.

Often in drug discovery the choice of the method is based on the practical issues specific to a given program chemistry. For compounds that are further on the development path, radiolabeled compound may be available and its use has obvious advantages. Prior to clinical studies, it is recommended that protein binding be determined by at least two different methods. For compounds in the discovery phase, all three methods will require expensive liquid chromatography/tandem mass spectrometry (LC/MS/MS) based analytical support; this becomes particularly relevant because it is in this early phase that the binding studies conducted are most numerous. In addition to these direct techniques, some *in vitro* pharmacology assays may be performed in the presence and absence of plasma or purified plasma proteins to determine effects of binding on the potency. This approach is widely used in antimicrobial efforts[61] and has more recently also been applied for antiangiogenesis assays.[62]

6.5.1 Equilibrium Dialysis

The experimental method is depicted in Figure 6.3. Briefly, drug-spiked plasma or serum is placed in one compartment, which is separated by a semipermeable membrane from a second compartment containing buffer (typically phosphate buffer pH 7.4). The membrane is impermeable to macromolecules, and hence to drug bound to plasma proteins. Unbound drug in the plasma compartment diffuses down its electrochemical gradient and across the membrane until the unbound concentrations in both compartments equalize, and equilibrium is achieved. A 6-h period at 37 °C is usually sufficient for most compounds when using dialysis setups with 1-mL volumes for each half-cell, although the actual attainment of equilibrium may be determined if needed. At equilibrium, the bound fraction is given as:

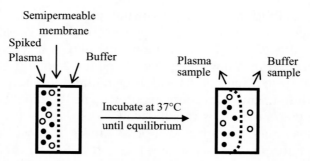

Figure 6.3. Equilibrium dialysis. Drug-spiked plasma is placed in one cell and buffer in the other; the two cells are separated by a semipermeable membrane. Unbound drug in the plasma compartment diffuses across the membrane down its electrochemical gradient until at equilibrium the unbound concentrations in the two compartments are equal.

$$\% \, f_b = 100 \times \frac{(C_{\text{Plasma}} - C_{\text{Buffer}}) \times (V_{\text{Plasma}} / V_{\text{Plasma,initial}})}{[(C_{\text{Plasma}} - C_{\text{Buffer}}) \times (V_{\text{Plasma}} / V_{\text{Plasma,initial}})] + C_{\text{Buffer}}} \quad (6.13)$$

in which C_{Plasma}, C_{Buffer}, V_{Plasma}, and V_{Buffer} are drug concentrations and volumes of the plasma and buffer compartments at the end of the incubation, and $C_{\text{Plasma,initial}}$ and $V_{\text{Plasma,initial}}$ are drug concentration and volume of plasma initially added into the plasma compartment. The volume terms are corrections for the osmotic volume shift that occurs during the course of the experiment because of the Donnan equilibrium: The presence of fixed charges on impermeable proteins and macromolecules in the plasma half-cell results in a net flow of ions and drug to the plasma compartment to ensure electrochemical neutrality at equilibrium. Osmotic flow of water accompanies this movement, and consequently the measured drug concentrations in the plasma and buffer cells must be corrected.[63,64] Where unlabeled compound is used, equilibrium dialysis typically requires quantitation of drug in two matrices, plasma and buffer.

When radiolabeled drug is available, a kinetic dialysis method can be used.[65] Here, plasma is placed in both compartments and into one of them radiolabeled drug is spiked. In this case, the rate of exchange of unbound drug is proportional to the unbound fraction in the sample. As the system is already at equilibrium at the start of the study, small dialysis times (30 min) are adequate.

Theoretically, nonspecific binding is not a major issue with use of the equilibrium dialysis method if adequate time is allowed for the system to reach equilibrium. However, studies show that pretreatment of filters with detergents, such as Tween 80 or benzalkonium chloride, can reduce the extent of such binding.[66] A potential concern is the dilution of both drug and potentially drug-displacing free fatty acids present in the plasma because they diffuse into the buffer compartment during the course of the study.[60] Because of the relatively long time required to attain equilibrium, it is better suited for *in vitro* rather than *ex vivo* determinations of protein binding, and it is less preferable for metabolically unstable compounds. The method is also used to study binding of drugs to purified AAG and HSA, brain homogenate, and subcellular fractions, such as liver microsomes.

In summary, equilibrium dialysis continues to the benchmark against which the other methods are assessed. Though traditionally cumbersome and time-consuming, equilibrium, dialysis can now be performed in 96-cell format and its use is increasingly becoming standard practice. A rapid equilibrium device has been described requiring shorter preparation and dialysis times and which is amenable to automation.[67] Bioanalysis can be simplified by mixing each buffer side study sample (say 50 μL) with an aliquot of blank plasma (50 μL), and similarly each plasma side study sample (50 μL) with an aliquot of blank buffer (50 μL). Calibration curve samples can be made in a similar mixture (50 μL blank buffer and 50 μL blank plasma) and the samples analyzed. This approach eliminates the need to prepare separate calibration curves in plasma and buffer matrices, generally works well in practice, and can save valuable analytical instrumentation time.[68] The volume correction term in Eq. 6.13 is generally not used with the 96-cell setup because of larger error associated with the quantitative withdrawal from the smaller volume cells (150 μL total volume) that is required to perform the correction.

6.5.2 Ultrafiltration

The ultrafiltration method is shown depicted in Figure 6.4. Briefly, drug-spiked plasma is loaded onto an ultrafiltration column–tube whose base is a semipermeable membrane that is impermeable to plasma proteins. The spike plasma is filtered across the membrane under centrifugal force or positive pressure and protein-free ultrafiltrate is generated at the bottom of the tube. In this case, the bound fraction is given as:

$$\% \, f_b = 100 \times (C_{\text{ultrafiltrate}})/(C_{\text{retentate}}) \tag{6.14}$$

Ultrafiltration is simpler and easier to perform than equilibrium dialysis and the entire study can be completed in 30 min. It has

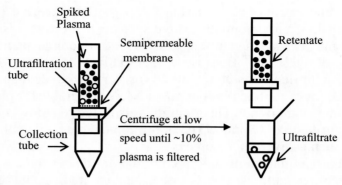

Figure 6.4. Ultrafiltration. Drug-spiked plasma is preincubated (37 °C, ~15 min), whereupon it is loaded onto a ultrafiltration tube and centrifuged at $500 \times g$ until <10% of the volume loaded initially is filtered out as ultrafiltrate in the collection tube.

traditionally been used when large numbers of compounds are involved, or when plasma samples are taken *ex vivo* after dosing. Because dilution of the sample does not occur with ultrafiltration, it is particularly suitable for drugs that show concentration-dependent binding after administration of therapeutic doses. The major concern with ultrafiltration is the extent of nonspecific binding of drug to the filter and tubes, and in contrast to equilibrium dialysis this will always lead to an underestimation of free-drug concentration. Presaturation of the membrane with drug solution can help reduce nonspecific binding;[2] other modifications of the basic ultrafiltration experiment to reduce nonspecific binding have also been described.[69] Spiked phosphate buffer, or better still, spiked plasma water is sometimes used to estimate the extent of nonspecific binding. Use of low centrifugal force–filtration pressures is recommended to reduce the "sieve effect" where water molecules are preferentially filtered compared to the larger drug molecules.[2] Also, the plasma pH (use of capped tubes to prevent loss of CO_2 is preferable) and temperature (temperature controlled centrifuges are preferable) have traditionally been more difficult to control when using ultrafiltration. These are now lesser issues. It is best to ensure that the volume of ultrafiltrate collected does not exceed 10% of the volume loaded in order to prevent concentration effects. Recently, ultrafiltration devices in 96-well format have also become available.

6.5.3 Fluorescence Measurements

Dansyl asparagine[70] and dansyl sarcosine[71] are probes that are reported to bind at HSA site I and II and they differ in their fluorescence characteristics in the free and protein-bound states. These fluorescent analogs can be used as probes using discovery compounds as displacers in order to determine their relative affinity for the proteins.

Fluorescence studies with nonfluorescent drugs can also give useful information.[72] Both albumin and AAG have an intrinsic fluorescence that is quenched upon drug binding. Human albumin contains a solitary tryptophan residue that alone is responsible for its ultraviolet (UV) fluorescence; this greatly enhances the utility of spectroscopy for studying its binding to drugs. A high-throughput method based on this principle has been described that can detect binding of drugs to albumin and AAG; results with this method were rank-order similar to those from equilibrium dialysis.[73] Intrinsic fluorescence of albumin and AAG also provide an avenue to assess the kinetics of binding. The extent of fluorescence quenching of the binding protein will be dependent on concentration of the added binding drug. Thus, the quench curve will provide an estimate of the on-rate; this, in conjunction with the equilibrium binding constant, will give a measure of the off-rate of the drug from the binding protein. If used to assess binding kinetics of different drugs, it is likely that only large differences in the off-rates would be distinguishable using this approach.

6.5.4 Other Methods

Ultracentrifugation uses a high centrifugal force ($100,000$–$450,000\,g$ for several hours) to generate a protein concentration gradient, based on buoyant density, across a tube containing plasma or protein solution. It is based on differential sedimentation of the plasma constituents that in turn is dependent on molecular mass. Thus, following ultracentrifugation of drug-spiked plasma, the protein is concentrated along a gradient at the bottom of the tube and plasma water at its top. Measurement of drug concentration in the carefully collected top fraction gives an estimate of unbound levels. Thermal agitation can cause bound drug to migrate back to the top of the tube and give artifactually high estimates of free concentration; temperature control is thus essential. Similarly, contamination of the pipet tip with the lipoprotein fraction (less dense than plasma water) can pose a problem. Limitations to the use of the method include requirement of an expensive high-speed ultracentrifuge, longer times for completion, and larger plasma volumes. Nakai et al. described the application of a fast microscale ultracentrifugation method using small volume of plasma ($200\,\mu L$) with a benchtop ultracentrifuge ($436,000\,g$ for $140\,min$); for 10 compounds they have shown an excellent correlation in protein binding determined in this manner with methods, such as equilibrium dialysis or ultrafiltration.[74] Despite its limitations, ultracentrifugation is probably the best method to measure free concentration of highly hydrophobic compounds where the other methods prove inadequate.

A second useful method is the use of column chromatography with HSA[75] and AAG columns to qualitatively discriminate drug binding. This approach does not require expensive LC/MS/MS resource. Compounds that bind HSA are retained on HSA columns, and the retention time is a measure of the binding affinity. In practice, retention time data of standard compounds whose binding is known through other methods are used to produce a retention time–% binding standard curve, which is then used to estimate the binding of unknown drugs whose retention time is measured.

Finally, surface plasmon resonance (SPR) biosensors have recently been applied to study drug–plasma protein binding.[76] The technology is particularly useful for mechanistic studies, including kinetics of the binding.

6.5.5 Dissociation Kinetics

The bound fraction f_b is the generally measured parameter for protein binding, but for some compounds this equilibrium parameter is insufficient to explain results of efficacy, PK, or toxicity studies. The lifetime of the bound complex, specifically the rate-determining dissociation rate, may be relevant in these cases (see also Sections 6.4.2 and 6.4.3). When the drug–protein complex dissociation rate is similar to the organ perfusion rate, sensitivity to changes in the dissociation rate is maximized. Tranter and co-workers[77] used HSA column chromatography and showed that the retention time for tryptophan reflects its equilibrium binding to the protein, while the shape–skewedness of the chromatogram reflects the kinetics of the binding process. In general, biophysical approaches using fluorescence and SPR lend themselves easily to the study of drug-binding kinetics.

6.5.6 Experimental Artifacts

Various factors can cause artifacts in *in vitro* protein-binding data, and MacKichen has written an exhaustive review on this topic over a decade ago.[2] Collection tubes (Vacutainer®) used for collection of blood samples prior to the 1980s contained the plasticizer tris(2-butoxyethyl) phosphate, which displaced the basic drugs alprenolol and impipramine from AAG and led to high and variable unbound fractions.[78] Thus, contact of blood with any plastic is a potential cause for concern. Use of the anticoagulant heparin can reduce apparent protein binding of various drugs (e.g., propranolol, lidocaine, quinidine, and verapamil)[79,80] because it releases lipoprotein lipase, which in turn increases free fatty acid levels that displace drugs bound to albumin.[81] Citric acid as an anticoagulant has been known to displace phenytoin, meperidine, and bretylium tosylate.[82] Use of serum instead of plasma can obviate these concerns. The physical conditions of plasma can be a source of variability. Storage at higher temperatures can release free fatty acid levels. The pH of plasma affects the binding value,[83] and it is recommended to record the plasma pH prior to start of the study. Changes in pH can alter binding through multiple mechanisms including changing the ionization state of the ligand[20] or that of the key residues in the binding site. The binding of warfarin to albumin is subject to the latter mechanism: albumin transitions from neutral to basic form over the pH range 6–9, and warfarin binds to the basic form to a threefold greater extent.[19] Finally, where purified albumin or AAG are used, variations in methods of their production may lead to debatable results,[84,85] and their purity is essential to determine.

6.6 EXAMPLES FROM DISCOVERY AND DEVELOPMENT

Protein binding is determined at various stages of the discovery and development process, and is often given high importance in the discovery phase. Its perceived importance for a therapeutic class is often driven by precedence: Compounds at an advanced clinical stage, whose effects have been shown experimentally to be modulated by protein binding, provide impetus for follower programs to give protein binding special attention. If it is known that binding is likely to be an issue, more data is generated earlier on a larger numbers of compounds to enable early structure–activity relationship (SAR) driven amelioration of the problem. Methods with larger throughput and less requirement of LC/MS/MS resource are preferred at this early stage. Figure 6.5 summarizes protein-binding data based on therapeutic class for 265 marketed compounds. It shows that most non-steroidal anti-inflammatory drugs (NSAIDs) are highly bound, as are diabetes drugs; however, clearly, generalizations cannot be made. The importance of protein binding for antimicrobial programs is well established. Recent interest has also revolved around anticancer and antiretroviral drugs, and AAGs role appears to be particularly important in this context.

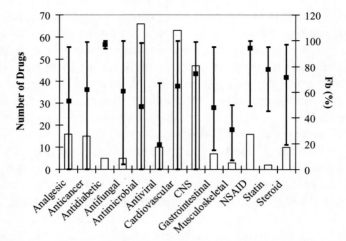

Figure 6.5. Summary of protein binding of marketed drugs. Bars indicate the number of drugs in each therapeutic class (left *y*-axis). Box and whiskers indicate the mean and range of the bound fraction for each class (right *y*-axis). Depicted is data for 265 marketed drugs. [*Source*: Thummel, K.E. and Shen, D.D., Appendix II, Design and optimization of dosage regimens: pharmacokinetic data. In Goodman and Gilman's *The Pharmacological Basis of Therapeutics* Eds.: Hardman, J.G., Lee, E.L, 10th ed., McGraw-Hill, **2001**.]

Protein-binding measurements are meaningful when made at concentrations relevant for pharmacology and safety. *In vivo*, protein binding can affect the efficacy and safety of a drug, and such effects would predominantly result from its effects on PKs and distribution. Protein binding also is important in the prediction of human PKs from preclinical data. In the following sections, examples relating to each of these points are discussed in turn.

6.6.1 Drug Efficacy

6.6.1.1 Antimicrobials. Antimicrobials as a therapeutic class has been longest and best studied in terms of relevance of protein binding. For antimicrobials, there is substantial evidence from preclinical efficacy studies that unbound concentrations in tissue govern efficacy, and that unbound concentrations in plasma correlate with those in tissue. This makes plasma protein binding a meaningful parameter to follow. Important clinical examples of this phenomenon cited by Wise[41] and Muller et al.[42] include therapeutic failures of fusidic acid and ceftrioxone in the treatment of gonnorhoea. In a series of elegant studies,

Derendorf and co-workers employed *in vivo* microdialysis in humans to directly measure unbound levels in the tissue. These were correlated with predictions of tissue concentrations based on drug concentrations in plasma; excellent concordance was observed for several compounds including cefodizime,[86] cefpirome,[86] pipericillin,[87,88] and tazobactam.[89] Such studies have underscored the value of measuring plasma protein binding for antimicrobials, and consequently it is routinely measured during antimicrobial discovery efforts.

6.6.1.2 Anti-HIV Compounds.

There is currently strong interest in assessing the importance of protein binding for HIV compounds. Protease inhibitors (e.g., amprenavir, saquinavir, ritonavir, and nelfinavir) are typically >90% bound and bind AAG.[90] A cross-study analysis of three phase-1 studies of amprenavir in HIV-positive and –negative subjects has shown a significant inverse relationship between AAG concentrations and the apparent total clearance (CL/F) of the drug.[91] Also in this study, black subjects had significantly lower AAG levels compared to white subjects and a higher amprenavir CL/F. In transgenic mice with elevated AAG levels, the volume of distribution and systemic clearance of saquinavir is reduced.[92] *In vitro*, SC-52151, a urea-based peptidomimetic protease inhibitor has an IC_{90} versus the enzyme of <100 ng/mL, which increases over 15-fold in the presence of physiologic concentrations of AAG.[93] Importantly, AAG levels show particularly large variability in infected individuals and this can affect efficacy and PKs.[26,27] Nonnucleoside reverse transcriptase inhibitors bind albumin, and an example is efavirenz (>99% bound). While strong attention is being paid to protein binding of anti-HIV compounds, it is still not entirely clear if low binding is a prerequisite for a successful drug.[9]

6.6.1.3 Anti-Cancer Compounds.

7-Hydroxy staurosporine (UCN-01), a protein kinase C inhibitor, provides a most remarkable case study for protein binding.[80–86] It binds AAG with very high affinity ($K_D \sim 1.25$ nM). Phase-1 studies showed that UCN-01 has a very small volume of distribution, a very slow clearance (17 mL/h), and a half-life in humans exceeding 200 h.[94,95] A subsequent PK study conducted over a 30-fold dose range showed a two- to three and one-half-fold increase in clearance and volume of distribution; AAG is a major determinant of the compound's unbound levels and explains, in large part, its PKs.[96]

Imatinib (Gleevec®, ST 1571) is a tyrosine kinase inhibitor developed for use against chronic myeloid leukemia. Preclinical studies provided evidence both for[97] and against[98] a role for AAG in modulating its efficacy. Indirect evidence came from a mouse model bearing human leukemic cell tumors: efficacy failed in animals with the larger tumors that had concomitantly higher AAG levels.[97] Subsequently, human studies suggested that AAG could serve as a biomarker for pharmacological resistance to imatinib.[99,100] A population PK study with imatinib has established a role for AAG binding *in vivo*, and pointed to the utility of a therapeutic drug monitoring approach that takes into account either circulating AAG levels or free imatinib concentrations.[101] For a different drug from this class, gefitinib (Iressa®, ZD1839), a molecule with promise against non-small-cell lung cancer, an *ex vivo* study suggests that it is highly protein bound in cancer patients (>97%).[102]

The histone deacetylase inhibitor, MS-275 (3-pyridylmethyl-*N*-{4-[(2-aminophenyl)-carbamoyl]-benzyl-carbamate), is currently in clinical trials for solid tumors and hematological malignancies. Its half-life in humans is longer (>50h) than in animal species (~1h), and this difference has been attributed in part to its higher plasma protein binding in human compared to preclinical species.[103]

6.6.1.4 *Central Nervous System Compounds.*

In most cases, unbound drug alone can cross the blood–brain barrier and be available for distribution into brain tissues.[104,105] Early *in vivo* brain microdialysis studies of the antidepressant diazepam in Wistar and analbuminemic rats showed that albumin does indeed modulate its entry into the brain.[106] Studies of *N*-methyl-D-aspartic acid (NMDA) receptor antagonists[104] in an *in situ* brain perfusion model in rat also supports the free-drug hypothesis at the blood–brain barrier. Equilibrium dialysis against a brain homogenate suspension yields an estimate of unbound fraction in brain. An assessment of 34 marketed drugs has revealed that the ratio of unbound concentration in plasma to unbound concentration in brain, estimated from the unbound fraction, provides a simple mechanism-independent assessment for central nervous systems (CNS) distribution of drugs.[68] Interestingly, however, low protein binding need not be essential for a CNS molecule. In other words, protein binding may be restrictive or nonrestrictive at the blood–brain barrier, and this is ultimately determined by other properties of the compound in question. An interesting example is provided by the small molecule antagonist of the corticotropin-releasing factor (CRF) type 1 receptor, DMP696. It is 98.5% bound in rat plasma, yet it occupies >50% of brain CRF-1 receptors at doses showing an anxiolytic effect.[107]

6.6.2 Drug Safety

6.6.2.1 Cardiac Safety. *Torsades de pointes* (TdP), a potentially fatal ventricular tachycardia, is an adverse effect observed in some non-cardiac drugs, and the condition is associated with prolongation of the QT interval and monophasic action potential duration. The TdP compound has caused several drugs programs to have been either terminated or marketed compounds to have been withdrawn; early assessment of the risk of TdP is thus an objective during development. The theories and methodology on the assessment of QT prolongation related cardiotoxicity will be discussed in Section 10.4 specifically. The importance of studying protein binding is worth mentioning here. An elegant preclinical PK–PD study with terfenadine, terodiline, cisapride, and E4031 in the telemetrized dog[108] has demonstrated that drug administration designed to achieve unbound levels that match unbound levels in humans produce significant effects on QT. These findings underscore the importance of (1) determining if there are specie differences in protein binding in human and the preclinical species and (2) using free levels to estimate the therapeutic margin.

6.6.2.2 Cytochrome P450 (CYP) Inhibition. *In vitro* CYP inhibition studies are routinely used to guide the design of drug–drug interaction studies in humans (details were discussed in Chapter 4). This is an important aspect of the safety assessment of a compound. *In vitro* CYP inhibition data can be used in place of *in vivo* data in case no inhibition is seen. Current practice is to use total plasma concentration as the relevant *in vivo* level to assess risk of an interaction when using *in vitro* CYP inhibition data; this is perhaps a safer assumption than correcting for f_u. The appropriateness of correcting for f_u has been a subject for discussion.[109] Though only free-drug enters the hepatocyte and inhibits the intracellular enzyme's active site, its concentration here thus far has been impossible to determine. Corrections for f_u are further complicated by the fact that since hepatocytes synthesize both albumin and AAG, their intracellular concentrations in these cells will be high; consequently, any intracellular drug is also subject to protein binding. Under these circumstances, use of total plasma levels rather than unbound ones seems justifiable.

6.6.2.3 Dose-Limiting Toxicity. Docetaxel, a semisynthetic taxene, binds extensively to both albumin and AAG and its unbound concentrations correlate well with its dose-limiting toxicity of neutropenia.[110]

Etoposide, a podophyllotoxin derivative, is another example of a drug whose unbound concentrations correlate well with its observed toxicity of myelosuppression. As described earlier, imatinab[111] and UCN-01[112] show concentration-dependent binding to AAG. If saturated protein binding is the major mechanism for dose-dependent change in clearance, then PK parameters based on unbound levels should be independent of dose. The unbound concentrations of imatinib are governed by AAG levels, and there is considerable interindividual variability in both normal subjects and cancer patients. Therapeutic drug monitoring of free-dug has value in this case from both efficacy and toxicity stand points.[101] Note, however, that for most anti-cancer drugs, variability in plasma protein levels contributes little to overall variability, and thus where necessary total exposure is most often considered for therapeutic drug monitoring and PK–PD relationships.

6.6.2.4 Nonlinearity. Because of the limited number of sites for binding, protein binding is invariably saturable for all drugs. If the drug concentration is much smaller than that of the protein to which it binds, then the free fraction will be relatively constant at different total drug concentrations. In general, therefore, saturability is more likely with AAG binding drugs because its molar circulating plasma concentration ($12–30\,\mu M$) is significantly lower than that of albumin ($600\,\mu M$). If protein-binding saturation occurs during dose escalation, then in the simplest case, total clearance would increase with an increasing dose resulting in less than dose proportional exposure; unbound clearance, on the other hand, would be relatively constant until the dominant clearance pathway for the drug starts showing saturation. It is important to measure protein binding across the relevant pharmacologic–toxicologic concentration range to have an understanding of the *in vivo* effects. In animal safety studies, *in vitro* determination across a 100-fold concentration range is important when setting doses for safety studies. In humans, knowledge of binding linearity in a relevant concentration range is important during phase-I studies, especially for compound with a low-therapeutic index.

6.6.3 Pharmacokinetic Predictions for Human

Allometry is used in PKs to relate PK parameters obtained in animal studies to body weight, and thus enable a prediction of human PKs. The approach assumes a general similarity in the biochemistry, anatomy, and physiology in the species used. Inclusion of protein binding in the scaling is likely to improve predictions for compounds that are highly bound and show big species differences in their unbound fractions. An example is UCN-01 for which f_u in rat is 1.75% and in human is <0.02%: Recently, Tang and Mayersohn showed that in this case the allometric prediction was improved by inclusion of protein-binding data.[113] Earlier studies had shown a similar large species difference in camptothecin binding to albumin.[114] Mahmood,[115] for a variety of drugs, overall found no clear evidence for better human predictions for unbound clearance than for total clearance; in fact there is likely a greater variability in the unbound value. Use of unbound levels did, however, improve the human prediction for some compounds. Similarly, Obach et al.[37] in an analysis of 83 compounds that had reached the clinical phase found a slightly better prediction for the unbound CL than for total CL; it was, however, uncertain if this is of practical significance.

In contrast to allometric scaling, a physiologically based PK prediction involves correlation of *in vivo* clearance data from preclinical species with *in vitro* data in microsomes or hepatocytes from the same species. If this relationship has strong *in vitro* to *in vivo* predictability, then *in vitro* clearance data from human liver microsomes provides a qualitative first estimate for PKs in humans. In this exercise, the estimated clearance is obtained by correcting the intrinsic clearance for *in vitro* protein binding ($CL_{Hep,estimated} = f_{u,Bld} \cdot CL_{int}$). Thus, incorporating protein binding for predictions of human PKs can be critical in making a best estimate before the initiation of clinical studies. The prediction of PKs for humans will be specifically discussed also in Chapter 7.

6.6.4 Protein-Binding Displacement

For most of the last century, the significance of displacement interactions was overstated. Classic examples that were originally attributed to displacement include severe hypoglycemia in diabetics taking tolbutamide and sulfonamides concomitantly,[116] and potentiation of the warfarin effect by concomitant phenylbutazone.[117,118] It is now clear that these resulted instead from metabolic interactions. Moreover, it is also now well accepted that the displacement effects are unlikely to have clinical significance, except in the most limited cases.

Theoretically, a significant displacement response can occur only for a highly potent, highly protein bound, high-clearance drug given intravenously. The theoretical demonstration of this conclusion was provided previously by Lin and Lu[119] and Benet and Hoener,[120] and clinical demonstration recently was provided for the IV anesthetic propofol.[121]

Importantly, for orally administered drugs, however, displacement effects will not affect the unbound levels, and are therefore clinically insignificant. This finding is true regardless of whether the compound has low or high clearance, and it is also true for a low therapeutic index drug, such as warfarin. Thus, for an oral drug:

$$AUC_{total} = F \cdot Dose/CL = F \cdot Dose/f_u \cdot CL_{int} \qquad (6.15)$$

Rearranging, the unbound exposure is

$$AUC_{unbound} = AUC_{total} \cdot f_u = F \cdot Dose/CL_{1 int} \qquad (6.16)$$

Therefore, the unbound exposure in this case is independent of the unbound fraction.

The effect of displacement on the volume of distribution may, on the other hand, offer an alternative mode to achieving efficacy. This would be especially true for compounds with a small volume of distribution where an increase in free fraction will be associated with an increased volume of distribution. Studies in mice of the anti-cancer drug imatinib have addressed such an approach,[97] although development of an ideal displacer would be a challenge in its own right.

An interesting and classical example of a clinically significant displacement interaction is given by endogenous bilirubin.[122] A life-threatening encephalopathy is seen in infants given sulfizoxazole, which apparently increases the free fraction of bilirubin via displacement from the circulating bilirubin–albumin complex. The slow clearance pathway for bilirubin in infants (unlike that for most drugs in adults) cannot compensate for the increase in free fraction. Recent studies recommend measurement of free bilirubin in managing neonatal jaundice;[123] however, some practical considerations may affect the utility of the approach.[124]

6.7 SUMMARY

The free-drug hypothesis applies in virtually all cases. Plasma protein binding is routinely measured and used along with other data for decision making during lead optimization. Various methods are used to measure drug–protein binding and each has its advantages and limitations. For compounds in the development phase, it is best determined by more than one method, and with the use of a radiolabeled drug. In general, protein binding appears particularly important for antimicrobial, anti-cancer, and antiretroviral programs. Most rational criteria for protein binding are typically made for back-up programs, where some key learnings with lead compounds have already occurred.

The extent to which protein binding is an important issue will depend on the chemical series and ultimately the compound in question. Early in the discovery process there is a predisposition for various therapeutic areas to favor compounds that are not very highly bound. It must be understood, however, that protein binding is not a factor that can *a priori* be reasonably used by itself to make a decision on the fate of a compound (like, e.g., CYP inhibition). Its importance for a given compound depends on its PK characteristics like distribution, clearance, and concentration at the target site or organ. A mixed PK parameter, such as $t_{1/2}$ is proportional directly to volume of distribution and inversely to clearance. Higher unbound drug levels should increase both volume of distribution and clearance; these simultaneous effects would reduce any net effect on $t_{1/2}$ unless the effect on one of the two parameters predominates. All other things being equal, greater free-drug levels should result in improved efficacy (desirable), but simultaneously in greater toxicity as well (undesirable). Ultimately, the importance of protein binding for a given compound depends on which, if any, of efficacy, toxicity, or PKs becomes limiting in development.

REFERENCE

1. Trainor, G. L.; John, E. M. in *Annual Reports in Medicinal Chemistry*; **2007**, 42, 489–502, Academic Press.

2. MacKichan, J. J. in *Applied Pharmacokinetics*; Eds. Evans, W. E., Schwentag, J. J., Jusko, W. J., **1992**, 5-1–5-48, Lippincott Williams and Wilkins.

3. Nicholson, J. P.; Wolmarans, M. R.; Park, G. R. *Br. J. Anaesth.* **2000**, 85, 599–610.

4. Swaminathan, R. *Handbook of Clinical Biochemistry*; **2004**, Oxford University Press.

5. Peters, T., Jr. *Adv. Prot. Chem.* **1985**, 37, 161–245.

6. Rowland, M.; Tozer, T. N. *Clinical Pharmacokinetics: Concepts and Applications*; 2nd ed.; **1989**, Lea & Febiger.

7. Mehvar, R. *Am. J. Pharm. Educ.* **2005**, 69, 1–8 (Article 103).

8. Israili, Z. H.; Dayton, P. G. *Drug Metab. Rev.* **2001**, 33, 161–235.

9. Boffito, M.; Back, D. J.; Blaschke, T. F.; Rowland, M.; Bertz, R. J.; Gerber, J. G.; Miller, V. *AIDS Res. Human Retroviruses* **2003**, 19, 825–835.

10. Wasan, K. M.; Cassidy, S. M. *J. Pharm. Sci.* **1998**, 87, 411–424.
11. Bree, F.; Houin, G.; Barre, J. *Clin. Pharmacokin.* **1986**, 11, 336–342.
12. Kaysen, G. A.; Dubin, J. A.; Muller, H. G.; Mitch, W. E.; Levin, N. W.; Group, H. *Kidney Internat.* **2001**, 60, 2360–2366.
13. Takahashi, N.; Takahashi, Y.; Blumberg, B. S.; Putnam, F. W. *Proc. Natl. Acad. Sci. USA* **1987**, 84, 4413–4417.
14. Huss, K.; Madison, J.; Ishioka, N.; Takahashi, N.; Arai, K.; Putnam, F. W. *Proc. Natl. Acad. Sci. USA* **1988**, 85, 6692–6696.
15. Kragh-Hansen, U.; Campagnoli, M.; Dodig, S.; Nielsen, H.; Benko, B.; Raos, M.; Cesati, R.; Sala, A.; Galliano, M.; Minchiotti, L. *Clin. Chim. Acta* **2004**, 349, 105–112.
16. Ghuman, J.; Zunszain, P. A.; Petitpas, I.; Bhattacharya, A. A.; Otagiri, M.; Curry, S. *J. Mol. Biol.* **2005**, 353, 38–52.
17. Sudlow, G.; Birkett, D. J.; Wade, D. N. *Mol. Pharm.* **1975**, 11, 824–832.
18. Petitpas, I.; Grune, T.; Bhattacharya, A. A.; Curry, S. *J. Mol.Biol.* **2001**, 314, 955–960.
19. Petitpas, I.; Bhattacharya, A. A.; Twine, S.; East, M.; Curry, S. *J. Biol. Chem.* **2001**, 276, 22804–22809.
20. Ermondi, G.; Lorenti, M.; Caron, G. *J. Med. Chem.* **2004**, 47, 3949–3961.
21. Wilding, G.; Blumberg, E. S.; Vesell, E. S. *Science* **1977**, 195, 991–994.
22. Petersen, C. E.; Ha, C. E.; Harohalli, K.; Park, D. S.; Bhagavan, N. V. *Chem. Biol. Inter.* **2000**, 124, 161–172.
23. Callan, W. M.; Sunderman, F. W., Jr. *Res. Comm. Chem. Path. Pharmacol.* **1973**, 5, 459–472.
24. Kragh-Hansen, U. *Pharmacol. Rev.* **1981**, 33, 17–53.
25. Wong, B. K.; Bruhin, P. J.; Lin, J. H. *J. Pharm. Sci.* **1999**, 88, 277–280.
26. Oie, S.; Jacobson, M. A.; Abram, D. I. *J Acquired Immune Deficiency Syndrome* **1993**, 5, 531–533.
27. Boffito, M.; Sciole, K.; Raiteri, R.; Bonora, S.; Hoggard, P. G.; Back, D. J.; Di Perri, G. *Drug Metab. Disp.* **2002**, 30, 859–860.
28. Herve, F.; d'Athis, P.; Tremblay, D.; Tillement, J.-P.; Barre, J. *J. Chromat B: Anal. Tech. Biomed. Life Sci.* **2003**, 798, 283–294.
29. Merritt, C. M.; Easteal, S.; Board, P. G. *Genomics* **1990**, 6, 659–665.
30. Zsila, F.; Visy, J.; Mády, G.; Fitos, I. *Bioorg. Med. Chem.* **2008**, 16, 3759–3772.
31. Maruyama, T.; Otagiri, M.; Takadate, A. *Chem. Pharm. Bull.* **1990**, 38, 1688–1691.
32. Wasan, K. M.; Brocks, D. R.; Lee, S. D.; Sachs-Barrable, K.; Thornton, S. J. *Nature Rev. Drug Discov.* **2008**, 7, 84–99.
33. Simon, N.; Dailly, E.; Jolliet, P.; Tillement, J. P.; Urien, S. *Pharm. Res.* **1997**, 14, 527–532.

34. McIntosh, M. P.; Batey, A. J.; Coker, S. J.; Porter, C. J. H.; Charman, W. N. *J. Pharm. Pharmacol.* **2004**, 56, 69–77.

35. Fichtl, B.; Nieciecki, A. V.; Walter, K. In *Advanced Drug Research*; Ed, Testa, B., **1991**, 20, 117–166, Academic Press.

36. Lalak, N. J.; Morris, D. L. *Clin. Pharmacokin.* **1993**, 25, 370–374.

37. Obach, R. S.; Baxter, J. G.; Liston, T. E.; Silber, B. M.; Jones, B. C.; MacIntyre, F.; Rance, D. J.; Wastall, P. *J. Pharmacol. Exp. Ther.* **1997**, 283, 46–58.

38. Obach, R. S.; John, E. M. in *Annual Report on Medical Chemistry*; **2007**, 42, 469–488, Academic Press.

39. Lombardo, F.; Obach, R. S.; Shalaeva, M. Y.; Gao, F. *J. Med. Chem.* **2002**, 45, 2867–2876.

40. Lombardo, F.; Obach, R. S.; Shalaeva, M. Y.; Gao, F. *J. Med. Chem.* **2004**, 47, 1242–1250.

41. Wise, R. *Clin. Pharmacokinet.* **1986**, 11, 470–482.

42. Muller, M.; dela Pena, A.; Derendorf, H. *Antimicr. Agents Chemother.* **2004**, 48, 1441–1453.

43. Woodnutt, G.; Berry, V.; Mizen, L. *Antimicr. Agents Chemother.* **1995**, 39, 2678–2683.

44. Sparreboom, A.; Nooter, K.; Loos, W. J.; Verweij, J. *Netherlands J. Med.* **2001**, 59, 196–207.

45. Schafer-Korting, M.; Korting, H. C.; Rittler, W.; Obermuller, W. *Infection* **1995**, 23, 292–297.

46. Zeitlinger, M.; Claudia, C. W.; Heinisch, B. *Clin. Pharmacokin.* **2009**, 48, 23–28.

47. Myers, D. R.; DeFehr, J.; Bennet, W. M.; Porter, G. A.; Olsen, G. D. *Clin. Pharmacol. Ther.* **1978**, 23, 356–360.

48. Zaske, D. E. in *Applied Pharmacokinetics*; Eds. Evans, W. E., Schentag, J. J., Jusko, W. J., **1992**, 14-1–14-47, Lippincott Williams and Wilkins.

49. Isoherranen, N.; Lavy, E.; Soback, S. *Antimicr. Agents Chemother.* **2000**, 44, 1443–1447.

50. Rowland, M.; Benet, L. Z.; Graham, G. G. *J. Pharmacokin. Biopharm.* **1973**, 1, 123–136.

51. Wilkinson, G. R.; Shand, D. G. *Clin. Pharmacol. Ther.* **1975**, 18, 377–390.

52. Gillette, J. R. *Ann. New York Acad. Sci.* **1973**, 226, 6–17.

53. Iwatsubo, T.; Hirota, N.; Ooie, T.; Suzuki, H.; Sugiyama, Y. *Biopharm. Drug Disp.* **1996**, 17, 273–310.

54. Forker, E. L.; Luxon, B. A. *Am. J. Physiol.* **1985**, 248, G709–717.

55. Baker, M.; Parton, T. *Xenobiotica* **2007**, 37, 1110–1134.

56. Levy, G. *J. Pharm. Sci.* **1980**, 69, 482–483.

57. van Ginneken, C. A.; Russel, F. G. *Clin. Pharmacokin.* **1989**, 16, 38–54.

58. Rodrigues de Miranda, J. F.; Hilbers, C. W. *Mol. Pharmacol.* **1976**, 12, 279–290.

59. Rodrigues de Miranda, J. F.; Hilbers, C. W. *Pharm Weekblad* **1975**, 110, 1267–1280.

60. Barre, J.; Chamouard, J. M.; Houin, G.; Tillement, J. P. *Clin. Chem.* **1985**, 31, 60–64.

61. Yigong, G.; Difuntorum, S.; Touami, S.; Critchley, I.; Burli, R.; Jiang, V.; Drazan, K.; Moser, H. *Antimicrob. Agents Chemother.* **2002**, 46, 3168–3174.

62. Kruger, E. A.; Figg, W. D. *Clin. Cancer Res.* **2001**, 7, 1867–1872.

63. Tozer, T. N.; Gambertoglio, J. G.; Furst, D. E.; Avery, D. S.; Holford, N. H. *J. Pharm. Sci.* **1983**, 72, 1442–1446.

64. Boudinot, F. D.; Jusko, W. J. *J. Pharm. Sci.* **1984**, 73, 774–780.

65. Pedersen, A. O.; Hust, B.; Andersen, S.; Nielsen, F.; Brodersen, R. *Eur. J. Biochem.* **1986**, 154, 545–552.

66. Lee, K.-J.; Mower, R.; Hollenbeck, T.; Castelo, J.; Johnson, N.; Gordon, P.; Sinko, P. J.; Holme, K.; Lee, Y.-H. *Pharm. Res.* **2003**, 20, 1015–1021.

67. Waters, N. J.; Jones, R.; Williams, G.; Sohal, B. *J. Pharm. Sci.* **2008**, 97, 4586–4595.

68. Kalvass, J. C.; Maurer, T. S.; Pollack, G. M. *Drug Metab. Disp.* **2007**, 35, 660–666.

69. Taylor, S.; Harker, A. *J. Pharm. Biomed. Anal.* **2006**, 41, 299–303.

70. Yamasaki, K.; Maruyama, T.; Kragh-Hansen, U.; Otagiri, M. *Biochim. Biophys. Acta* **1996**, 1295, 147–157.

71. Epps, D. E.; Raub, T. J.; Kezdy, F. J. *Analytical Biochemistry* **1995**, 227, 342–350.

72. Epps, D. E.; Raub, T. J.; Caiolfa, V.; Chiari, A.; Zamai, M. *J. Pharm. Pharmacol.* **1999**, 51, 41–48.

73. Parikh, H. H.; McElwain, K.; Balasubramanian, V.; Leung, W.; Wong, D.; Morris, M. E.; Ramanathan, M. *Pharm. Res.* **2000**, 17, 632–637.

74. Nakai, D.; Kumamoto, K.; Sakikawa, C.; Kosaka, T.; Tokui, T. *J. Pharm. Sci.* **2004**, 93, 847–854.

75. Beaudry, F.; Coutu, M.; Brown, N. K. *Biomed. Chromat.* **1999**, 13, 401–406.

76. Day, Y. S. N.; Myszka, D. G. *J. Pharm. Sci.* **2003**, 92, 333–343.

77. Talbert, A. M.; Tranter, G. E.; Holmes, E.; Francis, P. L. *Anal. Chem.* **2002**, 74, 446–452.

78. Borga, O.; Piafsky, K. M.; Nilsen, O. G. *Clin. Pharmacol. Ther.* **1977**, 22, 539–544.

79. Wood, M.; Shand, D. G.; Wood, A. J. *Clin. Pharmacol. Ther.* **1979**, 25, 103–107.

80. Brown, J. E.; Kitchell, B. B.; Bjornsson, T. D.; Shand, D. G. *Clin. Pharmacol. Ther.* **1981**, 30, 636–643.

81. Giacomini, K. M.; Swezey, S. E.; Giacomini, J. C.; Blaschke, T. F. *Life Sci.* **1980**, 27, 771–780.

82. Jackson, A. J.; Miller, A. K.; Narang, P. K. *J. Pharm. Sci.* **1981**, 70, 1168–1169.

83. Hinderling, P. H.; Hartmann, D. *Ther. Drug Monit.* **2005**, 27, 71–85.

84. Gambacorti-Passerini, C.; Le Coutre, P.; Zucchetti, M.; D'Incalci, M. *Blood* **2002**, 100, 367–368.

85. Jorgensen, H. G.; Elliott, M. A.; Paterson, S.; Holyoake, T. L.; Smith, K. D. *Blood* **2002**, 100, 368–369.

86. Muller, M.; Rohde, B.; Kovar, A.; Georgopoulos, A.; Eichler, H. G.; Derendorf, H. *J. Clin. Pharmacol.* **1997**, 37, 1108–1113.

87. Nolting, A.; Dalla Costa, T.; Vistelle, R.; Rand, K.; Derendorf, H. *J. Pharm. Sci.* **1996**, 85, 369–372.

88. Nolting, A.; Dalla Costa, T.; Rand, K. H.; Derendorf, H. *Pharm. Res.* **1996**, 13, 91–96.

89. Dalla Costa, T.; Nolting, A.; Kovar, A.; Derendorf, H. *J. Antimicrob. Chemother.* **1998**, 42, 769–778.

90. Schon, A.; del Mar Ingaramo, M.; Freire, E. *Biophys. Chem.* **2003**, 105, 221–230.

91. Sadler, B. M.; Gillotin, C.; Lou, Y.; Stein, D. S. *Antimicr. Agents Chemother.* **2001**, 45, 852–856.

92. Holladay, J. W.; Dewey, M. J.; Michniak, B. B.; Wiltshire, H.; Halberg, D. L.; Weigl, P.; Liang, Z.; Halifax, K.; Lindup, W. E.; Back, D. J. *Drug Metab. Disp.* **2001**, 29, 299–303.

93. Bryant, M. et al. *Antimicr. Agents Chemother.* **1995**, 39, 2229–2234.

94. Fuse, E.; Tanii, H.; Kurata, N.; Kobayashi, H.; Shimada, Y.; Tamura, T.; Sasaki, Y.; Tanigawara, Y.; Lush, R. D.; Headlee, D.; Figg, W. D.; Arbuck, S. G.; Senderowicz, A. M.; Sausville, E. A.; Akinaga, S.; Kuwabara, T.; Kobayashi, S. *Cancer Res.* **1998**, 58, 3248–3253.

95. Sausville, E. A.; Arbuck, S. G.; Messmann, R.; Headlee, D.; Bauer, K. S.; Lush, R. M.; Murgo, A.; Figg, W. D.; Lahusen, T.; Jaken, S.; Jing, X.; Roberge, M.; Fuse, E.; Kuwabara, T.; Senderowicz, A. M. *J. Clin. Oncol.* **2001**, 19, 2319–2333.

96. Sparreboom, A.; Chen, H.; Acharya, M. R.; Senderowicz, A. M.; Messmann, R. A.; Kuwabara, T.; Venzon, D. J.; Murgo, A. J.; Headlee, D.; Sausville, E. A.; Figg, W. D. *Clin. Cancer Res.* **2004**, 10, 6840–6846.

97. Gambacorti-Passerini, C.; Barni, R.; le Coutre, P.; Zucchetti, M.; Cabrita, G.; Cleris, L.; Rossi, F.; Gianazza, E.; Brueggen, J.; Cozens, R.; Pioltelli, P.; Pogliani, E.; Corneo, G.; Formelli, F.; D'Incalci, M. *J. Natl. Cancer Inst.* **2000**, 92, 1641–1650.

98. Jorgensen, H. G.; Elliott, M. A.; Allan, E. K.; Carr, C. E.; Holyoake, T. L.; Smith, K. D. *Blood* **2002**, 99, 713–715.

99. Larghero, J.; Leguay, T.; Mourah, S.; Madelaine-Chambrin, I.; Taksin, A. L.; Raffoux, E.; Bastie, J. N.; Degos, L.; Berthaud, P.; Marolleau, J. P.; Calvo, F.; Chomienne, C.; Mahon, F. X.; Rousselot, P. *Biochem. Pharmacol.* **2003**, 66, 1907–1913.

100. Le Coutre, P.; Kreuzer, K.-A.; Na, I.-K.; Schwarz, M.; Lupberger, J.; Holdhoff, M.; Baskaynak, G.; Gschaidmeier, H.; Platzbecker, U.; Ehninger, G.; Prejzner, W.; Huhn, D.; Schmidt, C. A. *Am. J. Hematol.* **2003**, 73, 249–255.

101. Widmer, N.; Decosterd, L. A.; Csajka, C.; Leyvraz, S.; Duchosal, M. A.; Rosselet, A.; Rochat, B.; Eap, C. B.; Henry, H.; Biollaz, J.; Buclin, T. *Br. J. Clin. Pharmacol.* **2006**, 62, 97–112.

102. Li, J.; Brahmer, J.; Messersmith, W.; Hidalgo, M.; Baker, S. D. *Invest. New Drugs* **2006**, 24, 291–297.

103. Acharya, M. R.; Sparreboom, A.; Sausville, E. A.; Conley, B. A.; Doroshow, J. H.; Venitz, J.; Figg, W. D. *Cancer Chemother. Pharmacol.* **2006**, 5, 275–281.

104. Rowley, M.; Kulagowski, J. J.; Watt, A. P.; Rathbone, D.; Stevenson, G. I.; Carling, R. W.; Baker, R.; Marshall, G. R.; Kemp, J. A.; Foster, A. C.; Grimwood, S.; Hargreaves, R.; Hurley, C.; Saywell, K. L.; Tricklebank, M. D.; Leeson, P. D. *J. Med. Chem.* **1997**, 40, 4053–4068.

105. Spector, R. *Pharmacology* **2000**, 60, 58–73.

106. Dubey, R. K.; McAllister, C. B.; Inoue, M.; Wilkinson, G. R. *J. Clin. Invest.* **1989**, 84, 1155–1159.

107. Chen, C. *Curr. Med. Chem.* **2006**, 13, 1261–1282.

108. Webster, R.; Allan, G.; Anto-Awuakye, K.; Harrison, A.; Kidd, T.; Leishman, D.; Phipps, J.; Walker, D. *Xenobiotica* **2001**, 31, 633–650.

109. Lin, J. H. *Drug Metab. Disp.* **1998**, 26, 1202–1212.

110. Baker, S. D.; Li, J.; ten Tije, A. J.; Figg, W. D.; Graveland, W.; Verweij, J.; Sparreboom, A. *Clin. Pharmacol. Ther.* **2005**, 77, 43–53.

111. Gambacorti-Passerini, C.; Zucchetti, M.; Russo, D.; Frapolli, R.; Verga, M.; Bungaro, S. *Clin. Cancer Res.* **2003**, 9, 625–632.

112. Fuse, E.; Tanii, H.; Takai, K.; Asanome, K.; Kurata, N.; Kobayashi, H.; Kuwabara, T.; Kobayashi, S.; Sugiyama, Y. *Cancer Res.* **1999**, 59, 1054–1060.

113. Tang, H.; Mayersohn, M. *J. Clin. Pharmacol.* **2006**, 46, 398–400.

114. Mi, Z.; Burke, T. G. *Biochemistry* **1994**, 33, 12540–12545.

115. Mahmood, I. *J. Clin. Pharmacol.* **2000**, 40, 1439–1446.

116. Christensen, L. K.; Hansen, J. M.; Kristensen, M. *Lancet* **1963**, 2, 1298–1301.

117. Aggeler, P. M.; O'Reilly, R. A.; Leong, L.; Kowitz, P. E. *New Engl. J. Med.* **1967**, 276, 496–501.

118. Fox, S. *J. Amer. Med. Assoc.* **1964**, 188, 320–321.

119. Lin, J. H.; Lu, A. Y. *Pharmacol. Rev.* **1997**, 49, 403–409.

120. Benet, L. Z.; Hoener, B.-A. *Clin. Pharmacol. Ther.* **2002**, 71, 115–121.

121. Hiraoka, H.; Yamamoto, K.; Okano, N.; Morita, T.; Goto, F.; Horiuchi, R. *Clin. Pharmacol. Ther.* **2004**, 75, 324–330.

122. Silverman, W. A.; Andersen, D. H.; Blan, W. A.; Crozier, D. N. *Pediatrics* **1956**, 18, 614–615.

123. Wennberg, R. P.; Ahlfors, C. E.; Bhutani, V. K.; Johnson, L. H.; Shapiro, S. M. *Pediatrics* **2006**, 117, 474–485.

124. McDonagh, A. F.; Maisels, M. J. *Pediatrics* **2006**, 117, 523–525.

CHAPTER 7

PREDICTION OF THE PHARMACOKINETICS IN HUMANS

CHAO HAN
Centocor Research and Development Inc., Malvern, PA

RAMESH BAMBAL
Absorption Systems, Exton, PA

7.1 INTRODUCTION

It was highlighted in the introduction chapter and Chapter 2 that one of the three main purposes of conducting preclinical pharmacokinetic (PK) research is to prepare for the prediction of PK behavior of a drug candidate in humans. Our ultimate goal is to discover and develop safe and efficacious medicines for human. Being able to make a well-educated prediction about the PK behavior of a drug candidate in humans is invaluable to the whole processes of drug discovery and development. In addition to stressing the importance of selecting a safe and sensible First Time In Human (FTIH) starting dose based on predictions, there are also several other valuable points that should be discussed in this chapter. Our aim is to address the evaluation of developability in this book. Prior to our discussion of those aspects, noted that the results from a safety assessment study play a critical role in the selection of the FTIH dose. The in-depth discussion of safety assessment and selection of FTIH dose for clinical trial, however, is not a main focus of this book. For these topics, one can refer to US Food and Drug Administration's (FDA's) guidance for selecting FTIH dose[1] and other available references.

During lead optimization of a drug discovery program, one of the ongoing processes is to fine-tune PK properties of the lead molecules to meet a desired profile. This desirable profile is normally closely related to and, therefore, defined by the biological target, potency of the molecule on the target, and proposed therapeutic approaches related to the target. In many cases, a commercial wish list has an impact on target product profile as well. This PK property could be further detailed as the exposure and time-concentration profile of a proposed drug candidate, which will directly link to the designing of the size and regimen of dose in pharmaceutical and clinical development perspectives. Before FTIH, the questions whether we have done well enough to make a molecule suitable for proposed therapy or treatment in drug discovery could not be answered definitively, unfortunately. The project and management teams would have to make decisions on whether to make further investment for a candidate based on available *in vivo* and *in vitro* preclinical data. A prediction of the PK profile in humans would be very helpful for the evaluation of whether a drug candidate is suitable for further development. Early predictions will also give the team some sense beforehand on how likely a molecule will reach desired exposure in humans, which will likely result in proposed pharmacological and therapeutic outcomes.

These results will also make its impact on the early stage of drug development. The size of the dose and hypothetical dose regimen in humans will be the basis of formulation designing in pharmaceutical development. Plans are formed accordingly on selection of the sizes of a pill, formulation, and so on. From a project team point of view a few very simple questions could be asked for reality checking (e.g., are the hypothetical doses practical?).

There are many different approaches to predict human clearance based on preclinical data. In addition to different allometric models, the metabolic clearance could be extrapolated from the *in vitro* rate of drug metabolism to the *in vivo* metabolic clearance. The discussions of using *in vitro* data to predict metabolic clearance in humans are very active areas of scientific research and discussion. This chapter will briefly discuss the basic concept of allometric scaling and some other classic approaches. We will also discuss the methods of using *in vitro* clearance to predict human metabolic clearance.

7.2 ALLOMETRIC SCALING

7.2.1 A Brief Introduction to the Mathematical Approach

Allometry in this regard is the study of a relationship between biological consequence, such as total body clearance or volume of distribution, and the size of the body. A simple allometric scaling equation is very often used to describe the relationship

$$Y = a * X^b$$

where, Y represents a specified biological function, such as the clearance; X is an independent variable related to body size, such as body weight; a is a factor defining the function; b is the exponent of the relationship.

A simple logarithm transformation on both sides of the equation reforms the exponential relationship into a linear relationship that we can deal with easily.

$$\log Y = b * \log X + \log a$$

Here b is the exponent, which defines the relationship of, for example, body weight and a specific biological function. All we need to do next is to collect experimental data from a few animal species with different body size. Each species will give us a measurement of the function and their body weight. We should be able to obtain the value of exponent and offset by plotting the data sets (linear regression should be used for a formal approach). The measure of such a biological function then could be extrapolated to or predicted in other species with different body size (e.g., in humans) theoretically.

7.2.2 An Example

An example of allometric scaling could be taken from preclinical evaluation of N-tert-butyl isoquine (NTBI) and other novel antimalarials published by Davis et al.[2] In this study, the PK properties of NTBI was determined in four preclinical species, namely, mouse, rat, monkey, and dog (Table 7.1).

The clearance values were plotted against body weights on logarithm scale for each animal species accordingly (Fig. 7.1). Human clearance was predicted[2] based on an extrapolation of the linear relationship to be ~7 mL/min/kg for a postulated 70-kg man. The squared correlation coefficient was 0.978; the exponent was 0.84. The volume of distribution estimated at steady state was scaled in a similar manner in this publication.[2] A similar example can be found also in the evaluation of other drug candidates.[3] These approaches are standard in the processes of evaluation of a molecule for further development.

TABLE 7.1. Pharmacokinetics of N-tert-Butyl isoquine Following Single Intravenous or Oral Administration to Animals[a]

Species	CL_b (mL/min/kg)[b]	$t_{1/2}$ (h)	F (%)
Mouse	17	3.3	~100
Rat	26 ± 5	8 ± 4	89 ± 12
Monkey	14.5 ± 0.7	11 ± 3	~100
Dog	6.3 ± 1.6	48 ± 3	68 ± 18

[a]Reference 2.
[b]Blood clearance = CL_b.
$t_{1/2}$ = elimination half-life; F = oral bioavailability.

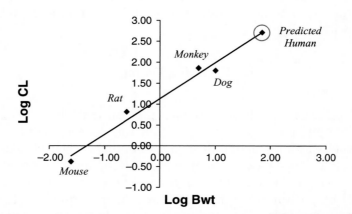

Figure 7.1. Simple allometric scaling of NTBI based on the published data. The body weight used in the plot was based on average weight of the species published by Davies and Morris (1993)[4] for a demonstration purpose. CL = clearance; Bwt = body weight.

7.2.3 The Biological Assumptions

It is very important to recollect the assumptions behind the mathematical relationship discussed earlier. The mathematical approach described briefly in the previous sections is based on the assumptions of biological, physiological, and anatomical *similarities* between animal species and humans.[5,6] The fact on which the assumption was based appeared to be obvious. Decades of scientific research on basic physiology of the circulation and biological events in different species, especially among those animal species with different body size, has lead us to a much better understanding of the rate of biological processes (e.g., metabolism). The rate of metabolism in different species and related homodynamic indexes were studied carefully. When the ratio of organ blood flow to organ mass was closely examined, it was found that it falls into a certain relationship.[6] Observing this from a different angle, it appears that the ratio is higher in smaller mammalian animal species, which also have a faster metabolic rate. The rate can be scaled up for a species with different body size based on the relationship. The observation seemed readily applicable to the fate of xenobiotics or drugs that are, by general understanding, eliminated largely via the liver and kidneys.

7.2.4 Fine Tuning for Better Accuracy of the Prediction

Upon review of published clinical and preclinical data for a fair number of agents, Mahmood et al.[7,8] indicated that a simple allometric approach is not always suitable for a reliable prediction. The authors suggested that some corrections to simple allometry could be necessary. For example, when the clearance value was corrected by brain weight or by mean life span (MLP) of the species, a better prediction was obtained for some of the agents.

Clearance (CL) correction by brain weight

$$CL \times BW = aW^b$$

where BW = brain weight; W = body weight.

Clearance correction by MLP

$$CL = a(MLP \times CL)^b / 8.18 \times 10^5$$

where MLP (years) = $185.4 \times BW^{0.636} \times W^{-0.225}$

The exponents of several marketed agents were collected and carefully examined. Based on published data, Mahmood et al.[7,8]

recommended that when the exponent from a simple allometric scaling is >0.7, a correction of the scaling should be made by the MLP. However, when the exponent from simple allometry is ≥1.0, the correction should be made based on brain weight for a greater prediction accuracy. Due to the limited size of the database of which the number of drugs had an exponent between 0.90 and 0.99, it is not clear which correction should be applied at this point.

It is known that small rodents (e.g., rat) have a relatively higher rate of biliary secretion.[4] When bile flow rate is normalized to the body weight or liver weight of the species, the index is strikingly higher than that of human. When biliary secretion of a compound becomes a significant elimination pathway, the allometry could potentially overestimate human clearance, especially when above-mentioned rodent species are used in allometric scaling. Mahmood and Sahajwalla[9] also suggested a correction of the allometry when biliary excretion is known to be involved in a significant way in the elimination of a drug. The relative factor for bile secretion is listed in Table 7.2.

In order to predict the clearance for a compound excreted significantly into the bile known in at least one species, simple allometric prediction and the exponent value should be established first. Corrected prediction with an appropriate correction method according to the value of the exponent is then chosen. The clearance in each species is corrected by the correction factor shown in Table 7.2; the allometry is performed again with corrected clearances.

These correction methods were applied in the prediction of clearance for drug candidates in humans.[2,3] The exponents and squared correlation coefficients of all methods were listed for comparison and evaluation. In addition, the linear regression was tested for significance of the slops from zero. The exponent of a simple allometry in these cases was >0.7. A correction method should be considered according to what Mahmood[7,8] suggested. Additional information (e.g., if the compound is also cleared via biliary excretion in a significant proportion, especially in rodents) will be required for making a further judgment on whether bile correction should be applied. *In vivo* animal experiment is likely necessary to generate the required information.

TABLE 7.2. Relative Bile Secretion in Different Animal Species[a]

Relative Bile Flow[b]	Mouse	Rat	Rabbit	Dog	Monkey
By liver weight	5.9	11.6	20	1.9	4.3
By body weight	20	18	24	2.4	5

[a]Bile flow data (see Ref. 4).
[b]Bile flow = mL/day/kg of liver or body weight; all numbers are relative to human's

Once an allometric scaling for a new chemical entity is made to predict PK behavior in humans, one would attempt to interpret the results for a decision-making process. Never should we take the biological assumption on which the allometry is based lightly. It is always very important and helpful to check surrounding experimental data carefully before interpreting the results and, do not intent to overinterpret the results. When information, such that the compound of interest is a specific substrate of a drug-metabolizing enzyme, drug-transporter, or biological or physiological process in one or some of the species, becomes available, one should examine the species used in allometric scaling carefully for potential species difference from humans. Selection of suitable species for an allometric scaling is essential to success. The decision on how to use the results from an allometry should be made accordingly.

Careful examination of the data from each species and their contribution to an overall outcome of allometric scaling is a good practice and should be adapted even if other information may not be readily available at the time. For example, check the correlation coefficient[2,3,10] that is a robust index of proposed correlation, to identify if there is any "outlire" species. Watch for the data set that generates a very high exponent value and seems not to fit into the basic biological assumption.[8] For example, check if the compound has much lower clearance in the mouse even than that in the monkey or dog. This relationship is apparently against the basis of allometry that smaller species should have a higher metabolic rate. An unreasonable low mouse clearance could likely result in an overestimation of the human clearance. The results, in this case, should be questioned and compared to the results from other methods. Surrounding data in the circumstances, such as the metabolic and elimination mechanism in related species, should be investigated.

Successful allometry usually depends on numerous factors including data quality, the number of species, and the number of individuals in each species used in the extrapolation, the similarity of the species used to human in terms of drug metabolizing enzymes and drug transporters that best related to the disposition of the compound. It is critical to identify appropriate scaling factors and correction methods based on the relationship of the data and other available information. Several publications are available with successful examples to enrich our experiences vicariously. The reality is we do not know if we did a good job or not before FTIH trial. The bottom line is to keep the biological assumption in mind, interpret and use the results properly, and strategically.

Several other approaches based on similar biological assumptions are also very interesting. Dedrick published his theories and scale-up approach in the early 1970s.[6] By using the scale-up theory from chemical engineering and based on physiological compartmental model, the author introduced the concept of using a chronological clock for different species. The author examined the PKs of several agents including methotrexate, thiopental, and cytosine arabinoside in several species. The PKs of these agents in the animals was very similar to that in humans when the concentration-time profiles were normalized by chronological time.[5] These works actually became the foundation of allometric scaling.

Wajima et al.[11] extended the successful experience further. The study normalized the concentration–time profile from an animal species by normalizing the concentration range using Css (concentration at steady state) and time domain by MRT (mean residence time). The C_{ss} and MRT estimates for humans were derived from the PKs obtained in animal species and an *in silico* model. The results were very interesting for the antibiotics investigated in the studies, namely, cefizoxime, cefodizime, cefotetan, and cefmenoxime.

These approaches can be readily applied with the concept of compartmental PK models (Chapter 2) and may provide more detailed information, such as the concentration–time profile. More values could be brought into the extrapolation from animal species and prediction of human PKs. Nonetheless, these models have not been popularly used in drug discovery and early development. The number of animals, number of samples, and selection of time points are very often limited due to experimental design and the knowledge about the test compound at the time. The quality and details of PK profiles in animal species in early discovery and development are also critical for being used in more complex models. The PK profiles derived from small animals sometimes depends on composite sampling, which is arguably a true representation of the PK profile. Insufficient information in earlier drug discovery could be one of the hurdles on employing more sophisticated modeling and mathematical manipulations.

7.3 INTRINSIC CLEARANCE

7.3.1 Measurement of Metabolic Capability

Hepatic metabolic clearance plays an important role in the elimination of most drugs or xenobiotics from the circulation. A correlation between *in vivo* clearance and the intrinsic capability of hepatic metabolism was first demonstrated by Rane et al.[12] in the rat. The value of intrinsic metabolizing capability was determined using enzyme kinetic parameters derived from incubations with 9000-g supernatant of liver homogenate. The enzyme kinetics follows Michaelis-Menten relationship defined by maximum reaction rate (V_{max}) and Michaelis-Menten constant (K_m) which is the concentration of substrate at one half V_{max}.

Under proposed linear conditions, intrinsic clearance[13] is defined as,

$$CL_{int} = V_{max}/K_m = \text{Rate of metabolism/CE}$$

where CL_{int} is intrinsic clearance; CE is the substrate concentration at the site of enzymatic reaction.

Intrinsic clearance is a pure *in vitro* measurement of enzymatic activities toward its substrate assuming there is no physiological limitation, such as hepatic blood flow or drug binding within the blood matrix. The 9000-g incubation system is actually a multienzyme system containing cytochrome P450s in the microsomes, and soluble cytosolic enzymes (we will discuss briefly the difference of different preparation in following paragraphs). Therefore, K_m should be viewed as an apparent value from an enzymology point of view.

A conventional method for determining K_m values is made by assessing the rate of product (metabolite) formation at several substrate concentrations. In order to accomplish this, quantitative and qualitative assays are required for the measurement of metabolite concentrations from *in vitro* matrices. Such analytical methods themselves require that metabolites be definitively identified and authentic standards prepared. These methods and standards may be feasibly obtained during the late phase of drug development; they are not readily obtainable for each of the thousands of compounds typically studied in early drug discovery. For alternatives in drug discovery, overall intrinsic clearance estimates can be obtained by monitoring substrate loss versus time using the *in vitro* half-life approach.[14,15] This approach involves measurement of substrate consumption at a single low concentration ($<K_m$ is preferred). This simple experimental design yields an estimate of CL_{int}, but not truly the V_{max}/K_m.

Typically for CL_{int} studies, a 0.5-μM test compound is incubated at 37 °C for 30 min in case of microsomes (may be up to 4 h for hepatocytes) in a pH-buffered medium containing either 0.5-mg microsomal proteins/mL or 0.2 million hepatocytes/mL incubation. Microsomal incubation additionally needs a reduced nicotinamide adenine dinucleotide phosphate (NADPH) generating system to start the reaction. At a designated time interval, aliquots are removed and quenched in a stop solution. The test compound is quantified in sample aliquots by liquid chromatography/tandem mass spectrometry (LC-MS/MS) analysis. Intrinsic clearance values are determined from the first-order elimination constant by nonlinear regression analysis.

Microsomal and hepatocyte CL_{int} are most commonly used in pre-clinical drug discovery to assess the metabolic stability of new chemical entities (NCEs). Microsomal preparation mainly contains the cyto-chrome P450s. The intrinsic clearance in microsomes is expressed as a micro L/min/mg microsomal protein. Fresh hepatocyte suspension is another commonly used system for the estimation of CL_{int}. The hepa-tocyte preparation preserves all the enzymes and cellular structures. It may be a better system to test Phase-II metabolism (see also related information in Chapters 2 and 5). In a case where the hepatocyte system is used, CL_{int} can be expressed in micro L/min/10^6 cells. These units are readily converted to a more readable format, based on the knowledge of hepatocyte counts or an average amount of microsomal proteins in a gram of liver tissue (e.g., mL/min/g liver) for making more relevant comparison with *in vivo* metabolic clearance. Most pharma-ceutical companies use empirical guidelines in drug discovery to rank order compounds during lead optimization and not for actual predic-tion of *in vivo* clearance. Generically, intrinsic clearance can be broadly classified as low (0.5–5 mL/min/g liver), moderate (5–8 mL/min/g liver), or high (>8 mL/min/g liver).

7.3.2 Estimation of *In Vivo* Clearance

Intrinsic clearance is a very useful index of hepatic metabolic clearance. However, overall *in vivo* hepatic clearance is not a simple function of the metabolic intrinsic clearance. There are two obstacles to overcome before we can make a valuable prediction. The first is the drug concen-tration at the site of action. Obviously, the drug concentration at the site is not readily and practically measurable. However, it is not too difficult to see that the concentration for a reasonably permeable com-pound would be proportionally related to the concentration in the circulation (e.g., blood concentration). Therefore, in most cases readily measured blood concentration can be used instead. Small molecule compounds are very often bound to plasma proteins and other proteins nonspecifically. Consequently, there is only a small portion of the com-pound free and available for the reaction (being permeable into the hepatocytes or reaching the enzymes). The importance of plasma protein binding in drug metabolism and PKs has been thoroughly dis-cussed in Chapter 6. In addition to the complexities of how readily a drug molecule can reach the reactions site, another limitation due to anatomical and physiological arrangement of the liver needs to be reflected. About a quarter of total cardiac output of the blood goes through the liver via the portal vein and hepatic artery. Inside the liver, the hepatocytes are arranged linearly in an array of ~18–20 hepatocytes in a sinusoidal space.[16] The liver is the most highly perfused organ; each hepatocyte is in contact with the capillaries by at least two faces if it is considered as a cube.[17]

Several mathematical models are established using such measured CL_{int} to predict the *in vivo* metabolic clearance. A "well-stirred" model was established by Rowland et al.[18]. As mentioned above, the liver is highly perfused and every hepatocyte is in direct contact with the capillaries (in the sinusoids). The organ could be imagined as a well-stirred system containing drug and metabolizing enzymes. A physiological limiting factor is then the blood flow to the organ, which brings the drug into this imaginary reactor. The relationship of CL_{int} and *in vivo* metabolic clearance is therefore defined with the consideration of all these factors

$$CL_H = \frac{Q_{H,B} \times f_u \times CL_{int}}{Q_{H,B} + f_u \times CL_{int}}$$

where CL_H is the predicted hepatic metabolic clearance; $Q_{H,B}$ is the hepatic blood flow; f_u is the unbound fraction of the drug in the system, which can be represented by the unbound fraction of the drug in the blood.

Note that by definition this equation uses total hepatic blood flow, and predicts hepatic blood clearance. Due to historical and practical reasons plasma or serum drug concentration are usually measured from *in vivo* samples for PK analysis. A such determined plasma or serum clearance was sometimes mistakenly used to compare with estimated hepatic blood clearance, CL_H, without an appropriate correction by the blood partitioning factor.[19] Unbound fraction, f_u, is often measured in separated plasma in *in vitro* systems (Chapter 6). The value of such an *in vitro* determined free-fraction may not truly represent an actual value in blood *in vivo*.

Other models to predict *in vivo* clearance also are developed based on the consideration of the sinusoidal structure in the liver, such as the parallel tube model[20,21] and the dispersion model.[22] Ito and Houston[23] compared three different models and concluded that there is little evidence to show one model being superior to the others. The "well-stirred" model probably is used more often only due to its conceptual and mathematical simplicity.

7.3.3 Discussions

There have always been some discussions on which system, as microsomes versus hepatocytes, should be used to generate the CL_{int} data, or would result in a better prediction for *in vivo* metabolic clearance. There is no doubt that isolated hepatocyte preserves Phase-II drug metabolizing enzymes and cellular integrity in addition to CYP enzymes. Ito and Houston[23] also compared the prediction using hepatocyte and microsomal intrinsic clearance. Based on rat data for a set of ~30 compounds, the hepatocyte data seemed to yield a slightly better prediction. When the correlation was examined against a larger set of lead molecules, the prediction using hepatocyte data was arguably different from that obtained using microsomal data in the mouse and rat.[24] For marketed agents, Zuegge et al.[25] studied 22 extensively metabolized compounds and compared the results with observed clinical *in vivo* data. The results suggested that hepatocyte data might provide better prediction than microsomal data. From a practical standpoint, however, it should be realized that the source and the quality of fresh human hepatocytes could be variable. Interindividual variability may affect the result significantly, especially for those compounds that are a specific substrate of certain CYP isoformes[26] with known polymorphism or variable expressions. To generate a set of reasonably reproducible data using the hepatocytes from different donors is sometimes quite challenging. Baring with this concern, cryopreserved human hepatocytes do have some advantages. Same batch of pooled hepatocytes from several donors can be tested and used in many experiments. The results are more representative of the general population and are repeatable. Nonetheless, whether all cellular functions and enzyme activities are reasonably preserved in the cryopreserved hepatocyte is yet quite debatable.

The use of *in vitro* CL_{int} to predict *in vivo* clearance remains a challenging task. For preclinical evaluation of developability for a drug candidate, conducting experiments for CL_{int} in multiple species using both microsomes and hepatocytes is a common practice in many drug companies.[2,3] The underlining thought of such a practice is to hope that if a good *in vitro–in vivo* correlation or prediction can be observed in the preclinical species for a compound of interest, the prediction of human *in vivo* clearance could be done with a little more confidence by using the *in vitro* data generated in the same way. This kind of thought has been popularly accepted though it lacks strong support from vigorously designed and conducted research. Naritomi et al.[27] carefully investigated the prediction of hepatic metabolic clearances for eight marketed agents. It seemed that if hepatic metabolism is the major elimination pathway the results from prediction were quite encouraging. However, the information on whether a compound will be mainly metabolically cleared *in vivo* may neither be readily available before running the clinical trials, nor reliably predictable based on limited preclinical data. When a much larger data set (>100 agents) of published *in vitro* intrinsic clearance of marketed agents was investigated,[28] the results highlighted the paucity and variability of the prediction. It clearly exposed the limitation of *in vivo–in vitro* prediction for a decision-making purpose. McIntyre et al.[24] raised this concern in the process of lead optimization. Any too large false-negative predictions would potentially risk deselecting or down prioritizing a potentially developable compound, which may not be affordable or acceptable at this stage of the game. An accurate prediction of hepatic metabolic clearance in human in the perspectives relies on many factors. One must pay close attention to surrounding data and PK properties of the test compounds. The decision of whether a drug candidate will be further developed should never be made based on a single predicted factor.

7.4 PREDICTION OF "FIRST TIME IN HUMAN DOSE"

The prediction of FTIH dose based on preclinical *in vivo* and *in vitro* data has been clearly outlined in an FDA guidance.[1] In this section, our intention is only to bring this into the context of discussions related to allometric scaling and prediction of metabolic clearance. The following discussion is to exemplify the thinking process in the evaluation of developability rather than preparation for a clinical trial. For the latter purpose, one should carefully follow the FDA guidelines.

In the late stage of lead optimization in drug discovery, a pharmaceutical R&D organization will have to carefully examine the chance of success for proposed drug candidates. Here is an example that hopefully will help us to see these sophisticated thinking processes. Using the efficacious exposure in animal disease models and predicted human clearance from the above stated approaches, we can estimate a range of human efficacious doses if we assume that similar exposure in human would likely result in clinical efficacy.

In Chapter 2, we learned that

$$\text{Clearance} = \text{Dose}/\text{AUC}$$

Rearrange the equation and replace AUC with efficacious exposure (AUC_{eff}) from an animal pharmacological model, and clearance with predicted human clearances (CL_{pred}) we can estimate a human efficacious dose.

$$Dose = CL_{pred} \times AUC_{eff}$$

For a nonparental administered drug, the proportion absorbed or delivered should be considered,

$$Dose = CL_{pred} \times AUC_{eff}/F$$

where bioavailability, F, is the fraction of the dose being absorbed from nonparental route. The value could be estimated from preclinical PK studies.

A human equivalent efficacious dose (HED) can also be estimated from the animal model,

$$HED = \text{Animal efficacious dose} \\ \times (\text{animal body weight}/\text{human body weight})^{0.33}$$

(for reference see FDA guidance 2005[1] and Mahmood et al.[7])

From the fact that the calculations were based on allometric scaling and/or predicted human metabolic clearance, and an assumption that the results from animal models can be extrapolated to humans pharmacologically, we extend the predicted information to check how well we have done with an integrated consideration of potency and PKs in lead optimization processes.

REFERENCES

1. US Food and Drug Administration. Guidance for industry. Estimating the maximum safe starting dose in initial clinical trial for therapeutics in adult healthy volunteers. July **2005**.
2. Davis, C. B.; Bambal, R.; Moorthy, G. S.; Hugger, E.; Xiang, H.; Park, B. K.; Shone, A. E.; O'Neill, P. M.; Ward, S. A. *J. Pharm. Sci.* **2009**, 98, 362–377.
3. Xiang, H.; McSurdy-Freed, J.; Subbanagounder, G.; Hugger, E.; Bambal, R.; Han, C.; Ferrer, S.; Gargallo, D.; Davis, C. B. *J. Pharma. Sci.* **2006**, 95 (12): 2657–2672.
4. Davies, B.; Morris, T. *Pharm. Res.* **1993**, 10, 1093–1095.

5. Mordenti, J. *J. Pharm. Sci.* **1986**, 75, 1028–1040.
6. Dedrick, R. L. *J. Pharmacokinet. Biopharm.* **1973**, 1, 435–461.
7. Mahmood, I.; Green, M. D.; Fisher, J. E. *J. Clin. Pharmacol.* **2003**, 43, 692–967.
8. Mahmood, I. *J. Pharm. Sci.* **2004**, 93, 177–185.
9. Mahmood, I.; Sahajwalla, C. *J. Pharm. Sci.* **2002**, 91, 1908–1914.
10. Hassard, T. H. *Understanding Biostatistics.* Mosby Year Book. Toronto. **1991**, 121–151.
11. Wajima, T.; Yano, Y.; Fkumura, K.; Oguma, T. *J. Pharm. Sci.* **2004**, 93, 1890–1900.
12. Rane, A.; Wilkinson, G. R.; Shand, D. G. *J. Pharmacol. Exp. Ther.* **1977**, 200, 420–424.
13. Houston, J. B. *Biochem. Pharmacol.* **1994**, 47, 1469–1479.
14. Obach, R. S. *Drug Metab. Dispos.* **1997**, 25, 1359–1369.
15. Obach, R. S. *Drug Metab. Dispos.* **1999**, 27, 1350–1359.
16. Greenway, C. V.; Stark, R. D. *Physiol. Rev.* **1971**, 51, 23–65.
17. Greenway, C. V.; Lautt, W. W. in *Handbook of Physiology—The Gastrointestinal System.* Eds. Schultz, S. G.; Wood, J. D.; Rauner, B. B. **1989**, Chapt. 41, 1519–1564, Oxford University Press.
18. Rowland, M.; Benet, L. Z.; Graham, G. G. *J. Pharmacokinet. Biopharm.* **1973**, 1, 123–136.
19. Yang, J.; Jamei, M.; Yeo, K. R.; Rostami-Hodjegan, A.; Tucker, G. T. *Drug Metab. Dispos.* **2007**, 35, 501–502.
20. Winkler, K.; Keiding, S.; Tygstrup, N. in *The Liver. Quantitative Aspects of Structure and Function.* Eds. Paumgartner, G.; Preisig, R. **1973**, 144–155, Karger.
21. Pang, K. S.; Rowland, M. Parts I-III. *J. Pharmacokinet. Biopharm.* **1977**, 5, 625–699.
22. Roberts, M. S.; Rowland, M. *J. Pharm. Sci.* **1985**, 74, 585–587.
23. Ito, K.; Houston, J. B. *Pharm. Res.* **2004**, 21, 785–792.
24. Mcintyre, T. A.; Han, C.; Xiang, H.; Bambal, R.; Davis, C. B. *Xenobiotica* **2008**, 38, 605–619.
25. Zuegge, J.; Schneider, G.; Coassolo, P.; Lavé, T. *Clin. Pharmacokinet.* **2001**, 40, 553–563.
26. McHugh, C. F.; Davis, C. B.; Bambal, R. B.; Nguyen, D.; Jiang, D. X.; Bulgarelli, J.; McSurdy-Freed, J. E. *Comparison of Intrinsic Clearance of Novel-Antimicrobial Leads in Individual Human Liver Microsomes* AAPS Conference on Critical Issues in Discovering Quality Clinical Candidates, Philadelphia, **2006**.
27. Naritomi, Y.; Terashita, S.; Kimura, S.; Suzuki A.; Kagayama, A.; Sugiyama, Y. *Drug Metab. Dispos.* **2001**, 29, 1316–1324.
28. Nagilla, R.; Frank, K. A.; Jolivette, L. J.; Ward, K. W. *J. Pharmacol. Toxicol. Methods* **2005**, 52, 22–29.

PART II

INTEGRATION OF PHARMACEUTICAL DEVELOPMENT INTO DRUG DISCOVERY

CHAPTER 8

PHARMACEUTICS DEVELOPABILITY ASSESSMENT

LIAN HUANG, JINQUAN DONG, and SHYAM KARKI

Johnson & Johnson PRD, Raritan, NJ

Evaluation of Drug Candidates for Preclinical Development: Pharmacokinetics, Metabolism, Pharmaceutics, and Toxicology, Edited by Chao Han, Charles B. Davis, and Binghe Wang
Copyright © 2010 John Wiley & Sons, Inc.

8.1 INTRODUCTION

For over a decade, pharmaceutical companies have invested significant development effort into drug discovery programs to profile biopharmaceutical and pharmaceutical properties early for a lead compound. By doing so, certain desirable properties can be incorporated into molecular design so that the lead compounds that are most likely to survive in the development pipeline can be selected.[1-3] However, despite the research and development spending in the pharmaceutical industry had doubled from 1996 to 2004, the number of new drugs approved by the Food and Drug Administration (FDA) has fallen by more than one-half since 1996.[4] The attrition rate still remains high (89%) for the 10 biggest drug companies during 1991–2000.[5] A significant percentage of new chemical entities (NCEs) in clinical development does not reach the market because of insufficient properties related to physicochemical parameters like solubility, pK_a, log P, permeability, stability, crystallinity, hygroscopicity, particle size distribution, or surface area.[6,7] Despite increasingly sophisticated formulation approaches, deficiencies in physicochemical properties may represent the difference between failure and the development of a successful oral drug product. Consequently, physicochemical parameters have been incorporated into drug discovery programs, along with other properties, to rank the lead compounds and filter out unsuitable compounds.

A successful assessment of pharmaceutical developability not only includes generating the physicochemical properties, but also requires scientists with cross-functional knowledge and an overall picture of the development process to understand the impact of these properties on future development of this compound. It is extremely important to understand that the developability is compound specific and simple selection of a drug candidate by using a set of developability criteria could eliminate a potential billion dollar product. This chapter will focus on the most fundamental physicochemical properties of a drug candidate and discuss the considerations in utilizing these properties to assess the pharmaceutical developability so that a drug candidate with good "developability" characteristics can be nominated.

8.2 IMPACTS OF SOLUBILITY ON DEVELOPABILITY

Solubility is one of the key physicochemical properties of a new molecule that needs to be assessed and understood very early on in the drug discovery and drug candidate selection process, since only dissolved drug molecules in physiological intestinal fluids can be absorbed with oral delivery. The aqueous solubility is correlated with the solubility in the intestinal fluids, and therefore has potential contribution to bioavailability issues. A drug candidate with poor water solubility or dissolution rate can cause low and variable bioavailability, have more potential for food effect, and create challenges to deliver high doses for toxicological studies and develop parental formulations. Although the evolving formulation technologies have allowed many poorly water-soluble candidates to become the successful drug products, the cost and time spent in overcoming the bioavailability issue associated with poor water solubility could be overwhelming, and the attrition rate can be high.

The minimum solubility requirement for a drug candidate is dependent on therapeutic dose and permeability of the compound based on the Maximum Absorbable Dose (MAD) approach.[8] The MAD value is essentially the quantity of drug that could be absorbed for oral dosage forms. However, the MAD value should not be taken as an accurate absolute value for the absorbable dose. Rather, it can serve to assess the developability of the drug candidates. If the dose for a drug entering development is projected to be greater than the MAD value, incomplete absorption should be expected and additional formulation resources to the development team may be assigned. The MAD concept also provides a tool for rank ordering a series of potential drug candidates, for identifying the source of low absorption in a series of potential candidates, and for setting physical chemical targets for the medicinal chemists.[9] For a 1 mg/kg clinical dose that we commonly encountered, if a compound has a moderate permeability, solubility requirement is ~50 μg/mL; if the permeability is low, the solubility requirement increases to ~200 μg/mL. For a highly permeable compound, then a solubility of ~10 μg/mL is acceptable. The minimum acceptable solubility proportionally increases as the projected clinical dose increases.[10]

However, there are some examples of successful drug products on the market with poor-water solubility. One of the examples is Zocor (Simvastatin), a cholesterol lowering product, which is practically insoluble in water. About 68% of 123 oral drugs in immediate-release dosage forms on the World Health Organization (WHO) Essential Drug List have poor water solubility. Similar percentage holds true for the top 200 prescribed oral products in the United States.[11]

8.2.1 Solubility and Dissolution Rate

Solubility is an intrinsic material property that can only be influenced by change in crystalline forms and/or chemical modifications of the molecule, such as salt, complex, prodrug, or cocrystal formation. In contrast, dissolution is an extrinsic material property that can be influenced by various chemical, physical, or crystallographic means like complexation, particle size, surface properties, solid-state modification, or solubilization enhancing formulation strategies. The drug dissolution rate is described by the Noyes–Whitney equation:

$$dC/dt = (C_s - C) \cdot D \cdot S/h$$

where dC/dt is the dissolution rate, D is the diffusion coefficient, S is the surface area, h is the diffusion layer thickness, C_s is the saturated solubility, and C is the concentration of the drug in bulk solution. Apparently, factors such as drug diffusion coefficient, surface areas, diffusion layer thickness, saturation solubility, as well as the concentration of the drug in bulk solution all play their roles in the drug dissolution. It is clear that the dissolution rate determines the concentration of the drug in the gastrointestinal (GI) tract. However, this concentration is limited by solubility. High solubility and permeability are essential for a drug to have a good bioavailability. For drugs with high permeability, a high dissolution rate could enhance drug absorption by ensuring near saturated solubility of drug in the GI tract. Compounds with low solubility can still have good bioavailability if they have a high dissolution rate and can be readily absorbed so that the absorption will not be solubility limited, especially for low dose compounds. On the other hand, a compound with high solubility administrated in an oral solid dosage form is not guaranteed to have good bioavailability if its dissolution rate is very low. The dissolution rate issue usually can be mitigated using formulation approaches, such as solution formulation to remove the dissolution step, therefore, to eliminate the dissolution rate limiting step, particle size reduction to increase the surface area of the drug substance, and so on. For a truly solubility limited absorption, the formulation strategy should focus on not only increasing solubility in the dosage form, such as using co-solvents, complexations, and lipid-based formulations, but also inhibiting precipitation in the GI tract by adding surfactants and polymers in the formulations. So, formulation strategy should be based on what is the limiting factor for absorption, i.e. dissolution rate versus solubility limited absorption. An animal pharmacokinetics (PK) screening of comparing the exposures from suspension formulations with different particle size or suspension versus solution formulation can usually help us to understand if the poor bioavailability is caused by solubility limited absorption or dissolution rate-limited absorption.[12]

8.2.2 Impact of Solid-State Properties on Solubility

By definition, solubility is the concentration of the solute in a solution that is in equilibrium with the solute phase. The ability of a pharmaceutical solid to dissolve in a physiological fluid strongly depends on the crystal lattice energy of the solid. When the attraction force between the solute and solvent molecules overcomes the attractive force between the solute molecule and its neighboring solute molecule, the solute molecule is pulled into solution. Since lattice energies of physical forms (amorphous, polymorphs, or solvates) are responsible for the difference in solubilities and dissolution rates, the largest difference in solubility is observed between amorphous and crystalline materials.[13] The solubility difference between different polymorphs is typically <10 times, whereas the difference between amorphous and crystalline material can be up to several hundred times.[14] In the majority of cases, the solubility ratios of polymorphs (each form relative to the least soluble form) were <2 and the anhydrous forms were more soluble in aqueous media than the corresponding hydrate forms. The crystallinity of the compound contributes to many properties, including solubility and dissolution rate. However, the extent of impact of solubility on bioavailability of polymorphs is almost impossible to predict.[15] At the discovery stage, programs frequently yield amorphous compounds due to time pressures and the methods used to isolate them on small scales. The limited availability of a compound and the form changes from batch to batch create challenges for developability assessment. It is important to monitor the forms used in the early studies using a polarized light microscope or pXRD, and it is essential to report form information along with the solubility so that a proper developability assessment can be made.

Solubility experiments are often described using the terms "kinetic solubility" and "thermodynamic (equilibrium) solubility". The methods most often used in determining solubility in discovery and preformulation will be briefly summarized below.

8.2.3 Solubility Measurements

8.2.3.1 Shake-Flask Method. Solubility measurements using the shake-flask method are largely a labor-intensive procedure, and require long equilibration times of from 4h to several days. Usually, a 24-h equilibrium time is sufficient. Results obtained using this approach are "thermodynamic solubility". The compound is added to a standard buffer solution (in a flask) and the suspension is shaken as equilibration between the two phases is established. After filtration with microfilters or centrifugation, the concentration of the compound in the supernatant solution is then determined using an ultraviolet–visible (UV–Vis) spectroscopic method or high-performance liquid chromatography (HPLC) with UV detection. A solubility–pH profile can be obtained by repeating the measurement in parallel in several different pH buffers. The final pH of the supernatant depends on the buffering capacity of the buffer used, as well as the amount of drug dissolved, and is frequently recorded.

Determination of thermodynamic solubility is required in preformulation studies conducted after a compound has been selected as a lead. The traditional shake-flask method is widely used for this purpose.

8.2.3.2 Turbidity-Based Determination.

This method generates what is usually called "kinetic solubility". The method, popularized by Lipinski and others,[16–18] in part have met some high-throughput needs of drug discovery research. The turbidimetric method was developed to determine kinetic solubilities for NCE screening purposes, as it reduces the time and sample consumption when estimates of solubilities are needed instead of accurate values.[19] For turbidity-based determination, the compound is first completely dissolved in dimethyl sulfoxide (DMSO), or another suitable organic solvent, and then a small volume is added to an aqueous buffer. Turbidity due to formation of precipitates causes a change in the UV/Vis absorbance, and the inflection point in the absorbance curve can be used to estimate solute concentration at saturation. The appearance of precipitate is kinetically driven; therefore, there is a requirement for stepwise addition of solute to avoid false precipitation that could occur upon rapid addition.

The turbidity approach, although not thermodynamically rigorous, is generally used to rank molecules according to expected solubility. The first appearance of a precipitate is kinetically controlled. A multitude of polymorphic and/or amorphous forms of the same compound can be formed during solubility determination, and they can interconvert depending on solution conditions and time scales.[20] The strengths of the turbidity method are its speed and the small amount of drug candidate required, both of which make it suitable for high-throughput drug discovery screening. The shortcomings of the turbidity methodology are (1) poor reproducibility for very sparingly water-soluble compounds, (2) use of excessive amounts (>1% v/v) of DMSO in the analyte addition step, and (3) lack of standardization of practice.[20]

8.2.3.3 Potentiometric Method.

The potentiometric method[2,16,21] is more for a preformulation setting than a high-throughput discovery setting. An entire solubility–pH profile is deduced from the assay. The intrinsic solubility can be deduced by inspection of the titration curves, applying the relationship.[22] The approach usually takes several hours for a solubility determination; therefore, it is not commonly used in drug discovery labs. The pH of an aqueous solution of a compound is measured as equivalents of acid or base are added. Because UV absorption by a chromophore is affected by an ionizable center that is within a few bonds of the chromophore, the UV absorption varies with pH and is recorded using a diode array UV detector. The difference spectrum from the compound titration and a blank aqueous titration indicates the $pK_a(s)$ of a compound. When solubility of the compound in aqueous media is insufficient, cosolvents are added and titration at three cosolvent concentrations allows back-extrapolation to zero cosolvent concentration.

The potentiometric method eliminates the limitations of the shake flask (different buffer species used to maintain pH) and the turbidimetric methods (kinetic solubility). For a basic drug candidate, HCl was usually used for pH control regardless of its salt form since the chloride ion is the dominant anion throughout the GI tract. Therefore, the pH solubility behavior of the drug candidate in regions where the K_{sp} of the salt dominates solubility will be closer to the physiological conditions.

Since these "kinetic" solubility methods do not take into account the contribution of the crystalline lattice energy to solubility, whether a good correlation with the equilibrium method is really compound specific. For compounds that are not soluble due to high crystallinity, it is obvious that "kinetic" solubility will most likely differ significantly from equilibrium solubility. On the other hand, for compounds that are not soluble in water due to high lipiphilicity, the difference between the "kinetic" and equilibrium solubility may be smaller. The significance in differences in solubility results by different methods is obvious and difficult to predict. The "kinetic" solubility is not an intrinsic property of drug molecules. With the advancement in automation, the throughput of measurement for equilibrium solubility may not necessarily be a bottleneck in supporting lead optimization.[14]

8.2.3.4 pH Solubility Profile.

The solubility of the substance in an aqueous system is dependent on several factors, including composition of the aqueous media, temperature, pH, solid state (amorphous, crystalline, polymorph), counterions (salt formation), and ionic strength. Rather than single point determinations, a solubility profile of the substance is required to identify potential issues for drug precipitation *in vivo*. The pH profiling for weakly basic salts is especially of critical importance as their solubility will vary in the intestinal pH (typically pH 1–8) and precipitation may occur. The pH profiling should be performed in different biorelevant buffer systems to mimic the high concentrations of the most common counterions of pharmaceutical salts in gastrointestinal (GI) fluids. Organic counterions may increase aqueous solubility through decreased crystal lattice energy, lowered melting point, and increased hydrogen bonding of the salt counterions with water.[20] Consequently, different buffer systems may yield very different solubility values at a specific pH. The solubility profiling should also include any other bio-relevant dissolution media, like simulated gastric fluid (SGF) with and without enzymes, fasted-state simulated intestinal fluid (FaSSIF), and fed-state simulated intestinal fluid (FeSSIF) at pH 5.0 and 6.5.[23] This approach allows detection of a potential counterion exchange and formation of more stable–less soluble salts of a molecule that will lead to precipitation *in vivo*. The pH profile additionally provides the basic guidance to choose the right approach among potential solubilization strategies. Conversion of the molecule to other salts or hydrates needs to be taken into account and evaluated in the solubility profiling. Different salts of the substance can be formed dependent on the buffer systems, as well as their ionic strength.

Typical solubility media for drug candidate profiling can be found in Table 8.1.

In general, certain things must be considered in solubility determinations. These are (1) the purity of both the dissolved substance and the solvent must be high, (2) a constant temperature must be maintained, (3) complete saturation must be attained, and (4) accurate quantitative analysis of the saturated solution and correct expression of the results are imperative. It is important to characterize the solid state (precipitates) in equilibrium with solution during solubility determination.[24] Powder X-ray diffraction, Raman spectroscopy, infrared (IR), micros-

TABLE 8.1. Typical Solubility Media for Drug Candidate Profiling

0.1 N HCl
0.1 N NaOH
Buffers at pH 2, 4, 6, 8, 10; or titration method
Water (to equilibrium)
0.5% Methocel
SIF with or without enzyme
SGF with or without enzyme
FassIF
FessIF
20% HPßCD

copy [polarized light microscopy, environmental scanning electron microscopy (ESEM)], and thermal analysis are typically used for solid-state characterization.

Adveef[16] pointed out that certain surface-active compounds, when dissolved in water under conditions of saturation, form self-associated aggregates or micelles, which can interfere with the determination of the true aqueous solubility and the pK_a of the compound. When the compounds are very sparingly soluble in water, additives can be used to enhance the rate of dissolution.[24] If measurements are done in the presence of simple surfactants, bile salts, complexing agents (e.g., cyclodextrins or ion-pair forming counterions), extensive considerations need to be applied in attempting to extract the true aqueous solubility from the data.[16]

8.2.4 Determination of Dissolution–Solubility Limiting Absorption

Poor solubility of drug candidates can often be mitigated though various formulation strategies, including particle size reduction, salt formulation, cocrystals, solid dispersions, lyophilization, complexations with cyclodextrin, emulsions, cosolvent systems, and liposomes.

To support the early drug discovery program, experimental formulations are developed and studied for solubility and short-term stability. When aqueous solubility or dissolution of the substance is identified as an issue for the *in vitro* and *in vivo* testing, simple and effective formulation strategies are applied to secure the expected drug deposition in the *in vitro* and *in vivo* trials.

Particle size reduction is one of the first strategies to be investigated. Wet milling is used for particle size reduction and a particle size of ~200 nm is readily achievable. Should particle size reduction not lead to the expected concentration in the *in vitro* assay or *in vivo* exposure, formulations with solubilizing agents like cyclodextrins or micellar systems are evaluated. Other systems that are used are solvent- and surfactant-based formulations (e.g., microemulsions) or solid dispersions. These latter systems require substantial development times and might be limited due to potential excipient-related toxicity or unwanted effects on the test system.

General study design to access if the absorption is dissolution rate or solubility limiting is outlined in Table 8.2. Tier 1 studies are designed to have an initial PK reading on a particular compound. Typical PK parameters including oral bioavailability, C_{max}, T_{max}, $t_{1/2}$, distribution volume and system clearance of the compound are generally obtained

TABLE 8.2. Study Design for Biopharmaceutical Evaluation

	Test Arm	Routes[a]	Test Designs, (mg/kg)
Tier 1, initial PK	1	iv	Solution, (2)
	2	po	Solution, (10)
Tier 2, dissolution limiting?	3	po	Suspension, (10)
	4	po	Suspension (micronized), (10)
	5	po	Suspension (salts), (10)
Tier 3, solubility limiting?	6	po	Suspension, (10)
	7	po	Suspension, (25)
	8	po	Suspension, (100)

[a]Intravenous = iv.
[b]Peroral = po.

through Tier 1 tests. Detailed definitions and their interpretations have been discussed in Chapter 2. Tier 2 studies, comparing the PK results for the compound before and after particle size reduction, are designed to assess if dissolution rate is a limiting absorption. In this Tier 2 study, various salts are also tested in order to study if there is any advantage over the neutral form of the compound. Tier 3 studies are designed to examine if the compound exhibits solubility-limiting adsorption, which is typically evidenced by less than linear dose-proportional response in absorption or saturation. The *in vivo* experiments also help to evaluate the overall physicochemical properties, which will be further discussed in Chapter 9, in addition to the solubility. This approach will also provide very important information to other development functional areas, for example, designing the safety assessment study, which also will be discussed later in a related section.

Indeed, solubility is one of the most important pharmaceutical properties for a drug candidate. The solubility of an NCE will directly affect the probability of success in the future developments of a chemical entity, as it will influence *in vivo* PK performance, safety assessment, formulation, and even the designing of first time in human trial.

8.3 THE pK_a

More than 60% of marketed drugs are weak acids or bases, and can exist in either the ionized or un-ionized form, depending on the pH of the surrounding environment. The proportion of a drug that is un-ionized and thus passes easily through membranes can exert their pharmacological effect.[2,26] The pK_a is the negative logarithm of the dissociation constant of a compound and can be calculated from the Henderson–Hasselbalch equation:

$$pH = pK_a + \log[A^-]/[HA] \quad \text{(acid form)}$$

$$pH = pK_a + \log[B]/[BH^+] \quad \text{(base form)}$$

From these equations, pK_a is equal to the pH where one-half of the compound is ionized and one-half is un-ionized. The pK_a affects solubility, permeability, log D, and oral absorption by modulating the distribution of neutral and charged species. Acidic compounds tend to be more soluble and less permeable at high pH values, and basic compounds tend to be more soluble and less permeable at low pH values.

For a weak acid, an acid environment, such as is found in the stomach or in acid urine, favors the passage of drug across membranes. Therefore, a weak acid is absorbed more rapidly in the stomach than in the intestine. However, the increased absorptive area of the small intestine means that the largest total quantity of a weak acid is absorbed from the intestine rather than from the stomach. Aspirin is an acidic drug with a pK_a of 3.49. In the stomach, the pH is from 1–3; hence, most of the drug will exist in the un-ionized form and be better at passing through the lipid membranes (i.e., better absorbed at ~30% of the oral dose, the rest is absorbed in the small intestine).[27]

The *in situ* salt formation is a common practice at the discovery stage to enhance solubility for a poorly water-soluble compound and also provides information for future formulation strategies. Through consideration of the ionic equilibria of acids and bases, one may readily calculate the solubility product (K_{sp}) and the solubility of the salt formed *in situ* solely on the basis of knowledge of the pK_a value of the acid and the pK_b value of the base.[28] It has been demonstrated[29] that multiple counterions, added in predetermined amounts so as not to exceed the solubility product K_{sp} of any salt, provided significantly higher solubility than any single counterion.

In general, at the early discovery stage, only limited amounts of material are available for analytical characterization, several software packages and webserver are available for the calculation of pK_a values. Potentiometric titration[1,30] is widely used and respected for pK_a measurement, especially in development laboratories.

8.4 LIPOPHILICITY

Lipophilicity is widely used to make estimates for membrane penetration and permeability and also has significant impact on solubility and protein binding. Lipophilicity is often expressed as a partition or distribution coefficient (log P or log D) between octanol and aqueous phases. Highly lipophilic compounds (log $D > 5$) tend to have high potency due to nonspecific binding, but they are also more vulnerable to CYP450 metabolism, leading to high hepatic clearance, have low solubility, poor oral absorption, and high plasma–protein binding. A compound with moderate lipophilicity (log D 0–3) has a good balance between solubility and permeability and is optimal for oral absorption, cell membrane permeation in cell-based assays, is generally good for blood–brain barrier (BBB) penetration (optimal log D ~2), and has low metabolic liability. Hydrophilic compounds (log $D < 0$) have good solubility, but poor permeability for GI or BBB penetration, and are more susceptible to renal clearance. However, lipophilicity can be increased by increasing molecular size and decreasing hydrogen-bonding capacity.

Like pK_a, log P can also be calculated using software or an internal built *in silico* model at the discovery stage. Several high throughput methods are available for log P determination, including shake-flask,[30] and HPLC.[31] The traditional approach for determining lipophilicity is partitioning between water and octanol. When the partitioning is performed at a pH where the compound is completely in the neutral form, log P is determined. At a pH where the compound is partially ionized, log D is determined and the pH must be specified.

By using potentiometric titration, an additional feature of the GLpK_a instrument (Sirius) allows the measurement of log P, for partitioning between water and octanol. After the pK_a titration is completed, octanol is added and the sample is retitrated. Partitioning of the compound into octanol shifts the titration curve, from which the log P can be calculated.[1]

Forsamax (Aldendronate sodium) is another multi-billion dollar drug. Aldendronate sodium, the active component in Forsamax, is a white, crystalline, nonhygrosciopic powder. It is soluble in water. Unlike most drugs, the strong negative charge on the two phosphate moieties limits oral bioavailability, and in turn, the exposure to tissues other than bone is very low. As with all potent biphosphonates, low permeability of the intestinal epithelia toward highly polar and charged molecules impedes the effective absorption of many low molecular weight drugs. And its systemic bioavailability after oral dosing is low, averaging only 0.6–0.7% in women and in men under fasting conditions. Intake together with meals and beverages other than water further reduces the bioavailability. The absorbed drug rapidly partitions, with ~50% binding to the exposed bone surface; the remainder is excreted unchanged by the kidneys. However, the low permeability of Aldendronate did not prevent it from becoming a blockbuster drug.

8.5 PERMEABILITY

Permeability is an important factor for passage through cell membranes in cell-based assays, absorption through the GI tract, penetration through the BBB, and through other physiological barriers. Compounds intended for oral administration must have adequate intestinal permeability in order to achieve therapeutic concentrations. There are several transport mechanisms: transcellular passive diffusion, paracellullar, active/carrier-mediated, and efflux. The two most important pathways for drug absorption are transcellular passive diffusion and efflux transport by P-glycoprotein (Pgp) or multidrug-resistant proteins. The roles of membrane transporters in drug disposition were discussed in Chapter 3. Transcellular diffusion is driven by the concentration gradient, and is enhanced by "sink" conditions that bind (e.g., plasma protein) and remove (e.g., bloodstream) drug from the absorption side. The neutral form of the compound is the species that permeates through the membrane. Another route of drug permeation is active transport, which is mediated by transporter proteins. The extent of active transport depends on the transporter protein–ligand affinity. Active efflux opposes drug uptake and is mediated by another set of transporter proteins (e.g., Pgp). None of the high-throughput physicochemical methods for permeability can predict active influx or efflux.

Cell-based assays for permeability screening, such as Caco-2[32] for oral absorption, tend to be labor intensive, expensive, moderate throughput, and composed of multiple-transport mechanisms. Recent development of the parallel artificial membrane permeability assay (PAMPA) provides a simple, low-cost, high-throughput, and single-mechanism method for permeability screening.[1,33] Studies showed that PAMPA gave similar predictions for oral absorption as Caco-2.[6] The PAMPA measures only passive diffusion. This single mechanism process, in conjunction with cell-based permeability assays, allows the diagnosis of the root cause for poor absorption, to drive synthetic modification for property improvement. There is a trend in the industry to use PAMPA as the first line permeability screen and use the cell-based assays as secondary assays for mechanistic studies and diagnostic purposes.

The fundamental molecular components for permeability and solubility are molecular size and hydrogen-bonding capacity.[34] Changing one will affect the other. Increasing molecular weight and lipophilicity, to a certain extent, will increase permeability; however, this will decrease solubility. Increasing hydrogen-bonding capacity and charge will increase solubility; however, this will decrease permeability. So, for optimal oral absorption, the key is to find a balance between the different physicochemical properties. When the chemist has to choose between improving solubility or permeability, preference should be given to permeability, because solubility can often be improved through formulation. However, Caco-2 permeability data showed that Lipitor (Atorvastatin calcium), an annual sell of $12 billions blockbuster, has significant efflux with A to B 4.9×10^{-6} cm/s and B to A 35.6×10^{-6} cm/s. Lipitor lowers plasma cholesterol and lipoprotein levels by inhibiting HMG–CoA reductase and cholesterol synthesis in the liver and by increasing the number of hepatic low-density lipoprotein (LDL) receptors on the cell surface to enhance uptake and catabolism of LDL. Lipitor also reduces LDL production and the number of LDL particles. It also reduces LDL–C in some patients with homozygous familial hypercholesterolemia (FH), a population that rarely responds to other lipid-lowering medication(s).

8.6 STABILITY

A compound intended for oral administration needs to survive the intestinal environment and possibly the gastric environment for hours.[35] In addition, it should be stable in the solid state for years, in the final formulation and packaging. As time restrictions do not allow early stability tests to be performed in real time, accelerated stress conditions like higher temperature, increased moisture, light, and oxidative stress are usually employed. The choice of the exact set of accelerated conditions for the developability decision is a difficult balance between higher stress delivering a fast result and lower stress delivering a more reliable result. Typically, International Conference on Harmonization (ICH) accelerated conditions plus it uses higher temperatures and humidities,[36] as well as exposure to light and hydrogen peroxide (H_2O_2). These samples then need to be analyzed for their chemical and physical stability. Under normal circumstances, for candidate characterization, both solution and solid-state stabilities are evaluated.

8.6.1 Solution Stability

The choice of the accelerated stress conditions used in many descriptions of early stability tests are discussed in detail,[35] but the relevance of the analytical method used for analysis is not emphasized sufficiently. For small molecules, HPLC is the analytical technology of choice. The development of the analytical method used during preformulation and stability testing is obviously key to the quality of the overall data set. The method needs to be able to pick up degradation products from the different stress conditions, which often give qualitatively different degradation patterns. However, during late lead optimization, a well validated, stability-indicating HPLC method is not readily available. In our laboratory, a validated stability indicating method will not be available until the first GMP batch material becomes available. Therefore, a brief HPLC method development will be conducted for the purpose of pharmaceutical profiling of drug candidates. Method development usually started with a 30-min long generic gradient method with a diode-array (DAD) UV detector. Several common HPLC columns (Agilent Zorbax Eclipse XRD-C8, Waters Xetrra RP18, Supelco Discovery HS C8, etc.), are tested to evaluate their separation performances. Mobile phases are typically 0.05% TFA in water, and 0.05% TFA in acetonitrile. The mobile phase gradient, as well as detector wavelength, will be adjusted according to characteristics of the compound and its potential impurities and degradants. With the use of a DAD UV detector, the peak purity of any eluting component peak can be monitored. Usually, a working HPLC method can be developed within ~1 day with the minimum requirement that no coelution exists with the compound peak. More sophisticated techniques, such as LC/MS and automated method development systems, nowadays allow a good stability indicating method to be generated within ~1 week.[35]

For solution stability, obviously simulated biological fluids like gastric or intestinal fluids are crucial, but light and oxidation sensitivity of the compound in solution should also be determined (Table 8.3).

The aqueous solubility of a given compound needs to be considered when determining its stability in solution. Only the dissolved part of a molecule will be significantly stressed by the medium used, that is, the solution stability of poorly soluble compounds can easily be dramatically overestimated, if no cosolvent is used to increase the amount of compound dissolved. A 0.02-mg/mL sample of compound concentration is usually recommended. For compounds with limited aqueous

TABLE 8.3. Typical Solution Stability Conditions for Drug Candidate Profiling

Media	Test Conditions (24 h)
0.1*N* HCl	Ambient and 60 °C
0.1*N* NaOH	Ambient and 60 °C
Profile at pH 2, 4, 6, 8, 10	Ambient and 60 °C
SIF	Ambient and 60 °C
SGF	Ambient and 60 °C
FaSSIF	Ambient and 60 °C
FeSSIF	Ambient and 60 °C
Photostability	Ambient, bench
Peroxides	Ambient and 60 °C
Metal ions	Ambient and 60 °C

solubility, mixtures of water and an organic solvent are employed. In our laboratory, a maximum sample of 60% acetonitrile in water is used for this purpose. Aqueous solutions of 0.1 *N* HCl and 0.1 *N* NaOH are usually used for acid and base stress on drug candidates.

Photostability was usually performed by exposing the solution to ambient light, in accordance with ICH photostability guidelines.[37] The recommended exposures for confirmatory stability studies are an overall illumination of not <1.2 million lux hours and an integrated near-UV energy of not <200 W·h/m^2. For forced degradation studies, the samples should be exposed to at least two times the ICH exposure length to ensure adequate exposure of the sample.

Oxidation degradation can take place under an oxygen atmosphere or in the presence of peroxides. Free radical initiators may be used to accelerate oxidation. Generally, a free radical initiator and peroxide will produce all primary oxidation degradation products observed on real-time stability. For peroxide conditions, hydrogen peroxide reagent (up to 3%) can be used. The addition of metal ions to solutions of compound can indicate whether there is a tendency for the compound to be catalytically oxidized. Iron and copper ions are routinely found in compounds and formulation excipients.[38,39] In addition, light can also effect oxidation reactions. Light absorbed by a photosensitizer can react with molecular oxygen to form the more reactive singlet oxygen species.

8.6.2 Solid-State Stability

Solid-state stability testing includes temperature, humidity, and light as the most relevant stress factors. Solid-state processes are normally

TABLE 8.4. Typical Solid-State Stability Conditions for Drug Candidate Profiling[a]

Control at 5 or −20 °C
40 °C / 75% RH
60 °C / Ambient RH
Photostability, ICH

[a]About 4 weeks stress duration, 8 h for ICH photostability.

much slower than reactions in solution, and these tests can take several weeks. In addition to chemical stability, physical parameters like polymorphism need to be included in these studies.

Solid-state stability can be evaluated utilizing accelerated storage conditions at >40 °C and 75% relative humidity. The duration of exposure is dependent on compound sensitivity. If the thermal–humidity stress conditions produce a phase change, it is recommended to also run thermal–humidity conditions below the critical thermal–humidity that produces the phase change. Typical solid-state stress conditions for drug candidate profiling can be found in Table 8.4.

Arrhenius kinetics may be used to establish an appropriate temperature and maximum duration of thermal degradation studies. The duration of storage in a temperature-controlled room that is simulated by the study can be estimated by using an appropriate assumption of activation energy. Assuming a reaction with an activation energy of 15 kcal/mol, 18 months storage at 25 °C may be simulated by 77 days at 50 °C, or 20 days storage at 70 °C.[38] Deviation from Arrhenius kinetics is increasingly expected at >70–80 °C, and the impact of this should be considered during experimental design.

The criteria for the selection of molecules for development with respect to their stability is rather straightforward for the stability in physiological media,[35] but is difficult for all the other stress conditions. For example, the impact of stability issues on the developability assessment will be different, if a candidate is susceptible to light exposure compared to elevated temperature. High-throughput screening of the solution stability may be easily accomplished, but the impact of the solution stability issues on the developability of dosage forms requires additional studies including studying the effect of solid-state properties on stability. Choosing the right primary and secondary packaging materials, that is, eliminating the stability problem for the drug product can often tackle light sensitivity and moisture sensitivity. There are many formulation approaches available that can be applied by the formulation scientists to overcome chemical stability problems.[40,41]

It may be ideal to screen away all the compounds with any solution stability problems. Additionally, formulations that overcome certain stability challenges may provide additional intellectual protection and life cycle management opportunities. If a compound is chemically unstable as the crystalline material, the challenge to develop an oral dosage form will be very significant. Early selection of salt and crystal form including considerations for excipient compatibility and the impact of various processing parameters is crucial to the key decision making in assessing developability.

For most pharmaceutical degradation reactions, because of the importance of molecular mobility, reaction rates are typically the greatest in the liquid or solution states and least in the crystalline state, with intermediate rates occurring in the amorphous state. Salt formation will also impact a compound's chemical stability. Some factors that may contribute to the stability difference between a salt and its un-ionized form or between different salts include different microenvironmental pH and different molecular arrangements in a particular crystal lattice.

8.7 SOLID-STATE PROPERTIES

Solid-state properties including polymorphism, solvate, and salt formation can have profound impact on solubility and dissolution rate, therefore, bioavailability, stability, and processing feasibility that are essential to the successful development of drug candidates.[14] During the risk assessment related to crystal form issues, the fundamental question is what will be the consequence should a new thermodynamically more stable form be discovered? Typically, it will be high risk if a new stable form could lead to significant delay in the overall projected timeline or product failure. However, if impact on timeline and resources are minimum, the risk is low. Compounds that fall into the following categories are considered to be at high risk: (1) poorly water soluble compounds as defined by the FDA biopharmaceutical classification system; (2) compounds that would require one of the nonequilibrium methods or semisolid–liquid formulations to enhance dissolution rate–bioavailability, such as, amorphous, metastable polymorphs, and solid dispersion lipid-based formulations; (3) compounds with parenteral formulations formulated close to equilibrium solubilities at a given temperature.

The phase appropriate strategies should apply for the developability assessment of a drug candidate when studying solid-state properties.

During the lead identification and optimization phases, the main objectives of developability assessment are to identify the need for physicochemical property improvement, such as solubility and stability, and to profile them so that structural property relationships can be established. As discussed previously, only equilibrium solubility results are reliable enough for structure–property relationships. Thus the solid-state property studies should focus on monitoring solid-state form, mainly for checking if the material is amorphous or crystalline since the difference in solubility is most significant between crystalline and amorphous materials. Sometimes, small-scale crystal form screening may be necessary to discover the possibility of crystallization for representative lead compounds and possibly to identify the thermodynamically most stable form. Since the availability of the compound during these phases is typically in very small amounts, miniaturization of crystallization is essential. Our experience is that structure–property relationship building from a small but representative set of compounds with good quality data coupled with computational property prediction can often address the need for the quality data that are required for the purposes of developability assessment, yet does not sacrifice the speed and throughput. The risks for not studying the solid-state properties during these stages of discovery may involve variable (batch dependent) *in vivo* efficacy and/or PK results, poor structure solubility relationships, and identification of lead compounds with poor developability properties that are only realized after the crystal form impact on solubility is later brought into the equation during the candidate evaluation or preformulation stages. This will make it rather difficult to incorporate the desirable pharmaceutical properties into the molecular design.

Polarized light microscopy (PLM), powder X-ray diffraction (pXRD), differential scanning calorimetry (DSC), thermogravimetirc analysis (TGA), hot-stage optical microscopy (HSOM), and dynamic vapor sorption (DVS) are useful techniques to probe the solid-state properties of the drug candidate. Due to the limitation of any single technique, multiple techniques are frequently required to characterize a pharmaceutical solid.

Polarized light microscopy should be used as a rapid screening tool for characterizing a wide range of solid-state properties, such as crystallinity and particle size and habit. In most cases, it provided a quick and easy way to check if a material is crystalline.

Powder X-ray diffraction is one of the most important characterization tools used for pharmaceutical solids. The pXRD patterns can be used to identify crystalline forms and characterize crystalline structure of a pharmaceutical solid. Once a few milligrams of compound are available, pXRD patterns should be generated to keep a record to compare with future forms. The limitation of this technique is that a pXRD pattern cannot tell if the crystalline material is an anhydrate, a solvate, or a mixture of forms. It is difficult to assign forms solely based on pXRD pattern that only has subtle differences.

Thermal analyses in pharmaceutical analysis usually include DSC and TGA. Being widely used for preliminary characterization of a pharmaceutical solid, DSC can be a simple and rapid method of identifying the mixture of forms, understanding phase transitions, assessing thermodynamic stability of forms, and estimating the purity of materials.[42] Figure 8.1 depicts a typical DSC thermogram of a pharmaceutical solid. Starting from an amorphous phase, the glass transition temperature T_g was evident as a small endothermic decrease in baseline and is represented by the midpoint of the decrease measured from extension of the pre- and post-transition baselines. The T_g was followed by an exothermic event, which was assigned to the recrystallization into a metastable crystal form. The metastable form then melted, and the melted compound was further recrystallized into a more stable crystal form, which eventually melted at a higher temperature. With the introduction of modulated DSC with improved sensitivity, the determination of T_g became much easier, especially when the glass transition of an amorphous material was also accompanied by a large enthalpy of relaxation.

Thermogravimetric analysis measures the thermally induced weight changes of a sample as a function of temperatures. It is capable of

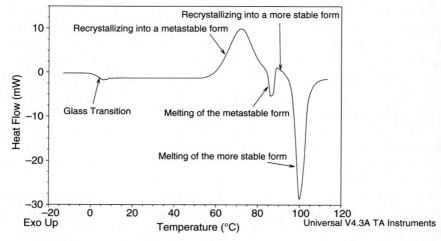

Figure 8.1. A DSC thermogram of a Johnson & Johnson drug candidate.

monitoring unbound and bound water or solvents, and compound decomposition associated with a thermal process. In conjunction with DSC and hot-stage optical microscopy, TGA provides an excellent approach for the determination of thermal properties of the pharmaceutical material. The combination of the TGA technique with mass spectrostrometry (MS) and infrared (IR) analysis provides the ability to not only measure the thermally induced weight change, but also chemically identify the volatile component during each weight-loss step.

Hot-stage optical microscopy is a useful instrument in monitoring phase transitions for a pharmaceutical solid and is used typically in conjunction with DSC and TGA to understand the nature of events leading to endotherms or exotherms on DSC traces or weight changes in TGA. Sometimes, the thermodynamically preferred polymorphic form can be ascertained from a simple bridging experiment where two polymorphic forms are placed on a microscope slide in contact with a common solvent.

The hygroscopicity of a drug material, the moisture uptake as a function of percent relative humidity, can be studied using a moisture sorption analyzer through dynamic vapor sorption technique. The instrument allows the measurement of the weight change kinetics and equilibration for small samples exposed to a stepwise change in humidity. A hygroscopicity evaluation should start with an independent determination of the initial moisture content (TGA, Karl Fischer, etc.). The testing sequence should then start with the instrument set at the initial moisture content and ambient humidity (~30% relative humidity, RH). Increasing the humidity to 95% RH in 5% increments, then descending to 5% RH, and returning to ambient–storage condition humidity over two cycles helps us to understand how a compound will respond to humidity.[43] X-ray analysis of the powder before and after this hygroscopicity analysis is also very important in detecting accompanying crystalline changes. Figure 8.2 depicts two typical DVS traces. It was observed in Figure 8.2a that the compound showed minimum water sorption at relative humidity <30%, however, at relative humidity >30%, the anhydrous form started to adsorb water and was converted to a hemihydrate. The desorption curve showed strong bonded water that was not removed even at 0% relative humidity. Variable hydrates in general are not a preferred form for development. A second J&J drug candidate, a variable hydrate, continuously absorbs moisture from 0 to 90% relative humidity, and the adsorbed moisture is not readily released when the relative humidity is decreased (Fig. 8.2b). A strict control on relative humidity will be essential to ensure successful development of the compound.

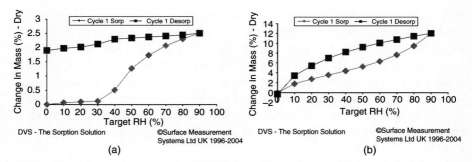

Figure 8.2. Dynamic vapor sorption of two Johnson & Johnson drug candidates.

Often a change in the compound crystallization process results in a change in crystal morphology with concurrent changes in powder flow. Low-magnification SEM (200–400×) can readily reveal particle size and crystal shape (morphology). Two of the commonly used particle-sizing methods are laser diffraction and image analysis using optical microscopy, each with its inherent limitations. For unmilled materials, where particle shape is usually not spherical, optical microscopy is particularly useful. Surface area analysis methods, such as Brunaur–Emmett–Teller (BET), also provide useful insight into changes in available surface area due to changes in chemical processing. The particle size recommendation for development is derived from the water solubility of the compound and the *in vivo* intestinal absorption rate constant, as well as the projected oral dose.[43]

Additional properties, including powder flow, tapped bulky density, tensile strength, and so on, are also important for process development. With this information, formulators know which properties they need to compensate for with excipients and processing to make a robust tablet or capsule.

8.8 CRYSTAL FORMS, SALTS, AND COCRYSTALS

8.8.1 Crystal Forms

Polymorphism is the property of molecules to exist in more than one distinct crystalline phase without any change in chemical structure. Polymorphs appear in a number of different structures as nonmixed polymorphs (free base or acid) or as mixed polymorph-like salts, cocrystals,[44] guest substances, hydrates, or solvates.[45,46] Different forms exhibit different physicochemical properties including stability and solubility, which, particularly for poorly water-soluble compounds, can lead to differences in bioavailability. Furthermore, some drugs may undergo transformation from a metastable form into a thermodynamically more stable form during processing, grinding, drying, or exposure to high humidity. In general, amorphous forms show better solubility characteristics, they normally have a better bioavailability compared to the crystal modifications. But the amorphous form normally shows higher hygroscopicity, reduced chemical stability, and the tendency to change into a crystal form, which generally is thermodynamically more stable.[47] This means that an amorphous compound with acceptable bioavailability might change into a poorly available modification by storage as a compound or the final product. Similar phenomena can be expected if we compare a metastable polymorphic form to the most stable thermodynamic form of a given compound.

Polymorphic forms can differ dramatically with respect to chemical stability and their physicochemical properties. Polymorph screens are used to learn about the different amorphous and polymorphic forms and the relevant solvates that a given compound can form, as well as to understand the physicochemical characteristics of the different forms found. The number of polymorphs and solvates found is generally proportional to the time and effort spent on polymorph mining. What is important are the conditions under which these forms are generated and the control we have over these conditions that is relevant. Insufficient characterization of possible polymorphic forms may lead to a more stable modification showing up as a problem in development or even in a marketed product.[48]

Polymorph screening is usually performed via recrystallization from various neat drug solutions. A typical procedure involves first dissolving the compound in a series of crystallization solvents; filtering the solutions through a syringe membrane filter; allowing for recrystallization through evaporation, temperature gradient, and cycling; and anti-solvent addition. For weak acids and bases, changing the pH of the solution is also often used as a recrystallization tool.[14] Since the crystallization results are often influenced by the presence of impurities, it is advisable to use the purest available material for polymorph screening. In general, the larger the scale of a crystallization step, the longer the processing time and the greater likelihood that one will generate the thermodynamically preferred form. Once a polymorph is found and characterized, additional polymorph evaluation experiments should be performed to understand its interrelationship with other forms of the compound.

Identifying the most appropriate form for development is essential for successful development. Generally, the most thermodynamically stable form should be chosen for development. Slurry tests in aqueous-based solvents are frequently used in identifying the most stable form. During the late lead optimization stage, a simple test of the drug in water could yield a good crystal form if the preparation is allowed enough time to come to equilibrium, usually in ~1 week.

8.8.2 Salts

In order to improve physicochemical properties of the compound, medicinal chemists traditionally preferred salts to weak bases or weak acids. However, only 20–30% of the new molecules form salts easily, and 70–80% remain challenging.[49] Selected salts of a molecule will be assessed in a salt screening following the same principle as polymorph screening to investigate the long-term stability, as well as its conversion to other, more stable salts and its precipitation in different aqueous and biorelevant media. With the increasing knowledge about the implications of polymorphs and salts in drug discovery, automated tools are being developed to standardize and implement these experiments as a routine process in drug discovery and lead substance selection.[50] For every salt form, the question of polymorphism needs to be investigated separately.

8.8.3 Cocrystals

Pharmaceutical cocrystals represent a new paradigm in compounds that might address important intellectual and physical property issues in the context of drug development and delivery.[51,52] In a pharmaceutical cocrystal, the compound is not modified covalently. Instead, it employs molecular recognition and self-assembly. This implication is important for streamline regulatory approval of new forms of compounds.

Currently, the preparation of cocrystals is mainly achieved by solution crystallization approaches, such as solvent evaporation, temperature gradient, and antisolvent addition. Additionally, crystallizations from the melt- and solid-state grinding methods have been employed. The solid-state grinding method was recently modified to include a very small quantity of solvent to wet the solids during grinding (solvent-drop grinding).[53]

8.8.4 Prodrugs

To overcome poor aqueous solubility or erratic bioavailability, chemical modification leading to a prodrug has successfully been used for several substances. The most commonly used prodrug approach is the incorporation of a polar or ionizable moiety into the molecule. The incorporation of *N*-acyloxyalkyl moieties of different chain length leads to a reduced crystal lattice interaction and decreasing melting point with the increasing number of methylene groups.[54] *In vivo* studies in dogs with the *N*-acyloxyalkyl derivatives of phenytoin confirmed a higher bioavailability in the fed state that did not correlate with decreasing water solubility.[55] Prodrugs also might reduce the presystemic metabolism of the substance in the GI tract or the release of the compound itself by enzymatic cleavage of the prodrug moiety close to the site of drug absorption.

8.9 DRUG CANDIDATE SELECTION

The process for bringing new drugs from the discovery laboratories to the marketplace is undergoing significant and rapid change. The change leads to a blurring of the traditional discovery–development interface. It becomes necessary to achieve the proper balance between the quantity of candidates brought into development and their quality as influenced by early consideration of development criteria along with receptor-based potency and specificity. It is also very important to properly balance between the risk and available resources in order to maximize the potential success. If developability criteria are considered at the time of lead selection and optimization, the compound attrition rate during clinical development should be decreased from the historical norm. Development scientists should ideally become involved in the drug discovery program in the early lead identification stages and then continue to provide input during *in vitro* and *in vivo* optimization.[56,57] Their objective is to address early on the various characteristics of the compounds from the chemical, as well as the pharmacological, toxicological, and biopharmaceutical point of view. The teams evaluate the ability of the substance to pass the various criteria to become an effective and safe medicinal product.[58] As a compound enters late lead optimization, much more attention is paid to the drug candidate profiling as they may determine potential issues during development. Lead candidate selection processes can be part of the development process at various stages between drug discovery and clinical development. The tools discussed in this chapter can basically be used at all stages of the drug discovery and lead optimization process (Table 8.5).

During the discovery phase, where a large number of substances are evaluated, some crude estimations based on maximum absorbable dose (MAD), molecular physical parameters, (e.g., rule-of-five),[17] and

TABLE 8.5. Typical Pharmaceutical Profiling Tests for "Drug Developability Assessment"

Assay	Tools
Solubility	Shake-flask; Turbidity; Potentiometric
pK_a	Potentiometric; Deduced from pH solubility profile
Lipophilicity (log P)	Shake-flask; Potentiometric
Permeability	PAMPA; Caco-2
Stability	
In solution	HPLC
Solid state	Stability stations, solid-state characterization and HPLC
Solid-state	
Characterization	DSC/TGA; pXRD; DVS; Microscopy; IR/Raman, etc.
Polymorph	Crystal-form screening, benchtop and automated
Salt	Salt screening, Benchtop and automated
Cocrystal	Cocrystal screening, Benchtop, and automated
Prodrug	

permeability data of structural related substances could raise alerts and provide directions away from structural areas known to cause absorption issues. The results from a PK screening in animals and CaCo-2 cells, together with solubility testing, can provide further guidance to the lead optimization program. Metabolism and PK studies in at least two animal species, as well as further solubility studies, will be performed. The decision-making process for entering in a clinical program includes a critical review of the tests performed and the consistency of the data resulting from these experiments that could reveal issues caused by the solubility characteristics of the substance. Compounds lacking sufficient aqueous solubility, especially when expected to be administered in high dose may not display their toxicological profiles as they do not achieve the calculated concentration in the toxicological assay. If a compound forms stable and less soluble forms (e.g., salts) with physiological fluids or food components, the potential risk for drug precipitation in the GI tract needs to be considered. The physical properties must also be addressed from a processing point of view. During synthesis and manufacturing in a large commercial scale, the hygroscopicity, amorphicity, crystallinity, and polymorphism of a substance need to be controllable and manageable in an industrial environment.

Aqueous solubility is one of the most important characteristics of pharmaceutical solids in developmental research, because it frequently has a direct effect on bioavailability. Hence, the key challenge during the developability assessment is often the decision making. Once the deficiencies in physicochemical properties have been identified, a decision needs to be made whether the compound should be sent back to chemistry for structure modification or continued for preclinical and clinical evaluation. In the best-case scenario, this information can be used to fix the issue by medicinal chemistry and thereby successfully improve the quality of the clinical candidate.

When the solubility is used to predict the bioavailability, it is often found that there is a lack of correlation between solubility and bioavailability. Except for the reasons we already discussed, (i.e., dose, permeability, and mechanism of the actions), it is also important to separate the dissolution from solubility. For compounds with dissolution-, or solubility-limited absorption, variability in bioavailability is often observed and can be a critical selection criterion. Formulation strategies must be considered early on to decrease the intra- and intersubject variability. Understanding the different root causes for poorly or highly variable oral bioavailability of a compound is already a key asset for finding a solution. Limited compound solubility in the physiological conditions of the GI tract is well known to be one of the main root causes. Early assessment of and eventually experimental formulation work is conducted to secure the solubilized drug concentration in the preclinical assays. In the later stages of development, more precise determination of the aqueous solubility is necessary for designing appropriate formulations.

In many cases, a compound with good potency and selectivity, but poor aqueous solubility and therefore poor bioavailability, is still recommended as a drug candidate, hoping the evolving drug delivery technologies will fix the solubility problem in the drug development process. However, to overcome poor aqueous solubility or highly variable bioavailability by applying special solubility enhancement technologies into formulation development, sometimes, could be very time consuming and expensive. How to effectively balance the management of poor aqueous solubility and its associated high spending and time is extremely challenging.

Formulation techniques stabilizing amorphous material and/or metastable forms might be a chance for compounds that are not sufficiently bioavailable in their most thermodynamically stable form. These formulations in many cases are kinetic stabilizations of an unstable modification, and therefore bear the risk of recrystallization into a less favorable, but thermodynamically more stable, form. Therefore, extensive characterization of the relevant forms, their characteristics, and stability is mandatory if an approach like this is considered.

8.10 CONCLUSIONS

The lead candidate selection is a complex decision process that involves all disciplines. The selection process does not necessarily lead to the selection of one lead substance; it can also provide clear directions and recommendations for further lead substance optimization. The decision process will include an assessment as to whether the foreseen limitation of the lead compound can be easily solved by specific technologies or by drug delivery strategies that are commercially viable or can be successfully developed during the development timelines.

Obviously, the goal is to nominate a candidate with good "developability" characteristics in order to reduce attrition rates during development. This should help to keep development cost and time low since it avoids specialized drug development techniques.

The development of a successful new product is often the results of lots of learning from lots of failures. Many major pharmaceutical companies have adopted a "fail fast, fail cheap" concept. Drug candidates that are not likely going to make it to market are ruled out early before going to very expensive preclinical and clinical studies. Factors, such as potency, solubility, pK_a, lipophilicity, metabolic stability, absorption, excretion, protein binding, and toxicity, affect the performance of a drug intended for oral administration. These factors are intimately linked to each other and any chemical structural modifications to modulate one property selectively may adversely affect one or more of the other key properties. The concept of multivariate optimization, therefore, will not guarantee success of the candidate in the clinic, but it should increase the chances of success during development. Each of these factors must be weighed in addition to developability in choosing drug candidates and in setting the go/no go hurdles for the project. In an ideal situation, the lead selection and optimization process should first eliminate the poor compounds and from the remaining pool of acceptable compounds, the winner compound(s) should be picked.

The commercial successes of Zocor (Simvastatin), Lipor (Atovastatin calcium), and Forsamax (Aldendronate sodium) clearly demonstrated that deficiencies in physicochemical properties of a candidate should be a "warning flag", not a "stop sign" for development. It is very possible that compounds with the most favorable pharmaceutical profiles are not chosen due to other considerations; however, results of the pharmaceutical profiles can help identify development risks early, thus providing the opportunity for early initiation of development efforts to reduce delays. In parallel with the analytical characterization of the initial material of the compound, substantial efforts are invested into understanding and optimizing the crystalline structure and identifing a potential pseudo-thermodynamic stable form of the substance. These investigations are looking into the polymorphs, solvates, and salts formed by the substance under various conditions to identify the most suitable material for dosage form development, scaling up, and later manufacturing.

REFERENCES

1. Kerns, E. H. *J. Pharm. Sci.* **2001**, 90, 1838–1858.
2. Kerns, E. H.; Di, L. *Drug Delivery Today: Technologies* **2004**, 1, 343–348.
3. Rodrigues, A. D.; Lin, J. H. *Curr. Opin. Chem. Biol.* **2001**, 5, 396–401.
4. Berenson, A. "Drugs in '05: Much Promise, Little Payoff", *The New York Times*, **2006**, January 11.
5. Kola, I.; Landis, J. *Nature Rev.; Drug Disc.* **2004**, 3, 711–715.
6. Di, L.; Kerns, E. H. *Curr. Opinion Chem. Biol.* **2003**, 7, 402–408.
7. Venkatesh, S.; Lipper, R. A. *J. Pharm. Sci.* **2000**, 89, 145–154.
8. Johnson, K.; Swindell, A. *Pharm. Res.* **1996**, 13, 1795–1798.
9. Curatolo, W. *Pharmaceutical Science & Technology Today*, **1998**, 1, 9, 387–393.
10. Lipinski, C. A. in *Pharmaceutical Profiling in Drug Discovery for Lead Selection*, Eds. Borchardt, R. T.; Kerns, E. H.; Lipinski C. A.; Thakker, D. R.; Wang, B. H. **2004**, 93–126, AAPS Press.
11. Kasim, N. A.; Whitehouse, M.; Ramachandran, C.; Bermejo, M.; Lennernäs, H.; Hussain, A. S.; Junginger, H. E.; Stavchansky, S. A.; Midha, K. K.; Shah, V. P.; Amidon, G. L. *Mol. Pharmac.* **2004**, 1, 85–96.
12. Neervannan, S. *Expert Opin. Drug Metab. Toxicol.* **2006**, 2, 715–731.
13. Yalkowsky, S. *American Chemical Society*, Annual meeting, Washington, DC, **1999**.
14. Huang, L.; Tong, W. Q. *Adv. Drug Deliv. Rev.* **2004**, 56, 321–334.
15. Pudipeddi, M.; Serajuddin, A. T. M. *J. Pharm. Sci.* **2005**, 94, 929–939.
16. Avdeef, A. *Curr. Top. Med. Chem.* **2001**, 1, 277–351.
17. Lipinski, C. A.; Lombardo, F.; Dominy, B. W.; Feeney, P. J. *Adv. Drug Deliv. Rev.* **2001**, 46, 3–26.
18. Pan, L.; Ho, Q.; Tsutsui, K.; Takahashi, L. *J. Pharm. Sci.* **2001**, 90, 521–529.
19. Gaviraghi, G.; Barnaby, R. J.; Pellegatti, M. in *Pharmacokinetic Optimization in Drug Research; Verlag Helvetica Chimica Acta.* Eds.

Testa, B.; van de Waterbeemd, H.; Folkers, G.; Guy, R. **2001**, 3–14, Zürich and Wiley–VCH.

20. Blasko, A.; Leahy-Dios, A.; Nelson, W. O.; Austin, S. A.; Killion, R. B.; Visor, G. C.; Massey, I. J. *Monatshefte Chem.* **2001**, 132, 789–798.

21. Faller, B.; Wohnsland, F. in *Pharmacokinetic Optimization in Drug Research; Verlag Helvetica Chimica Acta.* Eds. Testa, B.; van de Waterbeemd, H.; Folkers, G.; Guy, R. **2001**, 257–274, Zürich and Wiley–VCH.

22. Avdeef, A. *Pharm. Pharmacol. Commun.* **1998**, 4, 165–178.

23. Marques, M. *Diss. Tech.* **2004**, 11, 16.

24. Giron, D.; Grant, D. J. W. in *Handbook of Pharmaceutical Salts Properties Selection and Use.* Eds. Stahl P.H.; Wermuth, C.G., **2002**, 158–159, Verlag Helvetica Chemica Acta/Wiley–VCH.

25. Venkatesh, S.; Li, J.; Xu, Y.; Vishnuvajjala, R.; Anderson, B. D. *Pharm. Res.* **1996**, 13, 1453–1459.

26. Wells, J. I. *Pharmaceutical Preformulation: The Physicochemical Properties of Compounds* **1988**, John Wiley & Sons.

27. Available at Thai, D. www.geocities.com/d.thai, Pharmacology Semester1, **1997**.

28. Tong, W. Q.; Whitesell, G. *Pharm. Dev. Technol.* **1998**, 3, 215–223.

29. Marra-Feil, M.; Anderson, B. D. *Pharm. Sci.* **1998**, 1, S–400.

30. Avdeef, A. *J. Pharm. Sci.* **1993**, 82, 183–190.

31. Yamagami, C.; Araki, K.; Ohnishi, K.; Hanasato, K.; Inaba, H.; Aono, M.; Ohta, A. *J. Pharm. Sci.* **1999**, 88, 1299–1304.

32. Artursson, P.; Palm, K.; Luthman, K. *Adv. Drug Deliv. Rev.* **2001**, 46, 27–43.

33. Kansy, M.; Senner, F.; Gubernator, K. *J. Med. Chem.* **1998**, 41, 1007–1010.

34. van de Waterbeemd, H.; Smith, D. A.; Beaumont, K.; Walker, D. K. *J. Med. Chem.* **2001**, 44, 1313–1333.

35. Schröter, C. *Amer. Pharm. Res.* **2006**, 9, 60–67.

36. Balbach, S.; Korn, C. *Int. J. Pharm.* **2004**, 275, 1–12.

37. FDA, *Guideline for the Photostability Testing of New Compounds and New Drug Products*, Federal Register, **1997**, 62, 27115.

38. Alsante, K. M.; Ando, A.; Brown, R.; Ensing, J.; Hatajik, T. D.; Kong, W.; Tsuda, Y. *Adv. Drug. Deliv. Rev.* **2007**, 59, 29–37.

39. Waterman, K. C.; Adami, R. C.; Alsante, K. M.; Hong, J.; Landis, M. S.; Lombardo, F.; Roberts, C. J. *Pharm. Dev. Technol.* **2002**, 7, 1–32.

40. Yoshioka, S.; Stella, V. J. *Stability of Drugs and Dosage Forms*, **2000**, Kluwer Academic Publishers, Plenum Publishers.

41. Guillory, J. K.; Poust, R. I. in *Modern Pharmaceutics*. 4th ed; Eds. Banker, G. S.; Rhodes, C. T. Drugs and the Pharmaceutical Sciences. **2002**, 139–166. 121; Marcel Dekker.

42. van-Dooren, A. A.; Muller, B. W. *Int. J. Pharm.* **1984**, 20, 217–233.

43. Fiese, E. F. *J. Pharm. Sci.* **2003**, 92, 1331–1342.

44. Vishweshwar, P.; McMahon, J. A.; Bis, J. A.; Zaworotko, M. J. *J. Pharm. Sci.* **2006**, 95, 499–516.

45. Brittain, H. G. *Polymorphism in Pharmaceutical Solids.* **1999**, Marcel Dekker.

46. Vippagunta, S. R.; Brittain, H. G.; Grant, D. J. W. *Adv. Drug Deliv. Rev.* **2001**, 48, 3–26.

47. Singhal, D.; Curatolo, W. *Adv. Drug Deliv. Rev.* **2004**, 56, 335–347.

48. Bauer, J.; Spanton, S.; Henry, R.; Quick, J.; Dziki, W.; Porter, W.; Morris, J. *Pharm. Res.* **2001**, 18, 859–866.

49. Serajuddin, A. T. M.; Pudipeddi, M. in *Handbook of Pharmaceutical Salts Properties Selection and Use.* Eds. Stahl, P. H.; Wermuth, C. G. **2002**, 158–159, Verlag Helvetica Chemica Acta/Wiley–VCH.

50. Rohl, A. L. *Curr. Opin. Solid State Mater. Sci.* **2003**, 7, 21–26.

51. Almarsson, Ö.; Zaworotko, M. J. *Chem. Comm.* **2004**, 17,1889–1896.

52. Remenar, J. F.; Morissette, S. L.; Peterson, M. L.; Moulton, B.; MacPhee, J. M.; Guzman, H. R.; Almarsson, Ö. *J. Am. Chem. Soc.* **2003**, 125, 8456–8457.

53. Zhang, G. Z.; Henry, R. F.; Borchardt, T. B.; Lou, X. *J. Pharm. Sci.* **2007**, 96, 990–995.

54. Stella, V. J.; Martodihardjo, S.; Terada, K.; Rao, V. M. *J. Pharm. Sci.* **1998**, 87, 1235–1241.

55. Stella, V. J.; Martodihardjo, S.; Rao, V. M. *J. Pharm. Sci.* **1999**, 88, 775–779.

56. Bailey, C. A.; Railkar, A.; Tarantino, R. *Books of Abstract, 211th ACS National Meeting, New Orleans, LA, March 24–28*, American Chemical Society, Washinton DC, **1996**, 211, 12.

57. Railkar, S.; Sandhu, H. K.; Spence, E.; Margolis, R.; Tarantino, R.; Bailey, C. A. *Pharm. Res.* **1996**, 13, S–278.

58. Bowker, M. J. in *Handbook of Pharmaceutical Salts Properties Selection and Use.* Eds. Stahl, P.H.; Wermuth, C.G., **2002**, 161–189, Verlag Helvetica Chemica Acta/Wiley–VCH.

PART III

PREDICTIVE SAFETY ASSESSMENT IN DRUG DISCOVERY

CHAPTER 9

SAFETY ASSESSMENT IN DRUG DISCOVERY

VITO G. SASSEVILLE, WILLIAM R. FOSTER, and BRUCE D. CAR

Bristol-Myers Squibb Research and Development, Princeton, NJ

9.1   INTRODUCTION

As a new chemical entity (NCE) advances from initial discovery through development to registration, cost grows exponentially with the final investment exceeding \$1 billion.[1,2] It is estimated that more productive discovery programs or better preclinical screens that

Evaluation of Drug Candidates for Preclinical Development: Pharmacokinetics, Metabolism, Pharmaceutics, and Toxicology, Edited by Chao Han, Charles B. Davis, and Binghe Wang
Copyright © 2010 John Wiley & Sons, Inc.

increase success rates from 1 in 10 to 1 in 3 would reduce capitalized total cost per approved drug by several hundred million dollars.[3] Thus, by enhancing efficiency and improving early prediction for development limiting toxicity, expenditures would be markedly reduced. Yet despite major strides in reducing pharmacokinetic (PK) and formulation liabilities by early predictive absorption, distribution, metabolism, elimination (ADME) assays, and more-predictive PK, safety continues to be the most significant cause of drug candidate attrition.[4,5] The following is a breakdown of combined clinical and nonclinical safety causes of attrition at Bristol-Myers Squibb Co. (BMS) between 1993–2006: cardiovascular (27%), hepatotoxicity (15%), teratogenicity (8%), immune-mediated toxicity (7%), and other causes of diminishing importance (Table 9.1).[5] Following the introduction of scientifically driven strategies and novel technologies, attrition due to toxicity has fallen considerably, without reducing compound number advanced into development. This ongoing experiment is occurring at several pharmaceutical companies, but will take several more years to evaluate whether it translates into more successful new drug application (NDA) filings.

Therefore, the opportunity exists for the toxicologist to significantly impact expenditures by the early prediction of potential toxicity–side effect barriers to development by aggressive evaluation of

TABLE 9.1. Breakdown of Combined Clinical and Nonclinical Safety Causes of Attrition at Bristol-Myers Squibb Company between 1993 and 2006

Target Organ/Liability Classification	Percent of All Advanced Molecules[a]
Cardiovascular	27.3
Hepatic	14.8
Teratogenicity	8.0
Hematologic	6.8
Central and peripheral nervous system	6.8
Retina	6.8
Mutagenicity and clastogenicity	4.5
Male and female reproductive toxicity	4.5
Gastrointestinal and pancreatic	3.4
Muscle	3.4
Carcinogenicity	3.4
Lung	2.3
Acute death	2.3
Renal	2.3
Irritant	2.3
Skeletal (arthritis/bone development)	1.1

[a]88 molecules assessed; note as categories are partially overlapping, the total is >100%. Adapted from Ref. 5.

development-limiting liabilities early in drug discovery. Improved efficiency in pharmaceutical research and development lies both in leveraging "best in class" technology and integration with pharmacologic activities during hit-to-lead and early lead optimization stages (Fig. 9.1).[6] A leading edge discovery stage toxicology testing paradigm should allow the discovery toxicologist to advance an NCE with no genotoxicity into preclinical development; no significant toxicologic perturbations at projected efficacious exposures; well-defined dose-limiting toxicity; projected margin; identification of toxicity biomarkers; and selection of the most appropriate species for toxicology testing. Toxicology activities should be completed concurrently with pharmacologic assessments so that negative and positive attributes are evident to the medicinal chemist, thus optimizing speed and efficiency in the decision to advance an NCE to full development.[7] When predictive toxicology assessments do not identify liabilities discovered in longer term studies, feeding an understanding of this information together with facile counterscreens is equally important to the Discovery chemists' backup strategy. This chapter focuses on the various

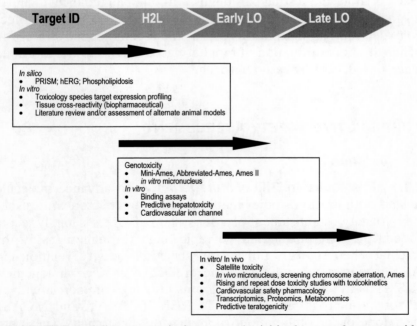

Figure 9.1. Timing of discovery toxicology assays/activities by stage from target identification (ID), through hit-to-lead (H2L), and early and late lead optimization (LO) phases of drug discovery. [Adapted from Sasseville et al. *Chem. Biol. Inter.*, **2004**, 150, 9–25. Ref. 6.]

strategies being applied to integrate toxicology in the drug discovery process and provides a greater understanding of the causes and timing of toxicology-driven attrition in drug development and how the discovery toxicologist can better interface with the pharmacologist and medicinal chemist. General practices, as well as innovative approaches and techniques for lead optimization and early preclinical development of small molecules, will be covered. Sections include *in silico* approaches to predictive toxicology, *in vitro* and *in vivo* screening approaches, the use of toxicogenomics, metabonomics, proteomics, and the application of alternative animal models (transgenic animals, gene knockdown–knockout models, nonmammalian species, etc.) currently being used in the industry for lead optimization and early preclinical development of small molecules. Biotechnology-derived pharmaceuticals, which include recombinant peptides and proteins, modified proteins, monoclonal antibodies, vaccines, gene-transfer products, cell-based and tissue-engineered therapeutics,[8] have different sets of toxicological concerns compared to small molecules. Due to the numerous and diverse types of biopharmaceutical products, it is beyond the scope of this chapter to discuss the details of typical safety concerns of each. However, where applicable, these differences will be discussed alongside small molecule testing paradigms. Although a guidance document (and an updated draft) for the nonclinical safety evaluation for biotechnology-derived pharmaceuticals exists,[9] the recommended strategy for preclinical safety evaluation of biopharmaceuticals is to use a rational, science-based, case-by-case approach.[8]

9.2   PREDICTIVE SAFETY ASSESSMENT

9.2.1   *In Silico*

9.2.1.1   *Predictive* **In Silico** *Mutagenicity.* To advance molecules into lead optimization studies that are well characterized with respect to genotoxicity, establishment of a tier system of assays is highly recommended. The first tier should be rapid, high throughput assay that medicinal chemists can utilize for structure–activity relationships (SAR) around structural alerts. The predictive *in silico* mutagenicity (PRISM) assays are modeling programs utilizing commercially available software programs, such as DEREK, TOPKAT, and MCASE, either alone or in combination to predict for genotoxicity. These programs compute the probability of the test compound to be mutagenic and can identify structural alerts within the test compound that may

lead to the compound's mutagenicity. Some or all of these computational models are utilized by both regulatory agencies and biotechnical–pharmaceutical companies to predict the mutagenic potential of compounds. In addition, models are also utilized for determining the potential risk of contaminants and degradation of drug substance in drug products at US Food and Drug Administration (FDA)–Center for Drug Evaluation and Research (CDER).[10] However, when used independently each of these systems have inherent limitations primarily because these model knowledge bases were mostly populated with bacterial mutagenicity data from nonpharmaceutical molecules.[11–13] When compared to the Ames Salmonella reversion assay, the individual *in silico* models have poor sensitivity for predicting an Ames positive test. Classification models have been developed to address this issue and to provide accurate prediction of genotoxicity.[14,15] A consensus model incorporating three unique classifiers correctly predicted 81.2% of the 277 polycyclic aromatic compounds and yielded a higher prediction rate on the genotoxic class than any other single model.[14] Utilization of a similar consensus model as a first tier test, can significantly reduce false-negative rates (false-negative rate <10%). In this paradigm, only positive predictions are confirmed in the more labor intensive second tier mutagenicity assays. With no compound requirement and a rapid turnaround time, PRISM provides an opportunity for almost instantaneous guidance in SAR around mutagenic potential and structural alerts. However, it is our experience that most mutagenic structural alerts are easily recognized by experienced medicinal chemists and the real benefit is in the ability to "educate" the systems by input of new data.

9.2.1.2 *Human Ether à go-go Related Gene (hERG).*

Several marketed compounds, including many nonsedating antihistamines (e.g., Seldane, Hismanal) have been withdrawn from the market due to reports of Torsades de Pointes (TdP), a fatal polymorphic ventricular tachycardia. Although the precise molecular mechanisms responsible for TdP are unclear, prolongation of the QT interval as recorded on an electrocardiogram (ECG) appears to always precede this lethal event.[16] The hERG (human ether à go-go related gene) channel corresponds to the α subunit of the delayed rectifier potassium current (I_{kr}) and is responsible for repolarization of the cardiac ventricle. This repolarization is manifested on the ECG as the T wave. When repolarization is delayed, the T wave is lengthened from the Q wave (ventricular depolarization) and leads to a prolonged QT interval. Mutations in the potassium channel encoded by hERG have been implicated in both congenital and acquired forms of long QT syndrome.[16] There are ample examples of small molecules from many classes of therapeutics including antihistamines, antibiotics, antipsychotics, and prokinetics, that inhibit the hERG channel. Due to the severe undesirable pharmacologic effects that may result from the interaction of small molecule inhibitors with the hERG channel, it is important to evaluate the potential of compounds to bind to the hERG channel early in the drug development process. As with PRISM, *in silico* models have been developed to predict hERG channel blockade by compounds.[17,18] However, the lack of a crystal structure of the hERG channel has impacted the development of these models and, as such they have a limited predictive value in screening large databases of compounds,[19] although application of models within validated chemical series may yield informative predictive data. Recently, more predictive quantitative structure–activity relationship (QSAR) models using a consistent sets of *in vitro* data have been developed, but *in silico* models are not substitutes for the gold standard *in vitro* and *in vivo* models, and their application in early discovery phases should only be used in streamlining which compounds go into second tier assays, such as binding and electrophysiology assays.[19,20] More detail on *in silico* modeling for hERG liabilities are provided in Chapter 10.

9.2.1.3 *Phospholipidosis.*

Drug-induced phospholipidosis is the excessive accumulation of drug or metabolites in the lysosomes of cells with inhibition of phospholipases and the formation of diagnostic paracrystalline arrays. This is a property of cationic amphiphilic (lipophilic) compounds with >50 marketed compounds showing this liability in nonclinical species,[21] though very few of these demonstrate phospolipidotic manifestations of clinical concern. While frequently this is an innocuous change that is considered to be an adaptive response, the risk-assessment is complex since biomarkers of phospholipidotic organ dysfunction are typically insensitive. The well-defined molecular properties underlying this toxicology lend themselves to development of *in silico* models, several of which are available and may be applied to the rank ordering of compounds for this liability in Discovery.[22]

9.2.2 *In Vitro*

Traditional toxicology testing paradigms examine drug candidates during late lead optimization in a select set of low throughput, labor-intensive, established "gold standard" assays. Identification of liabilities at this late stage can be costly and have serious implications to the development of a chemical class or series with a direct impact on development timelines. Liabilities detected earlier in the process give the medicinal chemists more time to assess other chemical series or classes and to develop SAR around a potential liability. In an attempt to reduce compound attrition during late lead optimization, novel high-throughput screening assays have been incorporated into testing paradigms early in the discovery process to identify potential liabilities and to select which compounds need earlier and more thorough evaluation in the more refined second and third tier assays, the type of assay commonly employed in late lead optimization.

9.2.2.1 *Toxicology Species Target Expression Profiling and Tissue Cross-Reactivity Studies.* Toxicology species target expression profiling is the process of identifying mRNA and/or protein expression patterns of drug targets in rat, dog, or nonhuman primate using real-time polymerase chain reaction (PCR) (TaqMan™), *in situ* hybridization, or immunohistochemical techniques.[6] Expression patterns for each target can be subsequently evaluated for concordance–discordance with the human expression profile. Comparative expression profiling, metabolite identification, and compound efficacy, together drive second species selection during preclinical development of small molecules. This technology is particularly relevant for novel target development. *A priori* knowledge of target expression patterns across species, positions the toxicologist to better judge the relevance to humans of novel pharmacology-related organ toxicity. In addition, this profiling enables one to identify potential anatomic sites for undesired target-mediated effects in a given test species and to develop an understanding of similarities and differences in the potential toxicity profile between two selected test species based on comparative target distribution profiles.

For biopharmaceuticals, cross-reactivity studies utilizing the clinical product in a routine immunohistochemical technique on a panel of cryopreserved tissues from human and toxicology species is required for aiding in the identification of relevant toxicological species, target distribution in human and toxicology species, and to show any unintentional reactivity toward tissues distinct from the intended target.[23] As these studies are expected to be performed according to good laboratory practice (GLP) and with the product intended for use in the clinic, these studies are generally conducted after candidate nomination for preclinical development as part of the first in human (FIH)-enabling battery of assays.[9] However, a limited panel of cells–tissues from human and test animal species can be utilized with the parent antibody earlier in discovery to help select relevant species.[9] Data garnered from flow cytometry results using the antibody is particularly useful in determining species cross-reactivity. In cases where an antibody does not cross-react with the target in non-human primate efficacy models or toxicology species, target distribution in these species with a homolog is recommended.

For target expression profiling and tissue cross-reactivity studies, comprehensive tissue sets from rat, dog, nonhuman primate, and humans are needed. The tissue lists are selected to reflect standard tissue lists employed in standard toxicologic pathology evaluation and as recommended in the biotechnology-derived pharmaceuticals draft guidance document.[9] Considerable cost savings in reagents and histotechnician time are realized by use of tissue microarrays for primary screens. For each species, microarray blocks can be generated containing full sets of tissues representing all distinct microanatomical regions in ~80 cores. Similar, but smaller frozen arrays consisting of 12–24 tissues per block, can also be generated.[6]

9.2.2.2 Genotoxicity. The typical GLP genotoxicity testing battery for small molecule therapeutics prior to conducting FIH studies in normal healthy volunteers are the reverse mutation assay in *Salmonella typhimurium* and *Escherichia coli* (Ames test), the *in vitro* chromosomal aberration assay using Chinese hamster ovary, mouse lymphoma, or human peripheral blood lymphocytes, and the rat or mouse *in vivo* bone marrow micronucleus assay.[24,25] Since many phase-1 clinical trials utilize normal healthy volunteers, a positive result in a genetic toxicology assay can adversely affect the clinical development of a drug.[10] Moreover, when positive, these assessments, which have implications in carcinogenesis and in teratogenesis, represent barriers to registration that are very difficult to manage for nonlife saving indications, unless the disease is disabling and in an indication where there is poorly met medical need.

For the development of cytotoxic chemotherapeutic agents, genotoxicity has historically not been a concern. These agents are frequently positive in clastogenicity or mutagenicity assays largely due to the DNA alkylating or nucleotide-substituting mechanisms of action.[26] Genotoxicity tests for such agents are still performed, not to protect the patient population, but rather to evaluate the potential hazards for those who may be environmentally exposed. Noncytotoxic targeted chemotherapeutic agents, which disrupt the cell cycle, are also frequently positive in clastogenicity assays, but should not be positive in mutagenicity assays. Given the risk–benefit of oncologic indications, genotoxic liabilities in cytostatic agents are likely to be tolerated; however, in the context of a chronic administration regimen, such features may be deemed undesirable in the future, especially as nongenotoxic alternatives become available.[26] Likewise, biopharmaceutical agents, which do not have the same distribution properties of small molecules are not expected to carry any genotoxicity liability and the standard battery of genetoxicity assays are not required.[9] In addition, testing for genotoxic impurities is not required. Consequently, these agents are not generally tested for genotoxic liabilities unless they contain protein- or immunoconjugates containing organic chemical liners or other substitutions that may have unknown properties.[9]

However, for development of compounds for nonlife saving indications, following first tier PRISM assays, shorter, higher throughput second tier assays should be used early in the discovery process (early-to-late lead optimization) to investigate SAR for compound optimization to avoid unwanted or unexpected genotoxic liabilities as determined by these assays.

Mutagenicity Assays. There are many non-GLP assays, which can serve as a reliable second tier screening assays, after PRISM, that are available to the discovery toxicologist as commercial assays for in-house use or via contract research organizations.

The SOS chromotest is a colorimetric bacterial assay for detecting DNA damaging agents. The assay is based on the premise that DNA damaging agents induce a set of SOS response or damage inducible genes. The assay utilizes *E. coli* K-12 and an operon fusion placing *lacZ*, the structural gene for β-galactosidase, under the control of one of these SOS response genes resulting in a direct colorimetric assessment of SOS response to DNA damage.[27] For 452 compounds assayed in the SOS chromotest, 82% gave a similar response in the Ames test indicating a close correlation between the two bacterial-based assays.[28] The capacity of the Ames test to identify carcinogens is higher than the SOS chromotest, but due to fewer false positives, the ability of the SOS chromotest to discriminate between carcinogens and noncarcinogens was better than the Ames test suggesting that the two assays can be used to complement each other.[28,29] At BMS, we have effectively utilized the high-throughput SOS chromotest for SAR around mutagenicity and to select which compounds or classes of compounds require more refined mutagenicity assessment earlier in the discovery process. In our experience, the major limitations for the colorimetric SOS assay are color and precipitation, which have been overcome via the application of luminescent endpoints.

The miniaturized-(mini-Ames) and abbreviated-Ames assays are relatively low-throughput plate-based assays using at least two *S. typhimurium* strains (TA98 and TA100) as used in the GLP Ames. The Ames II assay is a medium-throughput nonplate-based bacterial reversion assay that uses TA98 and the TA MIX (TA7001-7006).[30] Similar to the GLP Ames assay, all these assays use *S. typhimurium* strains that have been engineered to be histidine deficient and cannot survive in the absence of histidine. The assays measure a compound's mutagenicity by reverting the *S. typhimurium* strains back to the wild type and being able to produce histidine. The assays are performed with and without hepatic S9 from Aroclor 1254-induced male rats. Assay requirements range from 5 to 120 mg/compound depending on selected assay, number of strains used, and number of replicates. Due to compound requirement and limited throughput, it is suggested that the compound for these assays are first prioritized in the first tier PRISM. A concordance of 88–89.5% has been reported for the Ames II test as compared to the traditional GLP Ames plate test.[30,31] The Ames II assay typically requires 5 mg of compound, which is an amount that can be easily provided by medicinal chemists for rapid SAR. The medium throughput and low compound requirements make this an ideal second tier assay in support of discovery chemistry efforts. The mini-Ames requires 30 mg of compound and has the advantage of being plate based and using both TA98 and TA100. The high concordance of these assays to the GLP Ames assay generally precludes further advancement of a compound that is positive in these assays, with the caveat that a false positive could result from a mutagenic impurity.[10] Thus, to eliminate impurity derived false positives, it is suggested that the compound typically needs to have a purity of >95%. In addition, the compound typically needs to have a solubility >5 mg/mL. For compounds of continued interest, a third tier exploratory Ames assay using at least five tester strains is recommended prior to development candidate nomination to reduce the chance of any surprises in development.

Clastogenicity Assays. Once a lead series is determined, it is suggested that prototype compounds be run in clastogencity assays, such as the *in vitro* micronucleus assay or chromosome aberration assay. These assays determine a compound's ability to cause chromosome structural (clastogenic) and/or numerical (aneugenic) aberrations. The *in vitro* micronucleus assay is a widely used non-GLP assay to predict clastogenicity,[32] generally using less compound and having a faster throughput than the chromosome aberration assay. Multiple cell lines or lymphocytes can be used (e.g., CHL, CHO, V79, human lymphocytes, and L5178Y mouse lymphoma cells) in the *in vitro* micronucleus assay. Clastogenicity is determined in the *in vitro* micronucleus assay by the induction of micronuclei, which can be either chromosome fragments or whole chromosomes that were not able to migrate with the other chromosomes during the anaphase stage of cell mitosis.[33] Cells are treated with a concentration gradient of compound with and without hepatic S9 from Aroclor 1254 induced male rats. The strength of this assay is that <50 mg of compound are required, with the micronized *in vitro* micronucleus requiring <10 mg. As this assay is not automated and direct microscopic analysis of slides is necessary, turnaround time and throughput are limiting. Depending on the source, concordance between the *in vitro* micronucleus assay and the GLP chromosomal aberration test (metaphase assay) varies between 80 and 88.7%.[34,35] A reason for the discordance is that the micronucleus assay detects aneugenic materials while the chromosome aberration assay does not.[10] For compounds of continued interest, an exploratory chromosome aberration assay can be conducted to confirm an *in vitro* micronucleus positive result, but the cost, time involved, and good concordance between the two assays are deterrents and it is prudent to wait to conduct the GLP assay with refined material. Moreover, both of these assays have high sensitivities and low specificities, and thus false-positive results are common.[10] However, the usefulness of this screen is that it also identifies the need for *in vivo* assessment. A positive *in vivo* micronucleus although uncommon is usually *in vitro* positive. Thus, a positive *in vitro* micronucleus result predicts for either a chromosomal aberration positive or an *in vivo* micronucleus positive. A compound that is positive for *in vitro* chromosomal aberrations can delay or prematurely halt a drug development program, but can be a manageable issue in development providing that the compound is Ames and *in vivo* micronucleus negative. However, a compound that is positive for *in vivo* micronucleus creates a major development barrier and should be deprioritized. Hence, early identification of an *in vivo* micronucleus, although an uncommon occurrence, is a liability that should be ruled out early in the discovery process.

9.2.3.3 In Vitro *Binding Assays.* There are numerous options available to the discovery scientist in the form of novel in-house high-throughput platforms or via contract research organizations [e.g., MDS® Pharma, Cerep, Caliper (includes the former NovaScreen Biosciences)] to screen compounds for potential clinical liabilities via radioligand binding or enzyme assays.[4] These panels are designed to incorporate the most commonly occurring side effects of NCEs with GPCRs dominating the assay, but also including enzymes, transporters, nuclear receptors, and channels.[4] Generally, to save time, conserve compound, and to reduce costs, assays are run at one concentration ($\sim$10 μM) and it is recommended to reassess compounds and generate an IC50 value for inhibition of any target at $\geq$50%. Depending on the stage of discovery, this assay can be either used to rank order compounds in a chemical series, assist with SAR, or determine which second-tier assays are needed prior to compound advancement. Positive results should be followed up with definitive functional assays. For example, binding to cardiac ion channels, such as calcium channel L-type or sodium channel site 2, may be the first indication of potential cardiovascular liability and compounds displaying inhibition of these targets at $\geq$50%, should be examined in whole-cell patch-clamp to directly measure sodium and calcium currents. More details on whole-cell patch-clamp are provided in Chapter 10.

For those targets with IC_{50}s considered potent relative to drug pharmacology, the margin that is calculated from *in vitro* protein-free IC_{50} to the plasma unbound concentration of drug, typically at C_{max}, is determined. If an activity is considered a potential issue, such as potent phosphodiesterase 4 inhibition, typically one profiles additional related compounds and conducts focused second tier *in vitro* or *in vivo* studies to determine the potential impact of the liability. Typically, the profiling companies provide such services, but many can be performed in the Discovery environment. For example, a generic opioid receptor hit is defined by running IC_{50}s for binding of sigma, μ and κ receptors. A potent μ or κ activity may be followed by assessment of intestinal motility in the charcoal passage mode.

In addition to this classical ancillary pharmacology profiling, companies working with kinase inhibitors generally profile a selection of the kinome internally or with vendors, such as Ambit Biosciences' KINOME*scan*™. Placing kinase hits in perspective relative to unknown or potentially expected biology can be a complex undertaking.

9.2.2.4 *Predictive Hepatotoxicity.* *In vitro* cell viability assays have a central role in predictive toxicology, but interlaboratory variability in the quality of data has been an issue.[36] Recent advances in automation and information technologies have enabled pharmaceutical companies to develop fast and cost-effective *in vitro* screening assays to help predict clinical liabilities early in the discovery process.[4] For example, utilization of transformed human hepatotocytes in high-throughput assays can be useful first tier hepatotoxicity assessment. More labor intensive assays, such a primary animal and human cell *in vitro* assays, organ slices, and more recently, the use of multiorgan cell culture systems, are all particularly useful as second tier assays for evaluation of organ-specific toxicities and for investigative and mechanistic studies.[37,38] However, procurement and expense of human tissues and slow throughput remain major bottlenecks for the use of primary cells in discovery screening paradigms. Perhaps the best utilization of primary cells for predictive toxicology is in conjunction with gene expression profiling.[39,40] Although hepatocyte models have useful sensitivity and specificity for gauging the potential for human hepatotoxicity when the target is the hepatocyte, these models typically miss up to 30% of hepatotoxicants with alternate targets, such as the biliary epithelium. Robust *in vitro* models for prediction of biliary toxicity are currently not available.

9.2.2.5 *Cardiovascular Ion Channel.*
Safety pharmacology studies as defined by the ICH S7A guidance document are studies that investigate the potential undesirable pharmacodynamic effects of a substance on physiological function at the therapeutic and exaggerated exposures.[41] The objective of this document was to protect human clinical trial participants, as well as patients receiving marketed products from potential adverse functional effects of pharmaceuticals.

Of particular importance in safety pharmacology is the area of cardiovascular physiology (electrical conduction and hemodynamics), which is an integral and high profile component of the regulatory submission to support clinical trials, because of a heightened level of regulatory concern for the potential of drugs, such as terfenadine, to induce potentially fatal arrhythmias, namely, TdP. This arrhythmia has been associated with a specific electrocardiographic finding (termed the *prolonged QT interval*) that is secondary to inhibiting the potassium ion channel hERG. As such, a guidance document, ICH S7B, entitled "Nonclinical Evaluation of the Potential for Delayed Ventricular Repolarization (QT Interval Prolongation) by Human Pharmaceuticals", was created that describes a nonclinical *in vitro* and *in vivo* testing strategy for assessing the potential of a test substance to delay ventricular repolarization and proarrhythmic risk.[42]

The traditional gold standard to evaluate voltage-gated and other ion channels is manual patch clamping of cells with detailed cellular electrophysiology (EP) evaluation. In discovery, *in vitro* hERG channel assays and Purkinje fiber electrophysiology assays have shown very good concordance with the risk of prolonged QT interval in humans. This labor-intensive approach is clearly a bottleneck, especially when considering that on average, 50% of drug discovery chemistry efforts are developing SAR around ion channel activities. Thus, high-throughput, low-cost assays that are predictive of EP are ideal as first- or second- (after *in silico*) tier screens. To facilitate early assessment of a compound's potential to induce QT prolongation, a number of high-throughput and low-cost assays have been developed including radioligand binding, efflux, and fluorescence assays.[43–46] Recently, a 384-well, nonradiometric fluorescence polarization technology has been developed that is comparable to the more traditional radiometric assays and is predictive for functional hERG blockade as assessed by EP.[47] In addition, several higher throughput electrophysiology systems have been developed with a per person throughput approximately fourfold greater than the traditional approach.[48,49] Calibrating the relevance of *in vitro* findings from EP studies with *in vivo* electrocardiographic evaluation in relevant species is a critical step in assigning significance to EP data, particularly when interactions with multiple ion channels are demonstrated.[5]

Despite the focus on hERG channel interactions, drug-induced TdP, occurs rarely.[50] The relevance to risk assessment with hERG blockage compared to the risk assessment associated with the interactions of drugs with the cardiac myofiber Na^+ channel is minimal. While hERG binding predisposes an individual to a rare arrhythmia, Na^+ channel inhibition directly compromises cardiac output in a potentially already seriously compromised patient group. Through the authors' experience at BMS, hERG, and Na^+ channel interactions of compounds tested occur with a comparable frequency. It is important to remember that compounds can cause toxicity or even death by affecting any or all of the cardiovascular system components.[50]

Cardiovascular safety pharmacology is generally not considered a significant concern for biopharmaceuticals and specific studies are not usually required. However, first in person (FIP)-enabling studies should include appropriate safety pharmacology endpoints, such as electrocardiograms. More detailed safety pharmacology assessments are required if the mechanism of action to the product or observed toxicities suggest increased risk/concern. For example, there is emerging evidence of significant adverse cardiovascular effects of the breast cancer drug Herceptin®.[51]

Cardiovascular safety has become one of the most important developability criteria in drug discovery and development. Many assays and new technologies have been developed to predict ion channel related potential cardiovascular safety issues. The theories, related technologies, and their employment in drug discovery and development will be further discussed in Chapter 10.

9.2.2.6 Predictive Teratogenicity. Teratogenicity is a common cause of toxicology-based attrition ranking third after hepatic and cardiovascular toxicities.[52] Teratogenicity accounts for 8% of safety-related attrition at BMS (Table 9.1). As only limited reproductive toxicity studies, such as Segment II teratology studies, which comprise embryo fetal development in rats and rabbit, are initiated prior to FIP dosing, reproductive toxicity liabilities are usually not noted until 2 or 3 years into clinical development. At this stage of development, costs are high and such finding, depending on disease indication, can severely impact if not halt drug development efforts. As such, discovery strategies to address the potential for teratogenicity during late lead optimization are warranted. Such studies start with phenotypic assessment of genetically modified animals including gene-deleted or transgenic mice, extends to evaluation in zebrafish, organotypic, or stem cell culture with realtime PCR endpoints for important indicators of tissue differentiation, through to modified Segment I or II development and reproductive toxicology assessments in Discovery.

> *Phenotypic Assessment of Genetically Modified Animals.* Whether via a review of the existing literature or the actual evaluation of genetically modified animals, in-house or via a contract laboratory, a thorough phenotypic assessment for reproductive or developmental liabilities may be the first indication of potential teratogenic liability, and an indication for the more intensive *in vitro* profiling efforts on that particular class or series of compound.[52]

> *Rat Whole Embryo Culture Assay.* The rat whole embryo culture (WEC) assay is a useful screening assay for embryotoxic and teratogenic potential whereby rat embryos are collected at gestation days 9–11 and incubated with test article for ~48 h.[53] Morphological scoring of embryonic structures is then conducted to assess developmental liabilities. In a multinational validation study coordi-

nated by the European Centre for the Validation of Alternative Methods (ECVAM), the predictivity and precision of the rat WEC to identify embryotoxicants was considered high to excellent.[54,55] The BMS experience with this assay shows a predictivity for specific mammalian *in vivo* effects of >85%. For mechanistic investigations during the late organogenesis stage, a technique of culturing rat embryos between gestation days 12–15 was described, which provides toxicologists an opportunity for the mechanistic assessment of later developmental stages that is not available using the traditional embryo culture technique.[54]

Zebrafish Embryo Culture. The zebrafish (Danio rerio), which have most organ systems present in mammals, with the exception of lungs, prostate, mammary gland, and hair follicles, has recently emerged as a model for toxicological studies and drug discovery.[56–58] However, it has been more frequently and effectively utilized to study developmental biology and embryogenesis. The advantages of zebrafish embryos are many and include morphologic and physiologic similarity to mammals, small size (<1 mm in diameter) amenable to 96- and 384-well plating, rapid embryonic development, ability to absorb compounds through the water, and are optically transparent making it possible to detect functional and morphological changes in internal organs by light microscopy.[56–58] The BMS experience with this assay shows a predictivity for specific mammalian *in vivo* effects of >87, similar to that observed with the WEC. Recently, the zebrafish embryo model was modified to identify proteratogenic substances by combining it with an exogenous mammalian activating system (rat liver microsomes), and validation of this system is ongoing.[52,59]

Mouse Embryo Stem Cell Test. The mouse embryonic stem cell test (EST) is an *in vitro* assay that utilizes cultured mouse embryonic stem cells (D3 cell line) and differentiated mouse 3T3 fibroblasts.[60] Mouse blastocyst-derived pluripotent embryonic stem cells can be induced to differentiate into various cell types, including cardiomyoctes. The EST is a scientifically validated assay, based upon this feature, in that the embryotoxic potential of small molecules are evaluated for their ability to inhibit embryonic stem cells to differentiate into cardiomyocytes as compared to cytotoxic effects on these murine stem cells and mouse 3T3.[61,62] In an international ECVAM validation using *in vivo* results from a set of 20 reference compounds, the chemicals were correctly classified in 78% of the EST experiments.[63] Major advantages of this assay versus other *in vitro* embryotoxicity tests is that the EST utilizes permanent cell lines, as opposed to harvesting embryonic cells, tissues, or organs from time-mated pregnant animals, and the ability to differentiate into numerous cell types making it a good platform for exploring gene expression analysis and developmental processes.[62]

9.3   *IN VIVO* SAFETY ASSESSMENT

The conventional and more costly scenario commonly employed by pharmaceutical companies is to identify development limiting attributes during early development stages after significant investment in process chemistry during GLP regulated preinvestigational new drug (IND) activities and early clinical testing. In the case of small molecules, significant resource, time investment, and commitment to a chemical series have already taken place by this stage. Early prediction of potential toxicity–side effect barriers to development and delivery of an NCE with no genotoxicity; no significant toxicologic perturbations at projected efficacious exposures; well-defined dose-limiting toxicity, projected margin, and identification of toxicity biomarkers; and selection of the most appropriate species for toxicology testing during development are keys to the leading edge discovery stage toxicology testing paradigm. In support of this philosophy, the following practices drive the selection of compounds from late lead optimization for advancement to early development based upon toxicity profiling and eliminate compounds that have potential development limiting liabilities and insure a continuum of high-quality compounds into preclinical development.

9.3.1   Genotoxicity: *in Vivo* Erythrocyte Micronucleus

Positive results in the Ames assay and *in vivo* chromosome damage assays are relatively rare in IND submissions to the FDA–CDER.[10] As mentioned earlier, when these assays are positive, albeit rare, they have implications in carcinogenesis and in teratogenesis. As such, positive results in these assays represents a barrier to registration that are very difficult to manage for nonlife-saving indications, unless the disease is disabling and in an indication where there is poorly met medical need. Thus, any positive result in the *in vitro* clastogenicity assay(s) should be followed up with an *in vivo* micronucleus assay prior to advancement of a lead compound into IND enabling GLP studies.

The *in vivo* erythrocyte micronucleus assay is a test system, using either rats or mice, which detect two important forms of genetic damage, clastogenicity, and inhibition of spindle formation.[24] These types of genetic damage can be identified by examining the formation of micronuclei in polychromatic erythrocytes (PCE). Micronuclei are either chromosome fragments or whole chromosomes that were unable to migrate during cell replication. As a bone marrow erythrocyte matures into a PCE, the nucleus is extruded. However, micronuclei that may have been formed will remain in the PCE and can be visualized with appropriate staining. Chromosomal damage can be identified by an increase in the incidence of micronuclei formation in PCE. Ideally, compounds that are predicted to be clastogenic in the *in vitro* micronucleus assay should be quickly followed by an *in vivo* micronucleus assay. As compound requirements are high for this assay, this assay is limited to characterization of the lead candidate in late lead optimization or a sentinel molecule in early lead optimization. If bone marrow was archived as part of the rising dose satellite toxicity study, accelerated assessment performed in-house or via a contract lab with no additional chemical investment is possible. Positive results for *in vivo* clastogenicity signify an attribute potentially development limiting for a chronic use nonlife-threatening indication and should be deprioritized as early in the lead optimization phase as possible.

9.3.2 Alternative Animal Models

Genetically engineered mice include animals that have the activity of a specific gene removed (knock out), replaced (knock in), or the overexpression of a foreign gene (transgenic), and are used to investigate the molecular basis of disease, to screen novel targets for efficacy, and toxicity.[64] In the pharmaceutical industry, evaluation of knockout (KO) mice is firmly entrenched in target identification and validation. A retrospective evaluation of the 100 best-selling pharmaceuticals reports excellent correlation between drug efficacy and disease modulation as demonstrated by the respective target knockout.[65] However, the expense, time-intensive breeding, and redundancies leading to compensation of deficits, or in many instances embryonic lethality of a homozygous KO, preclude optimal use of these mice. Given the current time required to bring drug candidates and their backups to development, there can be adequate time for investigation of conditional knockout, adoptive transfer, adenoviral dominant negatives, and lentiviral-mediated RNA interference (RNAi) technologies yielding models much more closely approximating the administration of a pharmaceutical agent, and of potential use in pharmacology, as well as toxicology. The applicability of these models is exemplified in the scenario in which mice deficient in either the p65 (RelA) subunit of NF-κB or IKKβ die during fetal development via a TNF dependent mechanism.[66-68] However, chimeras in which lethally irradiated hosts were reconstituted with donor fetal liver stem cells from p65- or IKKβ-deficient mice survive, and have revealed a specific requirement for these molecules in development of T cells, B cells, and a role in regulating the production of granulocytes.[69] This mouse model accurately predicted NF-κB related pharmacologic effects observed at exaggerated dose levels during toxicity studies with an IKK2 inhibitor.[70] This example underscores the utility of adoptive transfer or conditional KO, the tissue or time-specific deletion of a gene, in instances in which potential redundancy or fetal nonviability may impair the usefulness of the unmodified knockout. Another useful application is to differentiate between on target pharmacology versus off-target drug-dependent lesions.[64] Observing drug effects in a KO devoid of the intended pharmacologic target would indicate an off-target effect. Phenotyping evaluations will often run concurrent with the early lead optimization phase and may even be initiated during the development phase in cases where there have been barriers to obtaining founder animals. While some predictive power is lost when these studies are conducted at later stages, phenotyping will, nonetheless, serve to corroborate existing efficacy, toxicology, and reproductive safety data. In addition, in programs where compounds do not block receptors in toxicology or efficacy species, it may be the only opportunity to assess inhibition of target function in a test species other than human. Phenotyping data can be formally reported and included in nomination documents supporting safety and efficacy of the compound.

It is beyond the scope of this chapter, which is focused on discovery toxicology, to discuss carcinogenicity risk assessment, but the role of transgenic mice in this endeavor will be mentioned for completeness. The gold standard carcinogenicity assessment for small molecules is the 2-year rodent bioassay performed in two rodent species. Genetically engineered mouse models of carcinogenicity testing include alterations that lead to either overexpression of an oncogene (e.g., rasH2, Tg.Ac) or abberrant DNA repair ($Xpa^{-/-}$) or deletion of a tumor suppressor gene (e.g., $p53^{+/-}$), which are genetic alterations that resemble certain spontaneous mutations that occur frequently in human neoplasms.[64] Since these mice develop more neoplasms and at a younger age than do wild-type mice, carcinogenicity testing can be completed in less time and at lower cost than the standard rodent bioassay.[71,72]

9.3.3   Satellite Toxicity Assessment

The aim of these studies is to identify potential chemical- or pharmacology-based toxicity during early lead optimization efficacy studies. By utilizing challenged animals in an ongoing efficacy study or unchallenged satellite animals (depending on the model) these studies facilitate lead selection with greatly improved efficiency with respect to consumption of chemistry-based resources. Ideally, these studies should be initiated during early *in vivo* efficacy studies by adding a full complement of toxicology endpoints including clinical observations, clinical chemistry, hematology, organ weights, macroscopic, and microscopic tissue examination. At least three animals per dose group on test for efficacy or on a similar subset of strain-matched satellite animals provide the tools to identify toxicity at efficacious exposures. Once target tissues are identified with a lead chemotype(s), it is generally acceptable to only examine target tissues in subsequent efficacy studies until the lead candidate is selected. In the absence of knockout data, these assessments may provide the first key evidence of *in vivo* pharmacologic effects associated with novel target antagonism or agonism. Another advantage is that structurally unrelated benchmark compounds are sometimes utilized in these studies that help to distinguish chemical toxicity versus exaggerated pharmacology. In addition, efficacy and/or toxicity biomarker identification can be delineated at this early stage. Early biomarker identification and/or refinement are crucial in order to determine applicability to the clinic. To support oncology discovery efforts, use of strain-matched, non-tumor-bearing satellite animals (at least three animals per dose group) is advised. Generally, a 10-fold dose over that obtained for efficacy is included. This provides an early read of exaggerated pharmacology effects, especially for novel targets, without access to genetically modified rodent models, as well as identification of target organs for additional toxicity studies. This early aggressive comparative approach may promote improved lead selection and augment SAR.

9.3.4   Rising Dose Tolerability

The purpose of the rising dose tolerability study is to establish the maximum tolerated dose for subsequent repeat-dose studies and to identify a tolerable range of doses from which allometric scaling may be used to select appropriate doses for non-rodent test species. Ideally these data are generated sufficiently early to facilitate dose selection for *in vivo* efficacy studies, thus minimizing resource wastage resulting from unexpected toxicity. Compound requirements are ~2.0 g for rats. To conserve resources, the following study design is suggested: One animal per sex are administered the test article in a dose escalating regimen. Dose limiting toxicity is confirmed by repetition with two animals per sex. Eight-point PK curves are generated and opportunity is presented to define dose-limiting toxicity as C_{max} or area under curve (AUC) driven. Bone marrow from a rising dose tolerance animals (rats) study can be collected and archived for future *in vivo* micronucleus assessment, as discussed above. If chemical resource is limited, the rising dose tolerability study can be eliminated and the dose selection for the repeat dose studies determined by 5- to 10-fold exposure exaggerations over projected human efficacious dose.

9.3.5 Repeat Dose Studies

During late lead optimization and prior to nomination of a compound for preclinical development, exploratory, non-GLP repeat dose study in rodents (mouse or rat), and when applicable a repeat dose study in dogs or non-human primates, should be designed to identify the maximum tolerated dose, target tissues, PK, and safety pharmacology profiles [e.g., central nervous system (CNS), renal], and projected safety margin. The number of days of dosing is flexible and should strive to achieve steady-state PKs. Dog and non-human primate studies can be conducted under non-GLP conditions, but in a manner suitable to utilize this data for dose ranging for IND enabling studies. To facilitate statistical analysis of clinical pathology and organ weight data, rodent studies should contain at least five animals/sex/group with three animals killed and examined at the end of the dosing phase and two animals/sex/group retained for reversibility. Eight-point PK curves are generated on the first and last day of dosing using two main study animals per time point. For non-rodent species, three-to-four animals per group are examined and toxicokinetic data is similarly obtained. The compound requirements are ~70–100 g to conduct both rodent and large animal toxicology studies. The philosophy of these studies is to establish a maximum tolerated dose. However, to conserve chemical an acceptable exposure exaggeration could be 5- to 10-fold over predicted human efficacious exposure, which should suffice to identify development limiting liabilities. Comparable findings across species at similar exposures suggest the potential for similar effects in humans at comparable exposure. If there is an effect observed in rats, but not in dog or non-human primate at similar exposures, the effect can be considered putatively rodent specific until further investigated. Generally, an effect in dog or non-human primates is considered more predictive for human findings. If the test agent has reached a steady state and there is minimal to no tissue accumulation of test article, then exacerbations of any observed changes in the short-term *in vivo* studies will be modest in the longer follow-up GLP nonclinical testing studies.

For biopharmaceuticals, examination of genetically engineered animals, a thorough review of the literature, and complete in-life and pathologic examination of *in vivo* efficacy models with the drug or surrogate help to define the pharmacology, but during late discovery, exploratory single-dose ranging studies in normal animals that focus on toxicology endpoints including PK/PD relationships, clinical pathology, and histopathology (when applicable), and immunogenicity are important adjuncts to facilitate FIP enabling studies. To be predictive of anticipated toxicities in humans, studies with biopharmaceuticals need to be conducted in a relevant animal species, which is defined as a species in which the biopharmaceutical has a similar biologic response to that observed in humans due to the expression of a responsive othologous drug receptor or antigen.[9] In particular, the high specificity for monoclonal antibodies means that most preclinical studies are conducted in non-human primates due to cross-reactivity, relevant pharmacology, similar immune systems, and similar PK.[23] The high target specificity of monoclonal antibodies translates into off-target effects are less of a concern, as compared to small molecules, and toxicologic findings are generally associated with exaggerated pharmacology. Thus, different from small molecule preclinical testing in which two species (rodent and non-rodent) are required; general toxicity of biopharmaceutical products can be assessed in only one species if that species has a cross-reactive or identical target to that in humans.[8,9]

A major safety concern for biopharmaceutical agents is immunogenicity during clinical studies. The generation of human antibodies to the therapeutic agent can have significant consequences regarding safety, as well as directly impacting PK. Immunogenicity is generally related to intrinsic properties of the protein, addition of conjugates to the protein (pegylation, etc.), or impurities either in the protein or its formulation (aggregates, fragments, etc.) and should be evaluated in all *in vivo* studies. Evaluating immunogenicity in a preclinical species has significant implications in the design of later studies to support clinical testing. The measurement of immunogenicity can be influenced by numerous factors including type of assay used, timing of sample collection, and interference from circulating drug.[8] Formation of neutralizing antibodies could limit usefulness of the species from chronic repeat-dosing studies as immunogenicity can eliminate the activity of the protein. Most often, non-human primates have been selected as toxicology species to minimize the chance for antibody response.[8] In some instances, this is overcome by the use of surrogate antibodies. In addition, neutralizing antibodies may also alter the PK, cross-react with other endogenous proteins, form immune complexes that deposit in tissues, or cause anaphylaxis or injection-site reactions. These are major concerns because experience unfortunately has shown that the extrapolation of immunogenicity from animal studies to humans is poor for all species. Other safety concerns that are of special note to human clinical studies are cytokine release reactions and anaphylaxis. Although anaphylactic reactions can occur with both small molecule therapeutics and biopharmaceuticals, the latter tend to be of greater concern, especially involving agents that are immunomodulatory in nature. Making this issue more complicated, anaphylaxis may be difficult to distinguish from cytokine release reactions.[73]

Although highly resource intensive, many serious adverse events are first detected in multiple-dose toxicity studies. Overall the predictive capacity of the various models discussed in this chapter are useful for detecting and eliminating approximately one-half of all toxicities, the remainder appearing in longer term studies. It is most important once having identified such an issue to reduce it to a practical and if possible, cell- or biochemical-based screen to allow SAR optimization away from such liabilities in Discovery. An iterative cycle of improving compounds is thus obtained.

9.3.6 Toxicokinetics and Effects on Metabolizing Enzymes

The exploratory repeat-dose safety assessment study with a preclinical development compound, in addition to providing safety margin assessment, provides a prospect on the status of hepatic metabolic enzymes, based on the toxicokinetic data observed. An increase in last day of dosing plasma exposure (AUC_τ) compared to that of Day 1 ($AUC_{0-\alpha}$) can be due to inhibition of cytochrome P450 values (CYP) responsible for the metabolism of the target compound, or a decrease could be via CYP induction or secondary bioaccumulation. For the definition of toxicokinetic–pharmacokinetic terms and their determination, the reader may refer to Chapter 2 for the details. Depending on the magnitude of activity, this can impact safety margins. Induction of CYPs activity can result in increased liver weight, but a more sensitive indicator is measurement of transcriptional expression of CYPs' protein. Note that increased liver weights can also occur with the increased expression of functionally nonactive CYPs due to enzyme inhibition and secondary compensatory induction. Thus, high-throughput activity measurement assays to determine the functional status of various CYPs may be warranted. Moreover, mechanism-based inhibition of CYP3A should be assessed to obtain clues as to activation of compounds to reactive metabolites that may lead to toxicity in multiple organs capable of metabolizing the compound. The CYP1A induction, mediated by the Ah receptor, can be predictive of increased tumorigenic potential for polycyclic aromatic hydrocarbons in higher species.[74] More detailed information regarding P450 induction and inhibition was discussed in Chapter 6. Drug metabolism and the generation of a potential reactive metabolite have been discussed from an angle of qualitative analysis in Chapter 5.

9.3.7 Cardiovascular Safety Pharmacology

The definitive cardiovascular safety pharmacology study is the conscious telemetrized dog or non-human primate model. If profiling in the first and second tier screening assays does not identify cardiovascular risk, compounds can be advanced directly into a definitive GLP telemetry study in support of regulatory filing. For a compound or class of compound that do not have a sufficiently large window between hERG and other cardiovascular ion channels and target IC_{50} margins, they should be profiled in exploratory *in vivo* ambulatory radiotelemetry implanted animals to assess the potential to prolong the QT interval and other cardiovascular parameters. The doses and concentrations used in this *in vivo* study should reflect 3×, 10×, and 30× of the projected efficacious therapeutic C_{max}. Depending on the indication, compounds that do not significantly alter cardiovascular parameters in telemeterized animals, at ≥10× projected efficacious therapeutic C_{max} may be progressed into further preclinical development. As the QT interval is inversely proportional to heart rate, several correction formulas have been used both nonclinically and clinically. For nonclinical studies, the Van de Water's correction formula for beagle dogs ([QT-0.87]*[$RR^{1/2}$-1]) and the Fridericia's correction formula for Cynomolgus monkeys (QT/$RR^{1/3}$) should be applied.

9.3.8 Systems of Biology Technologies

The introduction of transcriptional profiling of all late discovery and selected development compounds has provided early biomarker and mechanistic toxicology information, but current real impact on reducing attrition is limited. The application of metabonomics and proteomics has not impacted drug attrition, but has provided focused examples where risk assessment of safety liabilities is enhanced. The predictive capacity of the systems biology technologies is currently less well developed than their retroactive, judicious application to issues identified using traditional approaches. Thus, the applicability of the following technologies for predictive toxicology remains somewhat limited, however, these technologies can be integral to issue resolution and management. The specific evaluation of the issue, rather than the available technology, should dictate resolution of mechanistic and/or target organ related causes of drug attrition. Genomics technologies can be applied at multiple points in the nonclinical drug discovery pipeline from early *in vitro* assays through to samples from multiple-dose IND enabling GLP studies. Validation of assay procedures and assay interpretations for genomics methods at present are generally unavailable,[75] predisposing the use of findings toward company internal decision making around risk benefit of NCEs. In this role, each individual company assumes the risks of data over interpretation inherent in the new methods.[76] Nonvalidated uses of genomics can, however, make significant contributions toward characterization of the safety of NCEs.[77] Currently, key limiting factors for success in nonvalidated uses of genomics for safety assessment are the availability of sufficient historical data to place findings in perspective and availability of personnel knowledgeable in combining concepts from drug safety risk assessment and genomic data analysis. Over the long term, formal assay and interpretation validation efforts will be enabling of regulatory uses of genomic markers for diagnosis and prediction of toxicities, but currently these applications are largely unavailable.

Transcriptomics. The most advanced of the genomic biology technologies in application to reducing drug candidate attrition is transcriptomics. Example uses of the assay spanning multiple points of the drug discovery pipeline are given in the Table 9.2. Currently, to our knowledge, many pharmaceutical companies actively engage in transcriptomic activities in exploratory *in vitro* and *in vivo* studies during preclinical development, but for the most part avoid incorporation of transcriptomics into the IND enabling GLP studies and use for regulatory filings. This is primarily due to the lack of validated markers and methods. In lieu of such validation, transcriptional profiling of tissues from studies conducted in Discovery can provide a useful general biosensor for toxicity, and through reference to larger databases, such as those provided by Gene Logic (Gaithersburg, MD) and Iconix

TABLE 9.2. Example Uses of Transcriptomics

Model System	Location in Pipeline	Purpose of Transcriptomic Study
Rat primary hepatocytes	Lead evaluation to early lead optimization (LO)	Early identification of hepatoxicity *in vitro*
Repeat dose rat studies	Concurrent with LO efficacy studies	Identification of toxicity *in vivo*; ranking of competing candidate compounds in unchallenged satellite animals
Exploratory repeat dose rat and mouse studies	Late LO exploratory repeat dose studies with lead candidate(s) or range finding studies for definitive IND enabling GLP studies	Transcriptomic data is combined with traditional safety data for an integrated risk assessment
IND enabling GLP studies	Preclinical development	Characterization of candidate compound in pivotal GLP studies
Mechanistic *in vitro; in vivo*; rodent, non-rodent, single or repeat-dose studies	Preclinical through clinical development	Reactive mechanistic evaluations to refine assessment of a specific identified risk
Various	At any point.	Definitively predict human toxicity, submit data in regulatory filings

Biosciences (Mountain View, CA), transcriptional profiles may be assigned both diagnostic and mechanistic specificity. The introduction of transcriptional profiling to all late discovery and selected development compounds at BMS has provided early biomarker and mechanistic toxicology information, but current real impact on reducing attrition is limited.[77] Based on our experience with application of transcriptomics on NCEs, the kinds of benefits seen from the applications above include identification of pharmacologic response in the toxicity study, classification relative to candidate mechanisms of toxicity, characterization of transcriptional target organs and species, hypothesis generation around mechanisms of toxicity, and contribution to an integrated risk assessment across studies and assays.

Metabonomics. Metabonomics describes the profiling of body fluids for levels of small molecule endogenous metabolites, and the interpretation of these patterns as predictors of toxicity and disease.[78] Metabonomics is particularly attractive in that non-invasive sampling of body fluids (e.g., urine, plasma) is possible, and the sensitivity of nuclear magnetic resonance (NMR)- and mass spectrometry (MS)-based technologies requires low sample volumes; factors readily amenable to the clinic. This highly sensitive technology has been used successfully under controlled experimental conditions, to identify toxicity and disease, and provide information through which mechanisms of toxicity may be addressed. In a noncontrolled environment, influences ascribed to variation in environment, diet, and gastrointestinal flora can significantly affect the predictive value of studies.[79] Extrapolation to the more variable human test environment further tests the limits of the technology, though several clearly impactful studies of metabonomics in humans have been published.[80] Poor annotation of measured analytes is the major limiting factor in utilization of the NMR-based approach.[78] To accurately interpret metabonomic profile changes requires a precise understanding of the nature of measured endogenous metabolites. The current application of this technology in toxicology is limited to risk assessment, with predictive utility yet to be demonstrated on a larger scale.

Proteomics. Proteomics most commonly utilizes two-dimensional (2D) gel electrophoresis and MS in the global separation, quantitation, and functional characterization of expressed proteins in tissue samples.[81] As mRNA does not always reflect protein levels in tissues or the post-translational modifications of proteins, global protein expression pattern profiling provides complementary information to genomics.[80] Despite improved methodologies, the application of proteomics to predictive toxicology has lagged behind transcriptomics and metabonomics. The strengths of proteomics methods are the ability to detect post-translational changes, more directly relevant than mRNA analysis, and applicability of technology to clinical studies, while the weaknesses are throughput and annotation.[78] Thus, assessment of issues in biology is most advanced where well-annotated profiles of human samples or human cells are subject to analysis. To this end, the identification of clinical biomarkers of compound pharmacodynamics, efficacy, and disease are readily identified with this technology.[82] Providing a link from nonclinical to clinical proteomics is a nascent field. Peptide identification from non-human species is generally too slow to be of use in a practical timeframe for decision making in the Discovery environment. Focused extension of this approach, including protein arrays allowing facile specific protein identification and high content screening approaches, are quite valuable tools in the Discovery environment.

9.4   CHALLENGING AREAS IN PREDICTIVE SAFETY ASSESSMENT

Idiosyncratic or immune-mediated toxicities and biliary toxicity are events for which there are a paucity of validated predictive tools. These and many other toxicities are first observed in chronic multiple-dose toxicology studies. In general, the prudent application of predictive methodologies allows the removal of a large number of potential liabilities, but in the authors' experience, greater than one-half the toxicities observed are first noted in such longer term studies. To define and understand the mechanistic basis for findings from chronic studies allows the generation of facile counterscreens for Discovery chemists. The iterative nature of compound improvement depends on rapid communication of such issues between culturally disparate and often geographically separate groups in Development and Discovery environments. Effective communication is therefore key to rapidly establish the iterative cycle of improvement in compounds and their backups.

9.5   CONCLUSION

Identification of toxicity and side-effect liabilities early in drug discovery insures a continuum of high-quality compounds moving into preclinical development, thus significantly impacting expenditures associated with late-stage development attrition. This chapter focuses on the various strategies being applied to integrate toxicology in the drug discovery process and provides a greater understanding of the causes and timing of toxicology-driven attrition in drug development and how the discovery toxicologist can better interface with the pharmacologist and medicinal chemist. Implementation of an integrative discovery toxicology strategy encompassing general practices alongside innovative approaches from *in silico* to *in vivo* screening and the use of "omics" technologies during lead optimization and early preclinical development of small molecules provides this basis to predict and adequately manage potential causes of compound failure.

REFERENCES

1. DiMasi, J. A.; Hansen, R. W.; Grabowski, H. G. *J. Health Econ.* **2003**, 22, 151–185.
2. US Food and Drug Administration. Challenge and Opportunity on the Critical Path to New Medical Products, Department of Health and Human Services, Washington, DC, **2004**, 1–22.
3. DiMasi, J. A. *Pharmacoeconomics* **2002**, 20, 1–10.
4. Whitebread, S.; Hamon, J.; Bojanic, D.; Urban, L. *Drug Disc. Today* **2005**, 10, 1421–1433.
5. Car, B. D. *Am. Drug Disc.* **2006**, 1, 53–56.
6. Sasseville, V. G.; Lane, J. H.; Kadambi, V. J.; Bouchard, P.; Lee, F. W.; Balani, S. K.; Miwa, G. T.; Smith, P. F.; Alden, C. L. *Chem. Bio. Interact.* **2004**, 150, 9–25.
7. Alden, C. L.; Sagartz, J. E.; Smith, P. F.; Wilson, A. G.; Bunch, R. T.; Morris, D. L. *Toxicol. Pathol.* **1999**, 27, 104–106.
8. Cavagnaro, J. A. *Nat. Rev. Drug Discov.* **2002**, 1, 469–475.
9. Guidance for Industry S6 Preclinical Safety Evaluation of Biotechnology-Derived Pharmaceuticals. July 1997 (Draft Guidance August **2006**).
10. Jacobson-Kram, D.; Contrera, J. F. *Toxicol. Sci.* **2007**, 96, 16–20.
11. Snyder, R. D.; Pearl, G. S.; Mandakas, G.; Choy, W. N.; Goodsaid, F.; Rosenblum, I. Y. *Environ. Mol. Mutagen.* **2004**, 43, 143–158.
12. Richard, A. M. *Mutat. Res.* **1998**, 400, 493–507.
13. Pearl, G.; Livingston-Carr, S.; Durham, S. *Curr. Top. Med. Chem.* **2001**, 1, 247–255.
14. He, L.; Jurs, P. C.; Custer, L. L.; Durham, S. K.; Pearl, G. M. *Chem. Res. Toxicol.* **2003**, 16, 1567–1580.
15. Mattioni, B. E.; Kauffman, G. W.; Jurs, P. C.; Custer, L. L.; Durham, S. K.; Pearl, G. M. *J. Chem. Inf. Comput. Sci.* **2003**, 43, 949–963.
16. Keating, M.; Sangiunetti, M. *Cell* **2001**, 104, 569–580.
17. Ekins, S. *Drug Disc. Today* **2004**, 9, 276–285.
18. Wempe, M. F. *J. Mol. Structure* **2001**, 562, 63–78.
19. Arrigoni, C.; Crivori, P. *Cell Biol. Toxicol.* **2007**, 23, 1–13.
20. Seierstad, M.; Agrafiotis, D. K. *Chem. Biol. Drug Des.* **2006**, 67, 284–296.
21. Halliwell, W. H. *Toxicol. Pathol.* **1997**, 25, 53–60.
22. Pelletier, D. J.; Gehlhaar, D.; Tilloy-Ellul, A.; Johnson, T. O.; Greene, N. *J. Chem. Inf. Model* **2007**, 47, 1196–1205.

23. Chapman, K.; Pullen, N.; Graham, M.; Ragan, I. *Nat. Rev. Drug Discov.* **2007**, 6, 120–126.

24. International Conference on Harmonization (ICH), S2A: Specific Aspects of Regulatory Genotoxicity Tests for Pharmaceuticals, **1996**.

25. ICH S2B Genotoxicity: A Standard Battery for Genotoxicity Testing of Pharmaceuticals, **1997**.

26. Westhouse, R. A.; Car, B. D. Concepts in Pharmacology and Toxicology. in *Cancer Immunotherapy: Immune Suppression and Tumor Growth.* Eds. Prendergast, G. C., Jaffee, E. M. **2006**, Elsevier.

27. Quillardet, P.; Huisman, O.; D'Ari, R.; Hofnung, M. *Proc. Natl. Acad. Sci. USA* **1982**, 79, 5971–5975.

28. Quillardet, P.; Hofnung, M. *Mutat. Res.* **1993**, 297, 235–279.

29. Rosenkranz, H. S.; Mersch-Sundermann, V.; Klopman, G. *Mutat. Res.* **1999**, 431, 31–38.

30. Gee, P.; Sommers, C. H.; Melick, A. S.; Gidrol, X. M.; Todd, M. D.; Burris, R. B.; Nelson, M. E.; Klemm, R. C.; Zeiger, E. *Mutat. Res.* **1998**, 30, 115–130.

31. Fluckiger-Isler, S.; Baumeister, M.; Braun, K.; Gervais, V.; Hasler-Nguyen, N.; Reimann, R.; Van Gompel, J.; Wunderlich, H. G.; Engelhardt, G. *Mutat. Res.* **2004**, 558, 181–197.

32. Fenech, M. *Mutat. Res.* **2000**, 455, 81–95.

33. Norppa, H.; Falck, G. C. *Mutagenesis* **2003**, 18, 221–233.

34. Miller, B.; Pötter-Locher, F.; Seelbach, A.; Stopper, H.; Utesch, D.; Madle, S. *Mutat. Res.* **1998**, 410, 81–116.

35. Matsushima, T.; Hayashi, M.; Matsuoka, A.; Ishidate Jr. M.; Miura, K. F.; Shimizu, H.; Suzuki, Y.; Morimoto, K.; Ogura, H.; Mure, K.; Koshi, K.; Sofuni, T. *Mutagenesis* **1999**, 14, 569–580.

36. Pohjala, L.; Tammela, P.; Samanta, S. K.; Yli-Kauhaluoma, J.; Vuorela, P. *Anal. Biochem.* **2007**, 362, 221–228.

37. MacGregor, J. T.; Collins, J. M.; Sugiyama, Y.; Tyson, C. A.; Dean, J.; Smith, L.; Andersen, M.; Curren, R. D.; Houston, J. B.; Kadluba, F. F.; Kedderis, G. L.; Krishnan, K.; Li, A. P.; Parchment, R. E.; Thummel, K.; Tomaszewski, J. E.; Ulrich, R.; Vickers, A. E.; Wrighton, S. A. *Toxicol. Sci.* **2001**, 59, 17–36.

38. Li, A. P.; Bode, C.; Sakai, Y. *Chem. Biol. Interact.* **2004**, 150, 129–136.

39. Liguori, M. J.; Waring, J. F. *Expert Opin. Drug Metab. Toxicol.* **2006**, 2, 835–846.

40. Abel, S.; Yang, Y.; Waring, J. F. *ALTEX* **2006**, 23 Suppl: 326–331.

41. International Conference on Harmonization (ICH), Safety Pharmacology Studies for Human Pharmaceuticals, **2001**.

42. International Conference on Harmonization (ICH), Nonclinical Evaluation of the Potential for Delayed Ventricular Repolarization (QT Interval Prolongation) by Human Pharmaceuticals, **2005**.

43. Chiu, P. J.; Marcoe, K. F.; Bounds, S. E.; Lin, C. H.; Feng, J. J.; Lin, A.; Crumb, W. J.; Mitchell, R. *J. Pharmacol. Sci.* **2004**, 95, 311–319.

44. Diaz, G. J.; Daniell, K.; Leitza, S. T.; Martin, R. L.; Su, Z.; McDermott, J. S.; Cox, B. F.; Gintant, G. A. *J. Pharmacol. Toxicol. Methods* **2004**, 50, 187–199.

45. Dorn, A.; Hermann, F.; Ebneth, A.; Bothmann, H.; Trube, G.; Cristensen, K.; Apfel, C. *J. Biomol. Screen* **2005**, 10, 339–344.

46. Cheng, C. S.; Alderman, D.; Kwash, J.; Dessaint, J.; Patel, R.; Lescoe, M. K.; Kinrade, M. B.; Yu, W. *Drug Dev. Ind. Pharm.* **2002**, 28, 177–191.

47. Deacon, M.; Singleton, D.; Szalkai, N.; Pasieczny, R.; Peacock, C.; Price, D.; Boyd, J.; Boyd, H.; Steidl-Nichols, J. V.; Williams, C. *J. Pharmacol. Toxicol. Methods* **2007**, 55, 238–247.

48. Zheng, W.; Spencer, R. H.; Kiss, L. *Assay Drug Develop. Technol.* **2004**, 2, 543–552.

49. Guo, L.; Guthrie, H. *J. Pharmacol. Toxicol. Methods* **2005**, 52, 123–125.

50. Hamlin, R., *Tox. Pathol.* **2006**, 34, 75–80.

51. Routledge, H. C.; Rea, D. W.; Steeds, R. P. *Clin. Med.* **2006**, 5, 478–481.

52. Augustine-Rauch, K. A. *Current Drug Metab.* **2008**, 9, 971–977.

53. New, D. A. *Biolog. Rev. Cambridge Philos. Soc.* **1978**, 53, 81–122.

54. Liu, J. N.; Chan, H. M.; Kubow, S. *Toxicol. In Vitro* **2007**, 21, 53–62.

55. Piersma, H.; Genschow, E.; Verhoef, A.; Spanjersberg, M. Q. I.; Brown, N. A.; Brady, M.; Burns, A.; Clemann, N.; Seiler, A.; Spielmann, H. *Alter. Lab. Anim.* **2004**, 32, 275–307.

56. Rubinstein, A. L. *Expert. Opin. Drug Metab. Toxicol.* **2006**, 2, 231–240.

57. Kari, G.; Rodeck, U.; Dicker, A. P. *Clin. Pharmacol. Ther.* **2007**, 82, 70–80.

58. Zon, L. I.; Peterson, R. T. *Nature Rev.* **2005**, 4, 35–44.

59. Busquet, F.; Nagel, R.; von Landenberg, F.; Mueller, S. O.; Huebler, N.; Broschard, T. H. *Toxicol. Sci.* **2008**, 104, 177–188.

60. Spielmann, H.; Pohl, I.; Döring, B.; Liebsch, M.; Moldenhauer, F. *In Vitro Toxicol.* **1997**, 10, 119–127.

61. Seiler, A.; Visan, A.; Buesen, R.; Genschow, E.; Spielmann, H. *Reprod. Toxicol.* **2004**, 18, 231–240.

62. Seiler, A. E.; Buesen, R.; Visan, A.; Spielmann, H. *Methods Mol. Biol.* **2006**, 329, 371–395.

63. Genschow, E.; Spielmann, H.; Scholz, G.; Seiler, A.; Brown, N.; Piersma, A.; Brady, M.; Clemann, N.; Huuskonen, H.; Paillard, F.; Bremer, S.; Becker, K. *Altern. Lab. Anim.* **2002**, 30, 151–176.

64. Bolon, B. *Basic Clin. Pharmacol. Toxicol.* **2004**, 95, 154–161.

65. Zambrowicz, B. P.; Sands, A. T. *Nat. Rev. Drug Discov.* **2003**, 2, 38–51.

66. Beg, A. A.; Sha, W. C.; Bronson, R. T.; Ghosh, S.; Baltimore, D. *Nature (London)* **1995**, 376, 167–170.

67. Tanaka, M.; Fuentes, M. E.; Yamaguchi, K.; Durnin, M. H.; Dalymple, S. A.; Hardy, K. L.; Goeddel, D. V. *Immunity* **1999**, 10, 421–429.

68. Li, Q.; Van Antwerp, D.; Mercurio, F.; Lee, K. F.; Verma, I. M. *Science* **1999**, 284, 321–325.

69. Horwitz, B. H.; Scott, M. L.; Cherry, S. R.; Bronson, R. T.; Baltimore, D. *Immunity* **1997**, 6, 765–772.

70. Nagashima, K.; Sasseville, V. G.; Wen, D.; Bielecki, A.; Yang, H.; Simpson, C.; Grant, E.; Hepperle, M.; Harriman, G.; Jaffee, B.; Ocain, T.; Xu, Y.; Fraser, C. *Blood* **2006**, 107, 4266–4273.

71. Maronpot, R. R. *Toxicol. Pathol.* **2000**, 28, 450–453.

72. Alden, C.; Smith, P.; Morton, D. *Toxicol. Pathol.* **2002**, 30, 135–138.

73. Greenberger, P. A.; *J. Allergy Clin. Immunol.* **2006**, 117, Suppl. 2, S464–S470.

74. Waxman, D. J. *Arch. Biochem. Biophys.* **1999**, 369, 11–23.

75. International Conference on Harmonization (ICH), Terminology in Pharmacogenomics Draft Guidance, January **2007**.

76. Boverhof, D. R.; Zacharewski, T. R. *Toxicol. Sci.* **2006**, 89, 352–360.

77. Foster, W. R.; Chen, S.-J.; He, A.; Truong, A.; Bhaskaran, V.; Nelson, D. M.; Dambach, D. M.; Lehman-McKeeman, L. D.; Car, B. D. *Toxicol. Pathol.*, **2007**, 35, 621–635.

78. Guengerich, F. P.; MacDonald, J. S. *Chem. Res. Toxicol.* **2007**, 20, 344–369.

79. Robertson, D. G. *Toxicol. Sci.* **2005**, 809–822.

80. Lindon, J. C.; Holmes, E.; Nicholson, J. K. *Curr. Opin. Mol. Ther.* **2004**, 6, 265–272.

81. Gatzidou, E. T.; Zira, A. N.; Theocharis, S. E. *J. Appl. Toxicol.* **2007**, 27, 302–309.

82. Chapal, N.; Molina, L.; Molina, F.; Laplanche, M.; Pau, B.; Petit, P. *Fundam. Clin. Pharmacol.* **2004**, 18, 413–422.

CHAPTER 10

ASSESSMENT OF STRATEGIES UTILIZED TO MINIMIZE THE POTENTIAL FOR INDUCTION OF ACQUIRED LONG QT SYNDROME AND TORSADE DE POINTES

KHURAM W. CHAUDHARY AND BARRY S. BROWN
Department of Safety Pharmacology, GlaxoSmithKline, King of Prussia, PA

10.1 INTRODUCTION

Drug-induced prolongation of the QT_c interval (acquired long QT syndrome), can lead to the generation of a rare, but potentially lethal, tachyarrhythmia known as Torsade de Pointes (TdP). Of note, is the

Evaluation of Drug Candidates for Preclinical Development: Pharmacokinetics, Metabolism, Pharmaceutics, and Toxicology, Edited by Chao Han, Charles B. Davis, and Binghe Wang
Copyright © 2010 John Wiley & Sons, Inc.

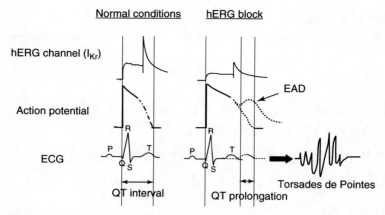

Figure 10.1. Compounds that inhibit I_{Kr}, the current encoded by the hERG gene, promote the prolongation of the cellular action potential and repolarization. Action potential prolongation manifests in the electrocardiogram (ECG) as a lengthening of the QT interval that can lead to the generation of early afterdepolarizations (EAD) and the potentially lethal arrhythmia known as Torsade de Pointes (TdP).[10b]

discovery of 50 compounds developed for noncardiac targets in the past two decades that cause QT prolongation and TdP.[1,2] With an estimated cost of >$800 million and >10 years of development in bringing a new drug to market, the ability to discharge this risk during the drug discovery process offers the prospect of bringing safer medications to patients in a more rapid, cost-effective manner.[3]

Thus far, all drugs that cause QT prolongation and subsequent generation of TdP, preferentially block the rapid component of the delayed rectifier potassium current (I_{Kr}), of the cardiac myocyte.[4–10a] Therefore, the propensity of compounds to bind to and inhibit the hERG potassium channel, the molecular determinant of I_{Kr}, has become a preclinical biomarker for QT prolongation and TdP (Fig. 10.1).[10b]

Compounds with potent hERG inhibiting properties, such as dofetilide, astemizole, and cisapride, are associated with clinical QT prolongation and have lead to incidents of TdP.[10–12] For a series of fluoroquinolone antibacterial compounds including sparfloxicin, Kang et al. found significant QT prolongation at free plasma concentrations near 15–30% of their respective hERG inhibiting IC_{50} values.[13] Further, retrospective analysis of 52 compounds of various chemical classes confirmed that those drugs implicated in causing a 10–20% increase in clinical QT measurements fall below a 30-fold safety margin with respect to their effective therapeutic free plasma concentration and their corresponding observed IC_{50} for hERG potency.[14]

Nonclinical Testing Strategy

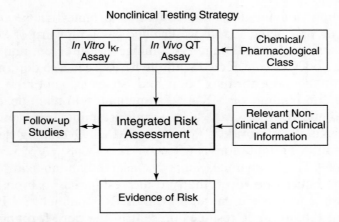

Figure 10.2. International Conference on Harmonization of Protocols risk assessment diagram for nonclinical evaluation of the potential for delayed ventricular repolarization by human pharmaceuticals.

As a result, the International Conference on Harmonization of Protocols (ICH) has issued a specific guidance (ICHS7B) suggesting that compounds, in a concentration range encompassing therapeutic exposure up to the limit of solubility, be assessed on the basis of their: (1) structural similarity to known torsadogenic agents; (2) effect on isolated cardiac ion channels, particularly hERG; (3) effect on cardiac action potential repolarization; and (4) effect on electrocardiogram *in vivo* (Fig. 10.2). However, there remains a lack of consensus on the methods to address this governance. In this chapter, we will discuss strategies most commonly used to profile the potential torsadogenic effect of preclinical drug candidates.

10.2   *IN SILICO* MODELING

In silico modeling of hERG inhibition involves computational approaches that are both channel structure (target) and phamacophore (ligand) based. Although the three-dimensional (3D) crystal structure of the hERG channel has not been identified, homology of the channel with bacterial KcsA and MthK channels allows for predictive modeling of compound-binding domains within the channel.[15–19] The hERG channel consists of a homotetrameric tertiary structure.[15,19,20] Each monomer is composed of a six transmembrane spanning domain protein with a pore loop and selectivity filter between the S5 and S6 domains. Unlike other voltage gated potassium channels, the S6 segment of the pore-forming domain does not contain a proline-rich sequence of amino acids, producing a large water filled cavity upward of 12 Å.[16]

Mitcheson et al., used alanine-scanning, site directed, mutagenesis in *Xenopus* oocytes transfected with the hERG gene, to determine the residues in the pore-forming loop and S6 transmembrane domain important for binding of MK-499, a methanesulfonanilide class III antiarrhythmic drug, as well as the antihistamine terfenadine, and gastric prokinetic cisapride.[19] Potency of MK-499 binding decreased with the following mutations: F656 > Y652 > G648 = V625 > T623 > S624 = V659. The K_v channels share a conserved amino acid sequence in the pore helices, however, the tyrosine residue at position 652 and phenylalanine at 656 are unique to the hERG channel.[7,21,22] It is suggested that the aromatic residues present in the pore-forming helices of the hERG channel are important in the binding of compounds. These amino acids provide a backbone for π–π interactions, π-stacking and hydrophobic interactions (F656), and cation-π (Y652) interactions with basic nitrogen groups present in many hERG blockers.[23–25] Although each of the above mutations caused a reduction in binding affinity of MK-499, a change in G648 and V625 did not dramatically reduce the affinity of cisapride and terfenadine for the channel; illustrating the diversity of common and unique binding interactions within the channel pore.[19,26]

Ligand-based *in silico* modeling requires the compilation of data from several known compounds in an effort to identify pharmacophores with inhibitory properties. This method provides structure–activity relationships and details of the binding pocket within the channel when structural information is scarce. Ekins et al. generated a pharmacophore model based on literature data from an initial set of 15 drugs with published electrophysiological hERG inhibiting properties.[27] The "general pharmacophore model" generated a correlation (R^2) of 0.90 versus observed potency of these compounds using patch clamp electrophysiology. The 3D-QSAR (quantitative structure–activity relationship) predicts the electrostatic and geometric interactions of drugs with the channel and allows for different molecular conformations of the inhibitor; hydrophobic, aromatic, and hydrogen-bonding interactions; as well as ionizable groups. Using this model, a potent hERG binding molecule is predicted to have four hydrophobic groups in the shape of a pyramid, containing a single positively ionizable feature at the apex (Fig. 10.3).[27] This model was subsequently tested with 22 drugs, mostly antipsychotics, and generated an R^2 value of 0.83.[27]

Several other QSAR models have been developed since these initial studies, including a Comparative Molecular Field Analysis model

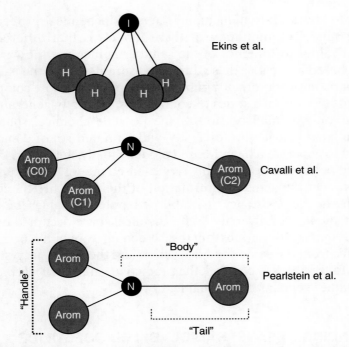

Figure 10.3. Pharmacophores with hERG inhibiting properties generated by the various ligand-based *in silico* modeling techniques. (Recanatini, M., E. Poluzzi, et al. (2005). *Med Res Rev* **25**(2), 133–166.)

(CoMFA) and a Comparative Molecular Similarity Indices Analysis model (CoMSiA).[17,18,28,29] The CoMFA model overlays novel compounds over the known structure of a potent hERG inhibitor, astemizole. This model predicts a pharmacophore with hERG inhibiting properties to have three aromatic moieties bound to an individual tertiary amine.[25,28] On the other hand, CoMSiA compares structures that have properties contributing to biological activity including steric, electrostatic, hydrophobic, and hydrogen-bond acceptors–donors utilizing 22 analogs of sertindole as a template.[17,18]

Both target- and ligand-based modeling approaches have provided insight on the promiscuity of the hERG channel for various molecules. The three most important lessons are (1) the F656 and Y652 amino acids of the S6 domain, which are unique to the hERG potassium channel, allow for interactions with structurally diverse drugs; (2) the large size of the intracellular pore cavity allows access to a multitude of pharmacophores; and (3) binding affinity may change based on the state (open vs closed) of the channel as the conformation of the pore is state dependent. A good *in silico* model should take all of these factors into consideration, including the physiochemical properties of the compound. The limitation of these models is that differences in published values for potency of the same drug increase the variability in ligand-based models, as these direct measurements are the backbone for comparison. Alternatively, published potency for most compounds reflects just one out of a series of compounds originally generated, and represents only a small portion of the possible chemical space. This leads to a lack of structural diversity, and a limited set of compounds to be used to generate a ligand-based model. Finally, the hERG channel remains to be crystallized and any target-based model we currently use may not reflect the actual conformation of the native hERG channel. Based on the inconsistency in published potency values of known inhibitors; the lack of diversity in the chemical space occupied by these reference agents; limitations on the screening capability of internal compounds from the same chemical series; and the lack of a crystallized structure for the hERG channel, the predictive value of *in silico* modeling techniques remains questionable.

10.3   BINDING ASSAYS: RADIOLABELED DOFETILIDE

The time and resources inherent in screening compounds for QT liability has necessitated the development of higher throughput assays.[30] Heterologous expression of the hERG gene in recombinant cell lines (human embryonic kidney cells and Chinese hamster ovarian tumor cells), as well as identification of potent inhibitors of the channel, including the Class III antiarrhythmic dofetilide, has aided in the characterization of channel properties.[9,31,32]

The [^3H]-dofetilide studies were first described by Chadwick et al.[31] as a means to "characterize drug-channel interaction at the molecular level". In this study, freshly isolated guinea pig and canine cardiac myocytes were incubated with radiolabeled dofetilide. Unlabeled dofetilde was able to displace the radioligand in a competitive manner, suggesting a high-affinity binding site for dofetilide. Further, hERG tail currents measured from guinea pig myocytes were inhibited by dofetilide with potency similar to that obtained from the displacement binding assay (IC_{50} of 44 vs 100 nM, respectively).

Diaz et al., conducted a thorough evaluation of the [^3H]-dofetilide displacement binding assay in both intact cells and membrane preparations from hERG trasfected HEK293 cells.[33] Both preparations produced similar K_d values for dofetilide (34.6 nM) and K_i values for 22 test compounds. However, isolated membranes provide a substrate more amenable to increased throughput and lack the low-affinity binding site for dofetilide present in intact cells, which may skew the observed potency of test compounds.[32]

Finally, 56 compounds were evaluated using the isolated membrane binding assay in comparison to published electrophysiological data for hERG inhibition.[33] Although a slight rightward shift in potency was observed in the dofetilide binding assay suggesting a decrease in sensitivity, a good correlation was detected between the two assays ($R^2 = 0.86$, Fig. 10.4).

The dofetilide displacement-binding assay has been employed by several pharmaceutical companies as a high-throughput preclinical screen to assess hERG liability. Although some might argue the physiological relevance of this nonfunctional assay, binding potency correlates very well with manual patch-clamp electrophysiology for many pharmacophores because compound-dependent current inhibition requires direct interaction with the intracellular channel vestibule.[34,35] However, it is important to consider the tolerance of the hERG channel-binding pocket to various pharmacophores when interpreting data from binding studies. It is plausible that a compound might bind to a site not occupied by dofetilide, thereby producing a false-negative result. Also, binding assays specifically address competitive displacement of ligands, but do not differentiate between activators or

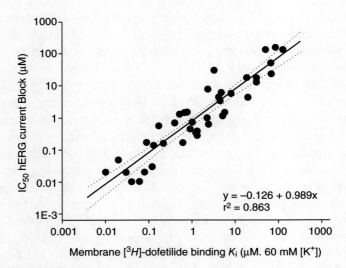

Figure 10.4. Comparison of [^3H]-dofetilide membrane binding K_i values at 60-mM [K^+]$_0$ to isolated whole-cell patch clamp IC$_{50}$. Dotted lines represent 95% confidence intervals.[33]

inhibitors of the channel. Finally, the predictive value of the dofetilide assay represent only a putative inhibition of the channel, as it is not a measure of functional current. Although published examples of a discord between dofetilide displacement potency and hERG inhibiting properties of a compound are difficult to find, personal experience suggests that the role of the displacement binding assay should not be to replace–circumvent a definitive functional assay in a testing strategy, but rather to identify those compounds in a series with potent hERG affinity.

10.4 UNICELLULAR PREPARATIONS

10.4.1 Fluorescence-Based Assays

The advent of fluorometric imaging plate readers (FLIPR) and availability of fluorescent probes have further enhanced the automation of hERG screening. Fluorescence-based hERG assays rely on opening–closing of the hERG channel and subsequent changes in membrane potential. These changes cause redistribution of the fluorescent probe from the extracellular environment into the cytosol.

Dorn et al. illustrated the advantages of the FMP dyes (fast responding electrochromic dye), over $DiBAC_4$ (slow responding Nernstian dye), including a 14-fold faster response time to changes in membrane potential, as well as a 300% change in absolute fluorescence after depolarization of the hERG expressing cells.[36] The FMP dyes display fluorescence kinetics that match changes in observed membrane potential, however, only a 10% change in fluorescence is induced by a 10-mV shift in membrane potential.[37]

Because fluorescent assays are useful for studying a variety of ion channels, emphasis has been placed on development and automation of the assay platform. Plate readers are now designed with 1536 wells, and can generate upward of tens of thousands of data points per day.[38] Although a functional assay, the lack of sensitivity of the fluorescence-based screen leads to a large number of false negatives: drugs that appear to have weak hERG inhibiting properties.[36,39] In general, potency values for potent reference agents have been reported to have a rightward shift of 5 to >100-fold in comparison to electrophysiological data. Limitations of this assay also include dye-compound interactions,[39] quenching and photobleaching of the dye, as well as sensitivity to background currents expressed in commonly used cells (HEK293).[34,40] Use of high $[K^+]_0$ buffer to induce depolarization is also problematic, as studies suggest changes in hERG binding affinity of compounds.[33,39]

Based on the confounding issues associated with fluorescent probes and their lack of sensitivity to variations in membrane potential, these assays are not often utilized in a traditional screening strategy for hERG liability.

10.4.2 Flux-Based Assays

Potassium channels are highly permeable to rubidium, an element not commonly found in biological systems.[41] The rubidium efflux assay, a technique that has been employed to study both ligand and voltage-gated potassium channels for decades, takes advantage of the property of the sodium–potassium pump to load the cytosol with rubidium.[42,43] Subsequent high $[K^+]_0$ depolarization of cells, and opening of potassium channels, causes the flow of rubidium ions down their chemical gradient: out of the cell. Originally described as a radioactive assay,[42,44] in its present form the assay utilizes nonradioactive rubidium measured by flame atomic absorption spectroscopy.[43] Since rubidium is ionized and detected by the spectrometer, contamination by cellular debris and other ions is not detected.

The rubidium efflux assay was able to rank known reference agents in order of hERG inhibiting potency quite accurately, albeit a 5–20-fold decrease in potency was observed when compared to patch clamp derived data.[35,39] In a measure of reproducibility, a Z′ factor of 0.80 was generated, validating its quality as a high-throughput screen. Using a sample set of 78 unknown compounds at 10 μM, Tang et al., were able to categorize compounds into highly potent and less potent groups in comparison to patch-clamp data. In a separate study, only 4 out of 19 compounds previously screened using patch-clamp electrophysiology tested positive for hERG blockade as measured by rubidium efflux.[35] Alternatively, the dofetilide displacement binding assay provided a coefficient of determination (R^2) of 0.90 in comparison to patch-clamp data for the same set of compounds.

Much like the fluorescence assay discussed previously, the rubidium efflux assay provides a functional means for the high-throughput screening of compounds. The plate handling and spectroscopy can be automated in such a way as to analyze upward of 700 compounds in duplicate per day.[44] However, many of the same limitations hold true for this assay including the use of high $[K^+]_0$ for depolarization and insensitivity of use or state-dependent blockers. Additionally, the use of Rb^+ as the charge-carrying ion reduces affinity of compounds for the hERG channel, and causes a reduction in channel inactivation that may further decrease compound potency.[45]

Both fluorescence and Rb^+ flux assays appear to lack sensitivity compared to direct measurement of channel function. Although one can assign scaling factors to observed potency values based on the shift in potency, this artificial manipulation of the data is based on a subset of known inhibitors. Any comparison to actual channel inhibition will still necessitate the manual measurement of channel function, and/or compilation of very large populations of known and unknown inhibitors. Thus, the indirect platforms may allow one to differentiate between various classes of compounds, but appear less useful for addressing actual inhibitory potencies. In addition, because the ICHS7B guidelines recommend measurement of channel inhibition over a therapeutic range, and up to the limits of solubility, the inherent rightward shift in potency associated with the fluorescence and Rb^+ efflux assays limits the experimental window of concentrations suggested in this guideline. The onus lies on the investigator to interpret these high-throughput assays in this context.

10.4.3 Electrophysiology Assays

Precise control of the sarcolemmal membrane potential, facilitated by the formation of a tight physical seal between a glass microelectrode and the cell membrane, allows for cycling of the hERG channel through various states. Binding of a compound to the inner vestibule of the channel is often a complex process dependent on activation and subsequent inactivation of the channel. For example, Class III antiarrhythmics, such as dofetilide, sotalol, as well as the gastric prokinetic cisapride bind to the channel in its open state, and inhibition is stabilized as the channel becomes inactivated.[46,47] Compounds can also exhibit frequency-dependent increases in their binding affinity and inhibition of the hERG current. Moreover, investigators can employ complex protocols to mimic the cellular action potential, thereby recreating the native stimulus for channel activation.[48]

The complexity of patch-clamp electrophysiology requires a specialized skill set that severely limits throughput. The availability of cell lines stably transfected with the hERG gene affords an increase in throughput while reducing variability between experiments, but estimates for the number of compounds screened per day remain modest. If measurement of the hERG current by conventional voltage-clamp electrophysiology is considered the "gold standard" of cardiotoxicity screening; automation of this assay provides the best means for high-throughput and high-fidelity screening. To that end, several companies have invested in the development of "planar" chip-based voltage-clamp platforms that multiply throughput by several orders of magnitude.

Whereas conventional electrophysiology uses a single micro-electrode, the IonWorks™ HT utilizes a polymer-based, 384-well, planar array to voltage-clamp cells. Compound addition is achieved by an automated pipetting head, which alternates with a voltage clamping electrode head.[49] Initial validation of this platform supported its utility as a functional hERG assay, as Z' vaules exceeded 0.5, and a success rate of 79% was observed. Although channel currents resembled those obtained by manual electrophysiology, and supraphysiological con-centrations of MK-499 caused complete channel block, a decrease in potency was observed for all compounds tested in comparison to manual electrophysiology. Furthermore, compounds tended to cause a "carry-over" effect due to adherence of compounds to the pipetting mechanism.

First, accurate voltage control is traditionally achieved by a high-resistance seal between electrode and cell. This platform allows for the use of cells with much "leakier" seals to the electrode ($100\,M\Omega$ vs $1\,G\Omega$ in conventional electrophysiology). Second, the voltage-clamping head and pipetting head function sequentially, causing a loss of voltage control between compound addition and current measurement. Finally, carry-over of compounds as they stick to the pipetting head, as well as compounds adhering to the plastic polymer of the plates, can lead to under/overestimation of the concentration exposed to the cells.

Alternatively, Molecular Devices Inc. (MDC), and Sophion Bioscience both have designed medium-throughput automated plat-forms with voltage-clamping capabilities analogous to manual electro-physiology. Each individual well is independently controlled by a separate high-impedance head-stage. This platform ostensibly allows for a user defined combination of 16 separate experiments. Average success of gigaseal formation was ~70% for Chinese hamster ovarian cells expressing the hERG channel, but differed depending on the cell line of choice.[50] A good correlation was observed for potency values generated by the PatchXpress (MDC) compared to published values for 12 compounds of various chemical classes ($R^2 = 0.87$), however, it was obvious that compounds with lipophilic properties tended to produce lower potencies because of nonspecific binding to plastic assay plates used for compound mixing and storage.[50] The QPatch (Sophion) platform provides similar seal success rate, and utilizes glass-coated microfluidics to resolve the confounding effects of lipophilic com-pounds binding to the plastic substrate.[51]

Automated voltage-clamp platforms require further validation with a larger subset of known hERG blockers, as well as novel chemical entities, as variability does exist in these assays.[52] A common complaint of investigators using planar patch technology is the difficulty with which an adequate seal is achieved with respect to the recombinant cell lines often used for hERG studies. The HEK293 cells are notorious for their ability to overexpress the hERG channel producing large outward tail currents. However, the assay platforms are not optimized for this particular cell line. Conversely, CHO cells form GΩ seals quite readily with planar patch electrodes, but do not express the channel as robustly.[50] Although the platforms are technically far less challenging than manually attempting current measurements, cell culture and harvest require quite a bit of technical optimization. Finally, it is estimated that fluorescence assays conducted utilizing the FLIPR cost roughly $0.20/data point, while planar patch-clamp electrophysiology can range from $2.00 to $10.00/data point. The cost alone will assuredly limit the use of this platform by smaller companies.

This section has highlighted several shortcomings of the automated patch-clamp platforms, but investment in and development of these assays are the future of cardiac ion channel screening. A novel approach by MDC to automating these platforms is called "population patch-clamp electrophysiology". In practice, patch-clamp measurement of current from cells actually measures the average current produced by the channels expressed in the cell membrane. Population patch-clamp measures the average current of up to 64 cells/well on a planar electrode containing 384 wells.[53] This strategy takes into consideration the lack of expression of the channel by some cells, and subtracts the leak current associated with empty holes in the well. The increased probability of cells forming seals in a 64-hole well leads to the successful measurement of current from upward of 95% of wells. It will be interesting to see if this novel approach is adopted–utilized in compound screening in the years to come.

These automated platforms allow us the flexibility to provide high-fidelity hERG channel data, but can be augmented to measure the function of various other ion channels, thereby providing a comprehensive screen of cardiac liability. They remain technically less challenging than manual electrophysiology, but retain the positive correlation established previously between hERG current inhibiting properties of compounds and prolongation of the QT interval.

10.4.4 Trafficking Assays

Drug-induced inhibition of hERG current is not the only mechanism by which QT prolongation can occur. Furutani et al. described a hypomorphic mutation in the G601 amino acid of the hERG channel that lead to a prolonged QT interval phenotype.[54] In fact, this mutation caused a decrease in cell surface expression of the channel, thereby implicating trafficking abnormalities in long QT syndrome. Studies have shown that compounds, such as arsenic trioxide (leukemia) and pentamidine (pneumonia), prolong QT interval not by acutely blocking the repolarizing hERG current, but by reducing the trafficking of functional channels to the cell surface over time.[55-57] This mechanism of QT prolongation is quite novel, but equally important as acute hERG inhibition with respect to its torsadogenic potential. Further, Wible et al. described a novel assay to address the trafficking liability caused by compounds, called HERG-Lite®.[58] In this assay 100 compounds of various hERG blocking properties were tested, and 40% of them produced trafficking abnormalities. Since this assay provides both acute block and trafficking defects as an endpoint simultaneously, it may prove to be an interesting alterative for some of the other high-throughput assays previously discussed.

10.5 MULTICELLULAR PREPARATIONS

10.5.1 *Ex vivo*

Although selective hERG blockade accounts for the majority of drug-induced arrhythmias in the clinical setting, it is well known that hERG is just one of >10 ion channels that shape the cardiac action potential[59] and that point mutations in any one of at least seven of these channels or their associated auxillary subunits or trafficking chaperones results in an inherited form of a cardiac rhythm disorder.[60] In addition, drug effects at other cardiac ion channels can elicit arrhythmias. For example, blockers of the cardiac sodium channel with slow dissociation kinetics (flecainide, encainide) have been recognized, since the termination of the Cardiac Arrhythmia Suppression Trials,[61] to be proarrhythmic, whereas compounds that "activate" the cardiac sodium channel by slowing its rate of inactivation (veratridine, DPI 201–106) are also arrhythmogenic.[62,63] Furthermore, drugs can exert multi-ion channel effects that can abrogate the functional consequence of their hERG inhibition. Perhaps the best example of this profile is verapamil, which inhibits hERG with a potency of 143 nM[64] but, owing to its block of calcium channels, possesses antiarrhythmic[65] rather than proarrhythmic activity. Thus, it is clear that any nonclinical assessment of torsadogenic or arrhythmogenic potential is incomplete and possibly misleading if it merely involves the evaluation of effects on hERG alone.

To assess drug effects on the cardiac action potential and/or its underlying ionic currents, investigators have long utilized dissociated myocytes, ventricular trabeculae, papillary muscles, or Purkinje fibers primarily from guinea pig, rabbit, or dog. Of these preparations, canine and rabbit Purkinje fibers have been evaluated most extensively for their ability to predict arrhythmogenic liability. In a study on the effects of 12 clinically utilized drugs, Gintant et al.[66] reported that 6 of 7 agents associated with QT prolongation or TdP in humans caused a >15% prolongation of action potential duration (APD) in canine Purkinje fibers (terfenadine was the lone exception), whereas 5 of 5 agents unassociated with either QT prolongation or TdP failed to prolong APD by >15%. The inability of the canine Purkinje fiber preparation to detect a change in APD in response to terfenadine may be related to the lower sensitivity of canine versus rabbit Purkinje fibers to drug-induced APD prolongation.[67] Accordingly, using rabbit Purkinje fibers, Aubert et al., demonstrated a significant prolongation of APD_{90} with terfenadine.[68] In this same study, however, verapamil was identified as a "positive" APD prolonging compound that showed effects similar to those of the torsadogenic agents, terfenadine and thioridazine. In aggregate, these results suggest that a homogeneous, isolated tissue preparation may be useful for identifying potential multi-ion channel effects, but its ability to predict arrhythmogenic liability appears somewhat limited.

The precise explanation for the limited ability of homogeneous cardiac tissue preparations to predict drug-induced arrhythmogenicity is uncertain. One possible explanation is that the most commonly studied preparations, papillary muscles and Purkinje fibers, do not contain M cells, the ventricular cell type that most influences the end of the QT interval and whose APD is most sensitive to both changes in heart rate and I_{Kr} blockade.[69] A second possible explanation is that drug effects on APD often differ between ventricular cell types, thereby making the correlation between drug effects on APD in a single-cell type and QT interval (let alone arrhythmogenicity) tenuous, at best.[70] A third possibility is that preparations, such as papillary muscles and Purkinje fibers, do not allow for the measurement of transmural dispersion of repolarization, a parameter considered to be better correlated with torsadogenic potential than changes in APD, a parameter routinely measured in these preparations.[71,72]

In recent years, several *ex vivo* preparations that retain the structural, electrophysiological, and pharmacological diversity of the ventricle have been tested for their ability to predict drug-induced QT prolongation or arrhythmogenic liability. Hamlin et al. assessed the effects of 39 compounds on the QTc interval of isolated, perfused guinea pig hearts.[73] In this study, all 26 compounds known to lengthen QTc clinically were shown to prolong QTc in the guinea pig Langendorff preparation and all 13 compounds known to not lengthen QTc clinically were without a significant effect. However, closer inspection of the results show that some drug concentrations required to prolong QTc appear clinically irrelevant. For example, a 1-mM concentration of erythromycin was required to show a significant QTc effect whereas, clinically, intravenous (iv) erythromycin attains a free plasma concentration of 1–10 μM. Similarly, 10-μM chlorpheniramine was needed to prolong QTc, whereas free therapeutic plasma concentrations are in the 2–10-nM range. In addition, clozapine appeared to be more potent than thioridazine whereas, clinically, both QT prolongation and TdP are clearly more problematic with thioridazine.[74] Thus, the utility of the perfused guinea pig heart to detect QT effects at meaningful drug concentrations and to differentiate between compounds within a given treatment class appears quite limited.

In contrast to the guinea pig, the rabbit Langendorff preparation appears to display a high degree of sensitivity and specificity for detecting drug-induced QT prolongation and arrhythmogenesis. With the use of an atrioventricular node-blocked, perfused rabbit heart, Milberg et al. demonstrated prolongation of QT interval, monophasic action potential duration at 50 and 90% repolarization ($MAPD_{50}$ and $MAPD_{90}$), early afterdepolarizations (EADs), and TdP with both erythromycin and clarithromycin at concentrations as low as 150 μM.[75] Interestingly, in the same concentration range (150–300-μM), azithromycin significantly prolonged QT interval, $MAPD_{50}$, and $MAPD_{90}$, but did not induce either EADs or TdP. The absence of an arrhythmogenic effect of azithromycin, in the presence of QT prolongation, was attributed to its lack of AP triangulation as reflected by little to no effect on the $\Delta MAPD_{90}/\Delta MAPD_{50}$ ratio. In a similar study, these investigators showed that although both sotalol and amiodarone prolong QT and MAPD to a similar extent, only sotalol induced EADs, TdP, and AP triangulation.[76] As has been proposed for drug effects in humans, these results suggest that QT prolongation, per se, is not necessarily pro-arrhythmic.[77] Thus, the rabbit Langendorff preparation appears well suited for not only differentiating between QT prolongation and arrhythmogenicity, but also detecting differences in arrhythmogenic potential between structurally related compounds at therapeutically relevant concentrations. The ability to differentiate between structurally related compounds is especially important in the lead optimization phase of drug discovery where the selection of a molecule to advance into the development process is often made between compounds of similar structure within a given chemotype.

Hondeghem and associates have also utilized the rabbit Langendorff preparation in their development of the SCREENIT procedure, a medium throughput, computerized system for the evaluation of pro-arrhythmic risk of new or existing chemical entities. The SCREENIT procedure, which has been validated in a blinded study of 14[78] or 31[79] compounds, determines the incidence of arrhythmias (ventricular tachycardia, ventricular fibrillation, or TdP) and evaluates drug effects on monophasic action potential conduction (upstroke velocity), duration at several levels of repolarization, triangulation of repolarization ($MAPD_{30}/MAPD_{90}$), reverse-use dependence of $MAPD_{60s}$, instability of beat-to-beat changes in $MAPD_{60}$ values, and dispersion of transmural repolarization as indicated by the $T_{peak} - T_{end}$ (T_{p-e}) interval in the ECG.[80] More recently, however, a blinded study of 55 compounds has demonstrated both false positives and false negatives utilizing the SCREENIT procedure.[81]

Another *ex vivo* model that retains the structural, electrophysiological, and pharmacological diversity of the ventricle is the arterially perfused, electrically paced left-ventricular wedge preparation. Since its development,[82] this model has been used extensively to define cellular mechanisms of arrhythmogenesis[83–86] and to assess the proarrhythmic potential of several drugs, including sotolol, azimilide, cisapride, and dofetilide.[84,87,88] Most recently, the rabbit ventricular wedge preparation was used in a blinded evaluation of 13 compounds to determine its suitability for predicting drug-induced QT prolongation and torsado-genic potential.[89] Each compound was assigned a TdP score that was based on its effect on QT interval, transmural dispersion of repolarization (TDR; measured as the T_{p-e}/QT ratio) and severity of phase 2 early afterdepolarizations. Of the compounds tested, 7 are known to be associated with QT prolongation and TdP in humans. All 7 of these drugs elicited a TdP score of 2.5 or greater at concentrations <100 times their free therapeutic plasma C_{max}. In contrast, the remaining 6 compounds, all of which are not torsadogenic in humans, elicited TdP scores of <2.5 (and, in some cases, negative values) over a similar relative concentration range. Thus, in this study, the rabbit-wedge preparation proved to be both highly sensitive and highly specific for the assessment of drug-induced QT prolongation and torsadogenic potential (Fig. 10.5).

In addition to its sensitivity and specificity, the rabbit-wedge preparation was able to accurately reproduce the relative risk of drugs within a given compound class. Accordingly, of the macrolide antibiotics

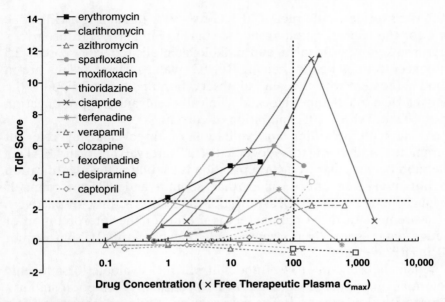

Figure 10.5. Effect of 13 reference agents on TdP scores recorded in the isolated rabbit ventricular wedge preparation with respect to their free (unbound) human therapeutic plasma concentration. Each compound was evaluated in a randomized, blinded manner.[89]

tested, azithromycin elicited TdP scores much lower than either clarithromycin or erythromycin. For fluoroquinolone antibiotics, moxifloxacin was less torsadogenic than sparfloxacin, for antipsychotics, clozapine was less torsadogenic than thioridazine, and for antihistamines, fexofenadine was less torsadogenic than terfenadine. The ability of a model to distinguish relative risk between compounds of similar structure is a highly desirable property within the pharmaceutical industry where decisions regarding selection of compounds for development are usually between similar structural entities. In support of these findings, Lu et al. reported that the rabbit-wedge preparation was superior to that of hERG current, rabbit Purkinje fiber, and rabbit Langendorff preparations in ranking the relative human risk for two fluoroquinolone (sparfloxacin and erythromycin), and two macrolide antibiotic (moxifloxacin and telithromycin) agents.[90]

Another striking feature of the data generated in the blinded validation study on the rabbit ventricular wedge preparation was the concordance between the hERG IC_{50} and the concentration at which known torsadogenic compounds elicited a TdP score >3. For example, the TdP score exceeded 2.5 for cisapride at ~20 nM. With a hERG IC_{50} of 45 nM,

20-nM cisapride would inhibit hERG by ~30% (assuming a Hill slope of 1 for the concentration–response curve).[6] Similarly, clarithromycin, erythromycin, sparfloxacin, and moxifloxacin elicited TdP scores >2.5 at concentrations below their hERG IC_{50} values. These results are in good agreement with the general observation that, when hERG is the only cardiac ion channel blocked, clinically relevant QT prolongation is associated with a 20% inhibition of current.[14]

Along with providing an evaluation of three clinically relevent parameters underlying torsadogenicity (QT interval, TDR, and EADs), the rabbit ventricular wedge preparation is useful for the identification of potential drug effects on cardiac sodium and calcium channels through its measure of QRS duration and contractility, respectively. Measurement of these parameters is useful for the interpretation of wedge data, especially for compounds that block hERG, but do not elicit TdP scores of >2.5.[91]

When choosing an *ex vivo* model in which to evaluate torsadogenic potential, an important characteristic to consider is temporal stability. Drugs with slow onset kinetics may require 30 min or more to elicit a steady-state response. Thus, if an investigator is interested in performing a standard concentration–response study involving four to five escalating concentrations, it may be necessary to work with a preparation that is stable for 4 h or more. The rabbit ventricular wedge preparation appears to satisfy this requirement,[92] whereas the rabbit Langendorff may not.[78]

In summary, aside from its technical difficulty and limited availability, the rabbit ventricular wedge preparation currently represents the best available *ex vivo* technique for assessing the risk for and potential mechanism of drug-induced arrhythmias, in general, and TdP, in particular. For all of the reasons stated above, this was the preparation of choice by an independent academic task force for preclinical, *ex vivo* evaluation of drug-induced TdP during the drug development process[93] and the model receiving the highest validation score from attendees of a British Society for Cardiovascular Research-sponsored conference on drug-induced TdP.[94]

10.5.2   *In vivo*

Although *in vivo* cardiovascular preparations are more labor intensive and require more compound and PK support than *ex vivo* studies, they offer the potential advantage of assessing hemodynamic, as well as arrhythmogenic, risk in the setting of plasma protein binding and intact autonomic nervous and liver metabolic systems. As with *ex vivo* studies, the selection of species for *in vivo* evaluation is an important consideration. Mice and rats are not appropriate species due to the insignificant role I_{Kr} and I_{Ks} play in their ventricular repolarization.[95,96] Studies in large animals, like dogs[97] or monkeys,[98] require large quantities of compound, are extremely labor intensive and, therefore, are usually performed only during the postcandidate selection, drug development process. Thus, the two species most widely utilized during the precandidate selection phase of drug discovery are guinea pigs and rabbits.

Testai et al.[99] examined the effects of nine reference agents on QT intervals in pentobarbital-anesthetized guinea pigs. When administered intravenously at doses of 0.1–10 mg/kg, all seven drugs known to be torsadogenic in humans elicited a dose-dependent prolongation of the QT interval and the corrected QT interval (using either the Bazett or Fridericia correction factors). Included in this group of positive standards were terfenadine and thioridazine, two compounds that are often false negatives in preclinical models.[98] The two non-torsadogenic compounds evaluated in this study (chlorprothixene and diazepam) had no significant effect on QT intervals. Thus, despite the fact that guinea pigs do not develop torsade or torsade-like arrhythmias and pentobarbital anesthesia may influence drug effects on repolarization and hemodynamics, this model demonstrated a high degree of sensitivity and specificity for the limited set of compounds investigated and, therefore, should be more broadly evaluated.

With the recognition that QT prolongation, per se, is not necessarily proarrhythmic,[77] Fossa et al.[100] developed a cardiac electrical alternans model in pentobarbital-anesthetized guinea pigs. In this model, drug effects on heart rate and blood pressure were evaluated at normal sinus rhythm, whereas $MAPD_{50}$ and $MAPD_{90}$ were measured while pacing at basic cycle lengths of 140–200 ms. To be able to relate drug-induced changes in hemodynamic or MAPD values to free plasma concentrations, separate PK experiments were performed. At a BCL of 150 ms, all four torsadogenic agents studied (E-4031, bepridil, cisapride, and terfenadine) induced a change in beat-to-beat $MAPD_{50}$ values (mean alternans) that exceeded vehicle controls by >10 ms at a free plasma concentration <100 times the known therapeutic concentration in humans. In the same study, neither verapamil nor risperidone increased mean alternans by >10 ms at any dose or BCL examined (Fig. 10.6). This same group of investigators has also shown that the anesthetized guinea pig electrical alternans model was capable of differentiating the relative arrhythmogenic risk of three antibacterial agents, moxifloxacin, erythromycin, and telithromycin.[101] Although more invasive and

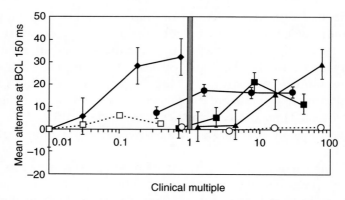

Figure 10.6. Effect of bepridil (♦), E-4031 (●), cisapride (■), terfenadine (▲), verapamil (□), or risperidone (○) on the mean alternans of beat-to-beat $MAPD_{50}$ recorded in anesthetized guinea pigs with respect to their free (unbound) human therapeutic plasma concentration.[100]

labor intensive than the model described by Testai et al.[99] the electrical alternans model gives a measure of drug-induced electrical instability that is likely to be of greater value than simply QT intervals alone. In agreement with this conclusion, Vos and his associates have demonstrated the superiority of evaluating beat-to-beat variability of repolarization (BVR) over the QT interval for predicting drug-induced TdP in an anesthetized, AV-blocked canine model.[102–105]

In addition to anesthetized guinea pig models, Hamlin et al. developed a novel conscious guinea pig model in which stable ECG recordings can be obtained without the need for anesthetics or chronic instrumentation.[106] Evaluation of three torsadogenic (sotolol, cisapride, and ketoconazole) and three nontorsadogenic (propranolol, verapamil, and enalapril) compounds showed that only the torsadogenic agents induced a significant prolongation of QTc following oral administration of clinically relevant doses of each drug. Should this model be shown to be able to discriminate between structurally related compounds and to provide a measure of compound exposure, it would be of greater interest even though its only outcome measure is QT interval.

The α-chlorolose-anesthetized, methoxamine-sensitized rabbit model, originally developed by Carlsson et al.,[107,108] appears to be most sensitive to the torsadogenic effect of selective hERG blockers. Lu et al. demonstrated that dofetilide and clofilium induced TdP in this model, but terfenadine and quinidine did not.[109] Similarly, Farkas and Coker reported that clofilium, but not erythromycin, was torsadogenic in this model.[110] In addition to yielding false negatives, this model appears prone to incorrectly predicting the relative liability of related compounds. For example, Anderson et al., reported that the arrhythmia induction rate for sparfloxacin was greater than that for grepafloxacin.[111] This result is in contrast to the clinical experience that has led to the classification by Redfern et al., of grepafloxacin as a Category 2 compound (withdrawn from the market due to TdP), whereas sparfloxacin is a Category 4 compound (isolated reports of TdP).[14] What is missing from most, if not all, of the studies with this model is adequate PK evaluation of the type so elegantly utilized by Fossa et al. in the guinea pig electrical alternans model.[100] Without that data, it is uncertain whether the α-chlorolose-anesthetized, methoxamine-sensitized rabbit model simply lacks sensitivity or if inadequate doses of test compounds were administered.

As with guinea pigs, an *in vivo* conscious rabbit model has been recently reported to have the capability of differentiating between torsadogenic and non-torsadogenic compounds on the basis of their effects on QTc intervals.[112] This model is worthy of further development especially in light of the fact that rabbits, as opposed to guinea pigs, develop drug-induced TdP.

In summary, the *in vivo* proarrhythmia model that currently seems most suitable for utilization during the drug discovery process is the guinea pig electrical alternans model established by Fossa and associates. This model has the advantage of (1) recording a measure of electrical instability shown to have predictive value in both perfused rabbit hearts[78] and anesthetized dogs[102], (2) requiring small-to-moderate compound supply, and (3) being amenable to concurrent PK evaluation. Validation of this model in a blinded study would significantly enhance the confidence in the predictive value of this preparation.

REFERENCES

1. Darpo, B. *Eur. Heart J. Suppl.* **2001**, 3(Suppl. K), K70–80.
2. Haverkamp, W.; Breithardt, G.; Camm, A. J.; Janse, M. J.; Rosen, M. R.; Antzelevitch, C.; Escande, D.; Franz, M.; Malik, M.; Moss, A.; Shah, R. *Cardiovasc. Res.* **2000**, 47(2), 219–233.
3. DiMasi, J. A.; Hansen, R. W.; Grabowski, H. G. *J. Health Econ.* **2003**, 22(2), 151–185.
4. Brown, A. M. *Cell Calcium* **2004**, 35(6), 543–547.
5. Gintant, G. A.; Su, Z.; Martin, R. L.; Cox, B. F. *Toxicol. Pathol.* **2006**, 34(1), 81–90.

6. Rampe, D.; Roy, M. L.; Dennis, A.; Brown, A. M. *FEBS Lett.* **1997**, 417(1), 28–32.

7. Sanguinetti, M. C.; Mitcheson, J. S. *Trends Pharmacol. Sci.* **2005**, 26(3), 119–124.

8. Snyders, D. J.; Chaudhary, A. *Mol. Pharmacol.* **1996**, 49(6), 949–955.

9. Zhou, Z.; Gong, Q.; Ye, B.; Fan, Z.; Makielski, J. C.; Robertson, G. A.; January, C. T. *Biophys. J.* **1998**, 74(1), 230–241.

10. a. Zhou, Z.; Vorperian, V. R.; Gong, Q.; Zhang, S.; January, C. T. *J. Cardiovasc. Electrophysiol.* **1999**, 10(6), 836–843. b. Hoffmann and Warner **2006**, *J Pharmacol Toxicol Methods* 53(2), 87–105.

11. Carmeliet, E. *J. Pharmacol. Exp. Ther.* **1992**, 262(2), 809–817.

12. Mohammad, S.; Zhou, Z.; Gong, Q.; January, C. T. *Am. J. Physiol.* **1997**, 273(5 Pt 2), H2534–2538.

13. Kang, J.; Wang, L.; Chen, X. L.; Triggle, D. J.; Rampe, D. *Mol. Pharmacol.* **2001**, 59(1), 122–126.

14. Redfern, W. S.; Carlsson, L.; Davis, A. S.; Lynch, W. G.; MacKenzie, I.; Palethorpe, S.; Siegl, P. K. S.; Strang, I.; Sullivan, A. T.; Wallis, R.; Camm, A. J.; Hammond, T. G. *Cardiovasc. Res.* **2003**, 58(1), 32–45.

15. Doyle, D. A.; Cabral, J. M.; Pfuetzner, R. A.; Kuo, A. L.; Gulbis, J. M.; Cohen, S. L.; Chait, B. T.; MacKinnon, R. *Science* **1998**, 280(5360), 69–77.

16. Jiang, Y. X.; Lee, A.; Chen, J. Y.; Cadene, M.; Chait, B. T.; MacKinnon, R. *Nature (London)* **2002**, 417(6888), 523–526.

17. Pearlstein, R. A.; Vaz, R.; Rampe, D. *J. Med. Chem.* **2003**, 46(11), 2017–2022.

18. Pearlstein, R. A.; Vaz, R.; Kang, J.; Chen, X. L.; Preobrazhenskaya, M.; Shchekotikhin, A. E.; Korolev, A. M.; Lysenkova, L. N.; Miroshnikova, O. V.; Hendrix, J.; Rampe, D. *Bioorg. Med. Chem. Lett.* **2003**, 13(10), 1829–1835.

19. Mitcheson, J. S.; Chen, J.; Lin, M.; Culberson, C.; Sanguinetti, M. C. *Proc. Natl. Acad. Sci. USA* **2000**, 97(22), 12329–12333.

20. Jiang, Y. X.; Lee, A.; Chen, J. Y.; Ruta, V.; Cadene, M.; Chait, B. T.; MacKinnon, R. *Nature (London)* **2003**, 423(6935), 33–41.

21. del Camino, D.; Yellen, G. *Neuron* **2001**, 32(4), 649–656.

22. Witchel, H. J.; Dempsey, C. E.; Sessions, R. B.; Perry, M.; Milnes, J. T.; Hancox J. C.; Mitcheson, J. S. *Mol. Pharmacol.* **2004**, 66(5), 1201–1212.

23. Lees-Miller, J. P.; Duan, Y.; Tsen, G. Q.; Duff, H. J. *Mol. Pharmacol.* **2000**, 57(2), 367–374.

24. Fernandez, D.; Ghanta, A.; Kauffman, G. W.; Sanguinetti, M. C. *J. Biol. Chem.* **2004**, 279(11), 10120–10127.

25. Aronov, A. M. *Drug Discov. Today* **2005**, 10(2), 149–155.

26. Keating, M. T.; Sanguinetti, M. C. *Cell* **2001**, 104(4), 569–580.

27. Ekins, S.; Crumb, W. J.; Sarazan, R. D.; Wikel, J. H.; Wrighton, S. A. *J. Pharmacol. Exp. Ther.* **2002**, 301(2), 427–434.

28. Cavalli, A.; Poluzzi, E.; De Ponti, F.; Recanatini, M. *J. Med. Chem.* **2002**, 45(18), 3844–3853.

29. Cramer, R. D.; Patterson, D. E.; Bunce, J. D. *Prog. Clin. Biol. Res.* **1989**, 291, 161–165.

30. Netzer, R.; Ebneth, A.; Bischoff, U.; Pongs, O. *Drug Discov. Today* **2001**, 6(2), 78–84.

31. Chadwick, C. C.; Ezrin, A. M.; O'Connor, B.; Volberg, W. A.; Smith, D. I.; Wedge, K. J.; Hill, R. J.; Briggs, G. M.; Pagani, E. D.; Silver, P. J. *Circ. Res.* **1993**, 72(3), 707–714.

32. Finlayson, K.; Pennington, A. J.; Kelly, J. S. *Eur. J. Pharmacol.* **2001**, 412(3), 203–212.

33. Diaz, G. J.; Daniell, K.; Leitza, S. T.; Martin, R. L.; Su, Z.; McDermott, J. S.; Cox, B. F.; Gintant, G. A. *J. Pharmacol. Toxicol. Methods* **2004**, 50(3), 187–199.

34. Murphy, S. M.; Palmer, M.; Poole, M. F.; Padegimas, L.; Hunady, K.; Danzig, J.; Gill, S.; Gill, R.; Ting, A.; Sherf, B.; Brunden, K.; Stricker-Krongrad, A. *J. Pharmacol. Toxicol. Methods* **2006**, 54(1), 42–55.

35. Chaudhary, K. W.; O'Neal, J. M.; Mo, Z.-L.; Fermini, B.; Gallavan, R. H.; Bahinski, A. *Assay Drug Dev. Technol.* **2006**, 4(1), 73–82.

36. Dorn, A.; Hermann, F.; Ebneth, A.; Bothmann, H.; Trube, G.; Christensen, K.; Apfel, C. *J. Biomol. Screen* **2005**, 10(4), 339–347.

37. Baxter, D. F.; Kirk, M.; Garcia, A. F.; Raimondi, A.; Holmqvist, M. H.; Flint, K. K.; Bojanic, D.; Distefano, P. S.; Curtis, R.; Xie, Y. *J. Biomol. Screen* **2002**, 7(1), 79–85.

38. Netzer, R.; Bischoff, U.; Ebneth, A. *Curr. Opin. Drug Discov. Devel.* **2003**, 6(4), 462–469.

39. Tang, W.; Kang, J.; Wu, X.; Rampe, D.; Wang, L.; Shen, H.; Li, Z.; Dunnington, D.; Garyantes, T. *J. Biomol. Screen* **2001**, 6(5), 325–331.

40. Yu, S. P.; Kerchner, G. A. *J. Neurosci. Res.* **1998**, 52(5), 612–617.

41. Hille, B. *Ion Channels of Excitable Membranes*. 3rd ed. **2001**, Sunderland: Sinauer. xviii, 814.

42. Weir, S. W.; Weston, A. H. *Br. J. Pharmacol.* **1986**, 88(1), 121–128.

43. Terstappen, G. C. *Anal. Biochem.* **1999**, 272(2), 149–155.

44. Cheng, C. S.; Alderman, D.; Kwash, J.; Dessaint, J.; Patel, R.; Lescoe, M. K.; Kinrade, M. B.; Yu, W. *Drug Dev. Ind. Pharm.* **2002**, 28(2), 177–191.

45. Rezazadeh, S.; Hesketh, J. C.; Fedida, D. *J. Biomol. Screen* **2004**, 9(7), 588–597.

46. Numaguchi, H.; Mullins, F. M.; Johnson, J. P. Jr; Johns, D. C.; Po, S. S.; Yang, I. C.; Tomaselli, G. F.; Balser, J. R. *Circ. Res.* **2000**, 87(11), 1012–1018.

47. Weerapura, M.; Hébert, T. E.; Stanley, N. *Pflugers Arch.* **2002**, 443(4), 520–531.

48. Kirsch, G. E.; Trepakova, E. S.; Brimecombe, J. C.; Sidach, S. S.; Erickson, H. D.; Kochan, M. C.; Shyjka, L. M.; Lacerda, A. E.; Brown, A. M. *J. Pharmacol. Toxicol. Methods* **2004**, 50(2), 93–101.

49. Kiss, L.; Bennett, P. B.; Uebele, V. N.; Koblan, K. S.; Kane, S. A.; Neagle, B.; Schroeder, K. *Assay Drug Dev. Technol.* **2003**, 1(Suppl. 1 Pt. 2), 127–135.

50. Tao, H.; Santa Ana, D.; Guia, A.; Huang, M.; Ligutti, J.; Walker, G.; Sithiphong, K.; Chan, F.; Tao, G.; Zozulya, Z.; Saya, S.; Phimmachack, R.; Sie, C.; Yuan, J.; Wu, L.; Xu, J.; Ghetti, A. *Assay Drug Dev. Technol.* **2004**, 2(5), 497–506.

51. Mathes, C. *Expert Opin. Ther. Targets* **2006**, 10(2), 319–327.

52. Guo, L.; Guthrie, H. *J. Pharmacol. Toxicol. Methods* **2005**, 52(1), 123–135.

53. Finkel, A.; Wittel, A.; Yang, N.; Handran, S.; Hughes, J.; Costantin, J. *J. Biomol. Screen* **2006**, 11(5), 488–496.

54. Furutani, M.; Trudeau, M. C.; Hagiwara, N.; Seki, A.; Gong, Q.; Zhou, Z.; Imamura, S.; Nagashima, H.; Kasanuki, H.; Takao, A.; Momma, K.; January, C. T.; Robertson, G. A.; Matsuoka, R. *Circulation* **1999**, 99(17), 2290–2294.

55. Kuryshev, Y. A.; Ficker, E.; Wang, L.; Hawryluk, P.; Dennis, A. T.; Wible, B. A.; Brown, A. M.; Kang, J.; Chen, X. L.; Sawamura, K.; Reynolds, W.; Rampe, D. *J. Pharmacol. Exp. Ther.* **2005**, 312(1), 316–323.

56. Ficker, E.; Kuryshev, Y. A.; Dennis, A. T.; Obejero-Paz, C.; Wang, L.; Hawryluk, P.; Wible, B. A.; Brown, A. M. *Mol. Pharmacol.* **2004**, 66(1), 33–44.

57. Cordes, J. S.; Sun, Z.; Lloyd, D. B.; Bradley, J. A.; Opsahl, A. C.; Tengowski M. W.; Chen, X.; Zhou, J. *Br. J. Pharmacol.* **2005**, 145(1), 15–23.

58. Wible, B. A.; Hawryluk, P.; Ficker, E.; Kuryshev, Y. A.; Kirsch, G.; Brown, A. M. *J. Pharmacol. Toxicol. Methods* **2005**, 52(1), 136–145.

59. Schram, G.; Pourrier, M.; Melnyk, P.; Nattel, S. *Circ. Res.* **2002**, 90(9), 939–950.

60. Priori, S. G.; Napolitano, C. *Circulation* **2006**, 113(8), 1130–1135.

61. *N. Engl. J. Med.* **1989**, 321(6), 406–412.

62. Milberg, P.; Milberg, P.; Reinsch, N.; Wasmer, K.; Mönnig, G.; Stypmann, J.; Osada, N.; Breithardt, G.; Haverkamp, W. E. *Cardiovasc. Res.* **2005**, 65(2), 397–404.

63. Kühlkamp, V.; Mewis, C.; Bosch, R.; Seipel, L. *J. Cardiovasc. Pharmacol.* **2003**, 42(1), 113–117.

64. Zhang, S.; Zhou, Z.; Gong, Q.; Makielski, J. C.; January, C. T. *Circ. Res.* **1999**, 84(9), 989–998.

65. Milberg, P.; Reinsch, N.; Osada, N.; Wasmer, K.; Mönnig, G.; Stypmann, J.; Breithardt, G.; Haverkamp, W.; Eckardt, L. *Basic Res. Cardiol.* **2005**, 100(4), 365–371.

66. Gintant, G. A.; Limberis, J. T.; McDermott, J. S.; Wegner, C. D.; Cox, B. F. *J. Cardiovasc. Pharmacol.* **2001**, 37(5), 607–618.

67. Lu, H. R.; Marien, R.; Saels, A.; De Clerck, F. *J. Cardiovasc. Electrophysiol.* **2001**, 12(1), 93–102.

68. Aubert, M.; Osterwalder, R.; Wagner, B.; Parrilla, I.; Cavero, I.; Doessegger, L.; Ertel, E. A. *Drug Safety* **2006**, 29(3), 237–254.

69. Antzelevitch, C.; Fish, J. *Basic Res. Cardiol.* **2001**, 96(6), 517–527.

70. Burashnikov, A.; Antzelevitch, C. *Cardiovasc. Res.* **1999**, 43(4), 901–908.

71. Akar, F. G.; Yan, G. X.; Antzelevitch, C.; Rosenbaum, D. S. *Circulation* **2002**, 105(10), 1247–1253.

72. Antzelevitch, C. *Heart Rhythm* **2005**, 2(2 Suppl.), S9–15.

73. Hamlin, R. L.; Cruze, C. A.; Mittelstadt, S. W.; Kijtawornrat, A.; Keene, B. W.; Roche, B. M.; Nakayama, T.; Nakayama, H.; Hamlin, D. M.; Arnold, T. *J. Pharmacol. Toxicol. Methods* **2004**, 49(1), 15–23.

74. Haddad, P. M.; Anderson, I. M. *Drugs* **2002**, 62(11), 1649–1671.

75. Milberg, P.; Eckardt, L.; Bruns, H. J.; Biertz, J.; Ramtin, S.; Reinsch, N.; Fleischer, D.; Kirchhof, P.; Fabritz, L.; Breithardt, G.; Haverkamp, W. *J. Pharmacol. Exp. Ther.* **2002**, 303(1), 218–225.

76. Milberg, P.; Ramtin, S.; Monnig, G.; Osada, N.; Wasmer, K.; Breithardt, G.; Haverkamp, W.; Eckardt, L. *J. Cardiovasc. Pharmacol.* **2004**, 44(3), 278–286.

77. Antzelevitch, C. *J. Electrocardiol.* **2004**, 37 Suppl. 15–24.

78. Hondeghem, L. M.; Hoffmann, P. *J. Cardiovasc. Pharmacol.* **2003**, 41(1), 14–24.

79. Hondeghem, L. M.; Lu, H. R.; van Rossem, K.; De Clerck, F. *J. Cardiovasc. Electrophysiol.* **2003**, 14(3), 287–294.

80. Shah, R. R.; Hondeghem, L. M. *Heart Rhythm* **2005**, 2(7), 758–772.

81. Lawrence, C. L.; Bridgland-Taylor, M. H.; Pollard, C. E.; Hammond, T. G.; Valentin, J. P. *Br. J. Pharmacol.* **2006**, 149(7), 845–860.

82. Yan, G. X.; Antzelevitch, C. *Circulation* **1996**, 93(2), 372–379.

83. Yan, G. X.; Antzelevitch, C. *Circulation* **1998**, 98(18), 1928–1936.

84. Yan, G. X.; Wu, Y.; Liu, T.; Wang, J.; Marinchak, R. A.; Kowey, P. R. *Circulation* **2001**, 103(23), 2851–2856.

85. Nam, G. B.; Burashnikov, A.; Antzelevitch, C. *Circulation* **2005**, 111(21), 2727–2733.

86. Yan, G. X.; Rials, S. J.; Wu, Y.; Liu, T.; Xu, X.; Marinchak, R. A.; Kowey, P. R. *Am. J. Physiol. Heart Circ. Physiol.* **2001**, 281(5), H1968–1975.

87. Di Diego, J. M.; Belardinelli, L.; Antzelevitch, C. *Circulation* **2003**, 108(8), 1027–1033.

88. Wu, Y.; Carlsson, L.; Liu, T.; Kowey, P. R.; Yan, G. X. *J. Cardiovasc. Electrophysiol.* **2005**, 16(8), 898–904.

89. Liu, T.; Brown, B. S.; Wu, Y.; Antzelevitch, C.; Kowey, P. R.; Yan, G.-X. *Heart Rhythm* **2006**, 3(8), 948–956.

90. Lu, H. R.; Vlaminckx, E.; Van de Water, A.; Rohrbacher, J.; Hermans, A.; Gallacher, D. J. *Eur. J. Pharmacol.* **2006**, 553(1–3), 229–239.

91. Wang, D.; Patel, C.; Cui, C.; Yan, G. X. *Pharmacol. Ther.* **2008**, 119(2), 141–151.

92. Chen, X.; Cordes, J. S.; Bradley, J. A.; Sun, Z.; Zhou, J. *J. Pharmacol. Toxicol. Methods* **2006**, 54(3), 261–272.

93. Fenichel, R. R.; Malik, M.; Antzelevitch, C.; Sanguinetti, M.; Roden, D. M.; Priori, S. G.; Ruskin, J. N.; Lipicky, R. J.; Cantilena, L. R. *J. Cardiovasc. Electrophysiol.* **2004**, 15(4), 475–495.

94. Pugsley, M. K.; Hancox, J. C.; Curtis, M. J. *Pharmacol. Ther.* **2008**, 119(2), 115–117.

95. Lees-Miller, J. P.; Guo, J.; Somers, J. R.; Roach, D. E.; Sheldon, R. S.; Rancourt, D. E.; Duff, H. J. *Mol. Cell Biol.* **2003**, 23(6), 1856–1862.

96. Regan, C. P.; Cresswell, H. K.; Zhang, R.; Lynch, J. J. *J. Cardiovasc. Pharmacol.* **2005**, 46(1), 68–75.

97. Toyoshima, S.; Kanno, A.; Kitayama, T.; Sekiya, K.; Nakai, K.; Haruna, M.; Mino, T.; Miyazaki, H.; Yano, K.; Yamamoto, K. *J. Pharmacol. Sci.* **2005**, 99(5), 459–471.

98. Ando, K.; Hombo, T.; Kanno, A.; Ikeda, H.; Imaizumi, M.; Shimizu, N.; Sakamoto, K.; Kitani, S.; Yamamoto, Y.; Hizume, S.; Nakai, K.; Kitayama, T.; Yamamoto, K. *J. Pharmacol. Sci.* **2005**, 99(5), 487–500.

99. Testai, L.; Calderone, V.; Salvadori, A.; Breschi, M. C.; Nieri, P.; Martinotti, E. *J. Appl. Toxicol.* **2004**, 24(3), 217–222.

100. Fossa, A. A.; Wisialowski, T.; Wolfgang, E.; Wang, E.; Avery, M.; Raunig, D. L.; Fermini, B. *Eur. J. Pharmacol.* **2004**, 486(2), 209–221.

101. Wisialowski, T.; Crimin, K.; Engtrakul, J.; O'Donnell, J.; Fermini, B.; Fossa, A. A. *J. Pharmacol. Exp. Ther.* **2006**, 318(1), 352–359.

102. Thomsen, M. B.; Verduyn, S. C.; Stengl, M.; Beekman, J. D. M.; de Pater, G.; van Opstal, J.; Volders, P. G. A.; Vos, M. A. *Circulation* **2004**, 110(16), 2453–2459.

103. Thomsen, M. B.; Volders, P. G.; Beekman, J. D. M.; Matz, J.; Vos, M. A. *J. Am. Coll. Cardiol.* **2006**, 48(6), 1268–1276.

104. Thomsen, M. B.; Beekman, J. D. M.; Attevelt, N. J. M.; Takahara, A.; Sugiyama, A.; Chiba, K.; Vos, M. A. *Br. J. Pharmacol.* **2006**, 149(8), 1039–1048.

105. Detre, E.; Thomsen, M. B.; Beekman, J. D.; Petersen, K. U.; Vos, M. A. *Br. J. Pharmacol.* **2005**, 145(3), 397–404.

106. Hamlin, R. L.; Kijtawornrat, A.; Keene, B. W.; Hamlin, D. M. *Toxicol. Sci.* **2003**, 76(2), 437–442.

107. Carlsson, L.; Almgren, O.; Duker, G. *J. Cardiovasc. Pharmacol.* **1990**, 16(2), 276–285.

108. Carlsson, L.; Abrahamsson, C.; Andersson, B.; Duker, G.; Schiller-Linhardt, G. *Cardiovasc. Res.* **1993**, 27(12), 2186–2193.

109. Lu, H. R.; Remeysen, P.; De Clerck, F. *J. Cardiovasc. Pharmacol.* **2000**, 36(6), 728–736.

110. Farkas, A.; Coker, S. J. *Eur. J. Pharmacol.* **2002**, 449(1–2), 143–153.

111. Anderson, M. E.; Mazur, A.; Yang, T.; Roden, D. M. *J. Pharmacol. Exp. Ther.* **2001**, 296(3), 806–810.

112. Kijtawornrat, A.; Ozkanlar, Y.; Keene, B. W.; Roche, B. M.; Hamlin, D. M.; Hamlin, R. L. *J. Pharmacol. Toxicol. Methods* **2006**, 53(2), 168–173.

INDEX

Evaluation of Drug Candidates for Preclinical Development: Pharmacokinetics, Metabolism, Pharmaceutics, and Toxicology, Edited by Chao Han, Charles B. Davis, and Binghe Wang
Copyright © 2010 John Wiley & Sons, Inc.

Printed and bound by CPI Group (UK) Ltd, Croydon, CR0 4YY

17/04/2025

14658879-0001